JAMES WONG

Eat Better the Easy Way

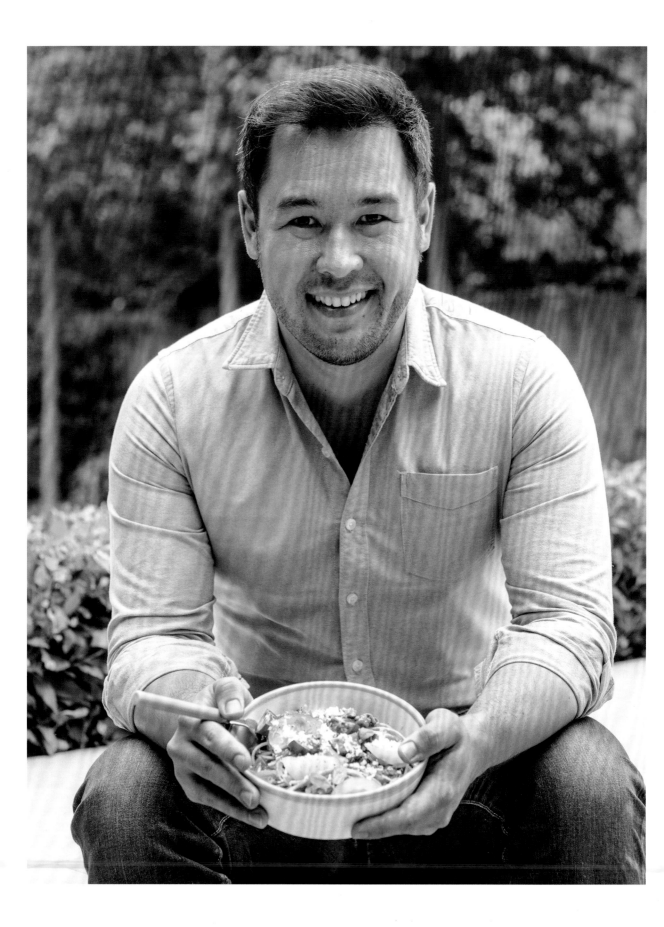

JAMES WONG

Eat Better the Easy Way

transform your health with plant-packed recipes and simple science

NUTRITION CONSULTANTS:
Rosie Saunt RD & Helen West RD

MITCHELL BEAZLEY

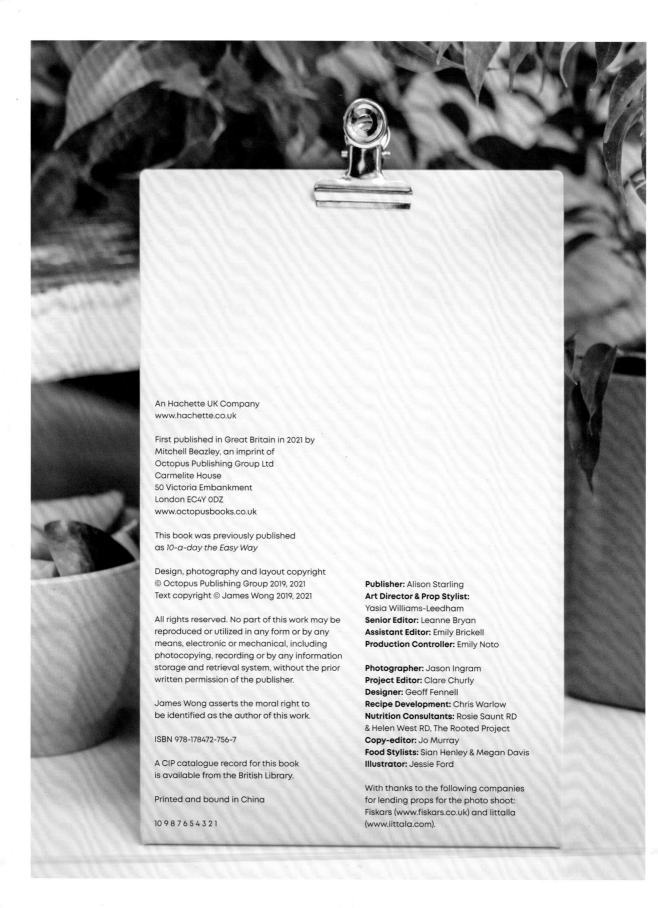

An Hachette UK Company
www.hachette.co.uk

First published in Great Britain in 2021 by
Mitchell Beazley, an imprint of
Octopus Publishing Group Ltd
Carmelite House
50 Victoria Embankment
London EC4Y 0DZ
www.octopusbooks.co.uk

This book was previously published
as *10-a-day the Easy Way*

Design, photography and layout copyright
© Octopus Publishing Group 2019, 2021
Text copyright © James Wong 2019, 2021

ISBN 978-178472-756-7

A CIP catalogue record for this book
is available from the British Library.

Printed and bound in China

10 9 8 7 6 5 4 3 2 1

Publisher: Alison Starling
Art Director & Prop Stylist:
Yasia Williams-Leedham
Senior Editor: Leanne Bryan
Assistant Editor: Emily Brickell
Production Controller: Emily Noto

Photographer: Jason Ingram
Project Editor: Clare Churly
Designer: Geoff Fennell
Recipe Development: Chris Warlow
Nutrition Consultants: Rosie Saunt RD
& Helen West RD, The Rooted Project
Copy-editor: Jo Murray
Food Stylists: Sian Henley & Megan Davis
Illustrator: Jessie Ford

With thanks to the following companies
for lending props for the photo shoot:
Fiskars (www.fiskars.co.uk) and Iittala
(www.iittala.com).

CONTENTS

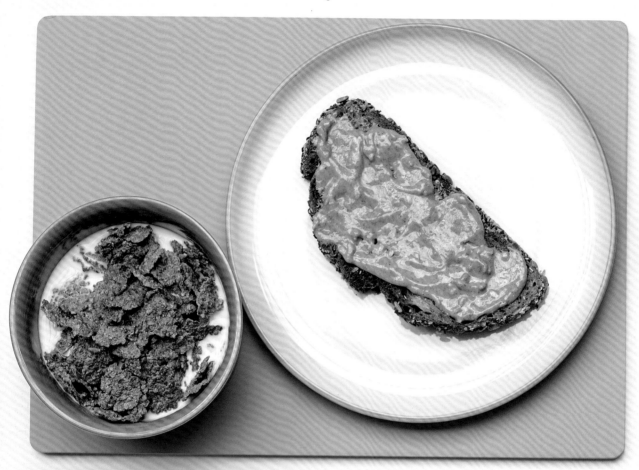

WHY EAT MORE FRUIT & VEG?

SO, I'LL LET YOU IN ON A LITTLE SECRET. THIS MORNING I TOOK A DOSE OF SOMETHING THAT COULD SLASH MY RISK OF HEART DISEASE BY NEARLY 25 PER CENT. The exact same treatment could also reduce my risk of a stroke in later life by a third and confer me protection against a range of common cancers. The latest research even suggests it is actually capable of cutting my risk of premature death from *any* cause by a whopping 30 per cent.

But this wasn't some kind of miracle pill or experimental treatment. It was simply, well, my breakfast. And it wasn't an awful 'superfood' green smoothie either, just cereal and toast, like millions of other people eat around the world. All I did differently was chuck a handful of berries on the cereal, slice a banana onto my toast and pour myself a glass of juice. That's it. Plain and simple.

These simple additions boosted my daily intake of fruit and veg by 3–4 portions in a single sitting. Repeated at each meal, this would add up to about 10 portions a day – double the minimum daily intake of the good stuff. Why is this relevant? Well, according to a growing body of international studies, little tweaks like this that get me beyond the 5-a-day minimum could confer significantly more protection against the greatest diseases that affect the Western world.

The amazing thing is, we are now discovering that the positive effects of fruit and veg consumption are cumulative. **For every extra portion of fruit and veg you enjoy, your statistical risk of stroke falls by as much as an additional 16 per cent,** and this is just one example. In fact, dietitians across the board agree that the simplest dietary change you

+1

+1

+1

Poor diet is responsible for almost **TWICE** as many premature deaths as lack of exercise, alcohol and drug use combined.

can make for good health is to consume more fruit and veg, especially when **as few as 1 in 3 Brits and only 1 in 10 Americans are making the *minimum* 5-a-day target.**

But no matter what the lab geeks say, is scaling up towards 10 portions of fruit and veg a day really plausible? As a plant scientist fascinated by nutrition (but who also loves a good burger and the odd ready meal), I decided to put its feasibility to the test during a year of self-experimentation, and with more than a little trepidation.

To my surprise, not only did my food bills go down, I also started eating a more varied, colourful and flavourful diet, and (here's the most important thing) I didn't have to cut anything out to get these benefits. Far from the Spartan restrictiveness of

living gluten-, dairy-, sugar- and carb-free, I just carried on eating all the normal, everyday foods I know and love, simply made more delicious with the added flavour, texture and colour of fruit and veg, both at home or on the run. **The only rule – 'eat pretty much whatever you like, as long as you get 3 portions of fruit and veg at each meal'** – isn't exactly hard to stick to either. Over the course of the year, I jotted down my recipe tweaks to everyday favourites that helped me reach my goal, along with some simple tips and tricks to help me along the way. And that's how this book started.

No gimmicks, no 'banned' foods or miserly portion sizes. Just 80 classic recipes made healthier (and tastier) by simply upping the fruit and veg in them, all backed by the most solid science available. **SO LET'S GET STARTED…**

THE SCIENCE
WHERE DID '5-A-DAY' COME FROM?

We all know that fruit and veg are good for us. Thanks to high-profile public health campaigns, we probably also have heard that we should enjoy at least 5 portions of them every day, too. **But where does this famous '5-a-day' figure come from?**

Back in the 1980s rates of diet-related chronic diseases around the world started to rise steadily, ironically triggered by increasing global prosperity. Populations that once struggled to feed themselves had been lifted out of famine and malnutrition but now began to suffer an increased risk of heart disease, stroke, diabetes and certain cancers as a result of the shift towards a more affluent diet. This prompted the World Health Organization (WHO) to undertake a landmark investigation reviewing the best scientific evidence to date, to come up with dietary recommendations that might help curb this global trend. Crunching the numbers, it found that fruit and vegetable consumption was one of the most important dietary factors associated with good health. In study after study, it was significantly associated with a lower risk of developing a range of chronic illnesses across the world, with people who consumed a minimum of about 400g (14oz) a day (the equivalent of five 80g/2¾oz portions) tending to have significantly better health than those eating lower amounts.

But, what many of us might not know is that even at the time of publication in 1990 these now-famous 5-a-day guidelines were not based on the level the science suggested was *optimal* for good health, but the *minimum* amount needed to enjoy a significant health benefit. It is surprisingly easy not to notice those two little words 'at least' when they precede '5-a-day', isn't it? It turns out that as so many people at the time were not consuming even half this minimum intake, governments around the world were

**UK
5
PORTIONS**

concerned that recommendations following the science to the letter and suggesting even higher levels might be too daunting a prospect for the public – one considered so unrealistic that the advice would simply be ignored. As a result, many governments chose to 'strike a balance' in their health education campaigns between clear, open science communication and, well, a narrative angle they thought the public would be more comfortable hearing. Welcome to the world of politics!

The degree to which individual governments focused on 'achievable' versus 'optimal' levels based on WHO's report explains why there is such a wide variation in the daily recommended intakes around the world. While France, the UK, Germany, the Netherlands and New Zealand, for example, suggest a modest minimum of 5 portions a day, in Denmark it is 6. Why? This number made for a catchier marketing slogan, as it sounds similar to the word for 'sex' in Danish: 'Sex every day'. No, really.

**JAPAN
7
PORTIONS**

In Australia and Japan, the number of portions is 7. In Canada, it is between 5 and 10, according to your age and sex. For me, as an adult male, for example, Canadian government advice of about 10 portions a day is twice the amount suggested in my native UK. In Greece, it is a generous average of 9 daily portions, but perhaps no one tops Italy, which despite not specifying an exact number of portions, recommends fruit and veg make up the largest component of your diet, more even than traditional dietary staples like rice, pasta and bread, which it ranks a mere second. That's a lot of fruit and veg!

**GREECE
9
PORTIONS**

DID THE '5-A-DAY' CAMPAIGN WORK?

So did the focus on more 'achievable' daily portions do the trick? Well, let's take a look at the evidence.

After millions of dollars of investment, years of work and some of the brightest marketing brains behind it, globally the current average fruit and veg consumption level is still much lower than the World Health Organization's minimum recommendation.

How much lower? Well, in Europe, this averages out at 2.7 portions a day, about half the minimum, and when it comes to our kids, as few as 6 per cent are getting enough. In the US, fewer than one in ten people achieves it, with an astonishing three-quarters not able to make the minimum of a *single* portion of fruit a day. The study that first reported this concluded that the typical American diet is in a 'worrisome state in the context of the obesity epidemic and alarming rates of other diet-related chronic diseases'. When the normally monotone language of academic papers reads like this, you know things are bad!

So, given that this focus on 'achievability' has only had limited success, I wonder if perhaps a more open, transparent approach that explains the *optimum* level might be more encouraging? Perhaps, rather than being daunting, realizing how far away current intakes are from what good science says is the optimum could be more motivating? It is possible this might be more effective than setting the bar lower, simply assuming the public would be put off by a more candid approach. Especially when it is revealed that even if you don't manage to make these more ambitious goals, *any* extra portion you sneak in above 5-a-day is linked to a measurable reduction in health risks.

The only study I could find that set out to compare the success of 'achievable' dietary goal-setting with more ambitious aims in relation to fruit and veg might just shed some light on this. Researchers at the Institute of Psychology at the University of Heidelberg in Germany set up a trial to test the hypothesis that what they called a 'realistic' goal of eating 'just one more' than usual intake would be more effective at increasing fruit and vegetable consumption than a 'challenging' 5-a-day goal. So what did they find?

It turns out that participants who were instructed to eat 5-a-day for a week dutifully did just that, effectively doubling their intake of fruit and veg. Likewise, a group instructed to eat 'just one more' also did pretty much exactly as they were told, boosting their intake to about 3.4 portions a day. Even with these surprisingly compliant volunteers, the 'just one more' group lagged far behind the 5-a-day group's number of portions. So it would be hard to argue that more modest goals are more effective at upping fruit and veg consumption than more ambitious ones, at least in an artificial, experimental situation like this.

But real life is not a lab experiment – what happened to these participants *after* the trial was over? Well, here's the really interesting thing. When researchers retested the participants a week after the end of the study, the 5-a-day group were still continuing to scoff on average 1 portion more than they had originally been eating, while the 'just one more' group had immediately gone back to their old ways.

OK, so this was a very small, short-term study, but its findings do provide some evidence to suggest that more ambitious goals not only may be far more effective motivators to increasing consumption towards healthy levels, but might also work better in the longer term.

So that is what I am setting out to do in this book – giving you the facts straight-up so that you can make well-informed decisions for yourself. If you struggle to get much further than 5-a-day, don't worry. **Every little bit extra counts. And I'll give you lots of tips and tricks to help you get to the 'optimal' levels that we'll look at next.**

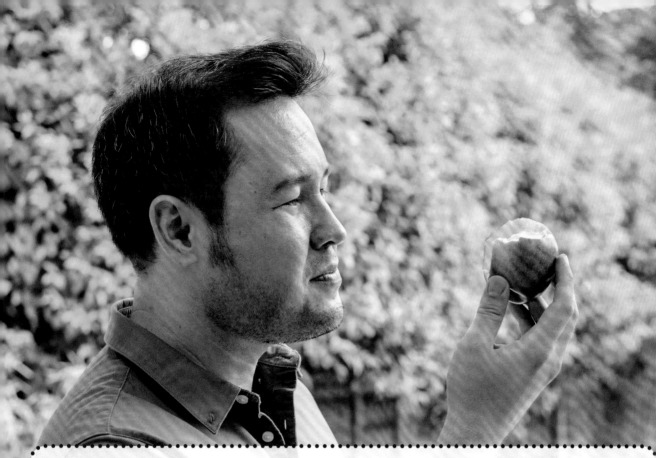

WHAT IS AN 'OPTIMAL' DAILY INTAKE?

So if 5-a-day is the *minimum* amount, what is the *optimal* daily intake of fruit and veg? After all, we have had a good 30 years to gather up more evidence on the impact of fruit and veg consumption since the initial World Health Organization (WHO) report was published.

Well, to answer this question, in 2017, an international team of scientists pooled together the results of 95 of the most well-designed observational studies from around the globe, involving an astonishing 2 million participants. Running the numbers, they found that while fruit and veg tended to have a bigger proportional impact when people who eat 1–2 portions a day were compared to those eating basically none, individuals who ate more – even beyond the 5-a-day recommendation – *continued* to benefit from every extra portion. And guess what? Those eating a generous 10-a-day enjoyed the very best state of health, with a 33 per cent decreased risk of stroke, 28 per cent lower risk of heart disease and 14 per cent lower risk of cancer. As a result of such research, it is now estimated that more than 5

million premature deaths every year are attributable directly to inadequate fruit and veg intake. (That's like the population of Norway. Every single year.)

Yet, even for those people who didn't go all out and manage 10 daily portions, every extra 200g (7oz) eaten a day (basically the equivalent of just one large apple) was associated with a statistical reduction in the risk of stroke of 16 per cent, an 8 per cent reduced chance of developing coronary heart disease and even a 10 per cent reduction in premature death from any cause. What's that they say about an apple a day? Considering the time, effort and cost it takes to eat an apple, these are some intriguing results when it comes to fighting the most common causes of early death in the Western world. Want a full breakdown? Here's what the research has turned up so far on a range of life-threatening conditions. Get ready for a flurry of stats.

HEART DISEASE

The most striking evidence we have for the potentially protective effect of fruit and veg consumption is for cardiovascular disease. This comes not only from studies that have identified that populations who tend to eat lots of fruit and veg also tend to have better heart health, but also from experiments that have shown that diets rich in fruit and vegetables can lower risk factors such as blood pressure and cholesterol.

In fact, WHO now reports that by increasing fruit and veg consumption to 7.5 portions a day, the global risk of heart disease could be reduced by some 31 per cent and stroke by 19 per cent. The effect appears to be so strong, that the organization estimates about 11 per cent of all deaths from heart disease and 9 per cent of deaths from strokes can be directly attributed to insufficient intake of fruit and vegetables.

The WHO findings echo those of another comprehensive review of the evidence published in 2017 that set out to estimate the optimum level of fruit and veg consumption. An international team of experts from the US, UK and Iran found a dose-dependent relationship for every extra portion of fruit and veg you eat. Add an extra couple of spoonfuls of veg to your daily diet and the extra portion this provides statistically reduces your risk of developing heart disease by around 5 per cent and stroke by 17 per cent, and amazingly this potential benefit appears to continue for every extra portion you add. Based on the calculations in the study, the benefits eventually seemed to plateau off, with the authors suggesting an intake of 9-a-day for heart health.

SO IS IT 7.5, 9 OR 10 PORTIONS A DAY WE SHOULD BE GETTING?

Well, while the exact stats do vary slightly between studies as you would probably expect, what they do repeatedly show is a consistent trend for fruit and veg conferring a protective benefit over and above the 5-a-day recommendation. Can't get 10? No worries. Just get more!

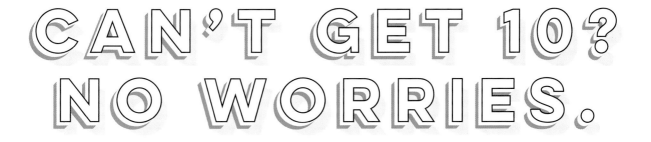

CAN'T GET 10? NO WORRIES.

JUST GET MORE!

CANCER

Let's make one thing clear from the start: cancer is complex. There are a huge number of potential factors that can increase your risk of developing the disease, many of which simply are not within your control, such as your genetics and your age. However, research has shown that lifestyle factors, including dietary patterns (such as how much fruit and veg you eat), can be one of them. So let's take a look at the what the evidence shows so far.

The largest and best-quality study to date on cancer and diet, published by the National Cancer Institute, found that during the study period **those who ate as little as the equivalent of an apple a day (200g/7oz of fruit or veg) experienced a 3 per cent reduction in risk of developing the disease**. Although this reduction was described as 'very small' by the researchers, it statistically increased for every extra 200g (7oz) participants tended to eat. **Those who ate the most (647g/1lb 7oz, or about 8 portions) had an 11 per cent lower total risk.**

While this percentage might not exactly constitute a 'miracle cure', let's look at what it *could* theoretically mean when it is applied. In the UK, about 360,000 people are diagnosed with cancer every year, a figure that is expected to rise significantly over the coming decades. These findings may suggest that by consuming 8 portions of fruit and veg a day, some 39,600 fewer cancer diagnoses could occur each year, at least in theory. That is more than four times the population of the City of London. Now, given that there are so many variables, it would be incorrect to think that people who get cancer did something 'wrong'. Sadly, the evidence suggests that sometimes people are just unlucky, no matter how healthy their lifestyles are. However, given that many risk factors are simply not within your control, the good news is that upping your fruit and veg consumption is one of the few things you *can* change (and very easily too) to help minimize your risk.

What if you can't make 8 portions? Well, other studies suggest that if half the US population increased their fruit and veg consumption by just a single portion a day, an estimated 20,000 cancer cases might be avoided each year. Reminder: a single portion is only half an apple a day.

It is also important to bear in mind that cancer is not 'one' disease, but a group of related diseases, each with different risk factors (including stuff like smoking, UV light etc.). So while the protective effects of fruit and veg consumption against overall risk of cancer in general may be more modest than that of, say, heart disease, for *specific* cancers the evidence can be much stronger. This is particularly likely to be the case, according to the research so far, for the following cancer types.

MOUTH & THROAT CANCER

The American Journal of Clinical Nutrition found that each portion of fruit or veg eaten a day was linked to an astonishing 50 per cent reduced risk of developing oral cancer during the trial period. Eat more than 1 portion and your statistical risk of developing the disease, at least according to this analysis, more than halves. Potentially eyebrow-raising stuff, especially if oral cancer runs in your family.

It is important to point out, however, that this impressive decrease was only partially echoed in other studies, such as those of WHO's 'Global Burden of Disease' report, which found the odds were for only a 20 per cent risk reduction. Frankly, however, either way it's a pretty great extra to all the other benefits fruit and veg might offer.

LUNG CANCER

While smoking is by far the most important risk factor for lung cancer, there does appear to be a dietary component behind the development of the disease, too. The evidence suggests that in general those who eat larger amounts of fruit and veg tend to be conferred some protection. One Dutch study found that this could be as high as a 40 per cent reduced rate. Other research suggests a much more modest association, however, with WHO reporting only a 12 per cent reduction in risk, so more investigation is clearly needed. But so far, the trend for a potential protective effect does seem pretty consistent.

LIVER CANCER

Interestingly, while high vegetable consumption was associated with a 28 per cent reduction in the risk of developing liver cancer, no protective association was found with fruit intake. This reinforces the importance of getting your portions from a wide variety of foods and not just relying on a handful of crops.

PANCREATIC CANCER

A review in the *European Journal of Cancer Prevention* found those eating the most fruit and veg were 27 per cent less likely to develop pancreatic cancer than those who ate the least.

STOMACH & BOWEL CANCER

In contrast to the risk of liver cancer, studies looking into the effect of diet on stomach cancer found that while vegetables did not appear to have a protective effect, fruit consumption was associated with a significant risk reduction (yet another reason why dietary diversity is so important). This drop in risk could be potentially as high as 19 per cent according to the WHO. It found a similar protective effect for gastrointestinal cancer in general, too, so much so it estimates insufficient intake of fruit and vegetables could be the key cause of 14 per cent of deaths from the disease worldwide.

BLADDER CANCER

People who ate the most fruit and vegetables were up to 19 per cent less likely to develop bladder cancer. This risk reduction was shown to be dose-dependent, too, with an 8 per cent decrease in risk for every 200g (7oz) eaten a day.

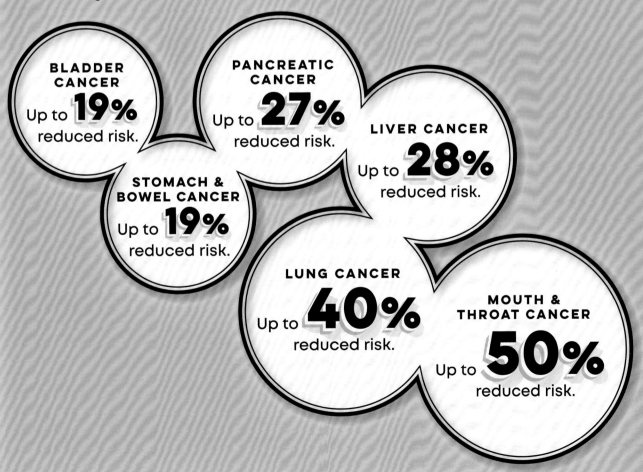

HEALTHY AGEING

Eating more fruit and vegetables is associated with a 21 per cent lower risk of developing cognitive impairment as we age, at least according to a big review of the evidence published in the *European Journal of Clinical Nutrition*. This wasn't a one-off finding either, and was echoed by a number of others, including China's Southwest Medical University, which found a 13 per cent statistical reduction in dementia risk for every extra daily portion you enjoy. Theoretically, a pretty persuasive potential offer in exchange for nothing more than a handful of berries on your morning cereal.

But aside from health and quality of life, could upping your fruit and veg intake also give you a *longer* life? That's exactly the question Swedish scientists aimed to investigate by tracking, over 13 years, the health of a good 70,000 middle-aged and old-aged people. They found that those eating 5 portions of fruit and veg lived a full 3 years longer than those who didn't eat any at all, and enjoyed a more than 50 per cent reduction in mortality risk at any given point during the trial period. **Even 1 portion of fruit a day was associated with living 19 months longer compared to those who ate none.** While these benefits appeared to plateau off at 5-a-day in this study, others have reported them to continue to accumulate.

One study at University College London, for example, analysed the deaths from all causes from a group of more than 65,000 people in Britain aged 35 and above over 7 years. It found that while **people who ate 3–5 portions a day were 24 per cent less likely to die before the end of the study period** than those who ate less than 1 portion, this continued to increase with each extra portion, peaking at a 33 per cent reduction in risk for people who tended to eat 7 portions or more.

DEPRESSION

The causes of depression are not fully understood, but it's thought that chronic psychological stress and cellular damage caused by chemicals called free radicals (found in stuff like pollution, cigarette smoke and even produced by your own body) could play a role in its development. Because of this, it's been suggested that **people who eat lots of fruit and vegetables** – which are themselves rich in chemicals known as antioxidants that have been demonstrated to be able to protect cells from the harmful effects of free radicals – **might be at lower risk of depression.**

To get to the bottom of this, a study in *The International Journal of Applied and Basic Nutritional Science* ran a comprehensive review of the evidence – the first of its kind, in fact, to compile all the research on the topic from all publications globally (an ambitious task). Gathering together studies that involved 450,000 participants, it found that any level of fruit and veg consumption was associated with protection against depression, but those who ate the highest levels had the most benefits. The most enthusiastic fruit and veg eaters showed as much as 14 per cent less likelihood of developing depression.

OK, it may be early days in our understanding of the causes of depression, this was a pretty modest reduction and some of the studies included in the review were of weaker quality, but given all the other potential benefits (and no real downsides) what have you got to lose?

COULD THIS ALL BE A COINCIDENCE?

People who tend to eat more fruit and veg also tend to engage in other healthy behaviours, like exercising more frequently, drinking less alcohol and being less likely to smoke. They tend to be more educated and wealthier, too, which may mean that in some countries they also have better access to healthcare. So could the link we observe between fruit and veg consumption and better health be a mere coincidence and not a genuine cause and effect relationship? After all, avid fruit and veg eaters are more likely to be wealthy, but it doesn't mean that simply eating a little more salad will boost your bank balance!

Well, this might be the case, but three key observations suggest that this association isn't simply down to chance. First, the relationship appears to be dose-dependent, meaning the more fruit and veg people eat, the more their health is likely to benefit. This result would be rather unlikely if there was no cause and effect link, although it could still be down to a statistical quirk if it had been reported by only one or two studies. Yet, the link is remarkably consistent, reliably appearing in hundreds of studies from across the world. Even when the results of all the studies are pooled together to even out any potential red herrings in the data, the same general pattern emerges time after time. That's hard to ignore.

Secondly, although the degree of benefit does vary between health conditions and between studies (as you would expect), the effect is generally too strong to put down to chance. Even when the results in these studies are adjusted to take into account the confounding factors of things like age, obesity, smoking, alcohol and activity level that might have skewed them, the same consistent link still shows up. Speaking of which, it is important to point out here that the very evidence we have to demonstrate the harmful effects of smoking, excessive alcohol consumption and even exposure to asbestos is from exactly the same types of studies that aim to find meaningful patterns between lifestyle factors and health risks.

Last but not least, there is a range of plausible mechanisms to explain *why* those who eat more fruit and veg also tend to be healthier according to pretty much every scientific measure. These foods contain a range of natural compounds that are known to do everything from improving gut health to lowering blood pressure and cholesterol, not to mention protecting cells from harmful free radicals, supporting the body's own detoxification system and even controlling appetite. So we have not only lots of evidence to suggest that fruit and veg *do* help improve health, but also a good idea of *how* they do it. And that's what we'll look at next…

HOW DOES IT ALL WORK?

Diets rich in fruit and vegetables may help improve health in a number of surprising ways, some of which science is only just beginning to reveal. Here's the very latest on what the lab geeks have uncovered about fruit and veg so far.

VITAMINS, MINERALS & PHYTONUTRIENTS

Let's start with a pretty simple one. Fruit and veg are excellent sources of key vitamins and minerals that are essential to life. As some of these are much harder to find in other foods, it probably comes as little surprise that diets rich in fresh plant matter are consistently linked to good health.

Take vitamin C, for instance. Of all the 4,000 or so known mammals, humans are one of a tiny handful of species whose bodies cannot manufacture their own vitamin C. Our extremely rare genetic inability to do this means that without a constant supply of the stuff we would soon succumb to scurvy and perish. Thanks a lot, evolution.

Now, it just so happens that the few other mammals that share this quirky trait (namely guinea pigs, fruit bats and monkeys) are also those that consume loads of fresh plant foods naturally rich in vitamin C, and this isn't a coincidence. Evolutionary scientists hypothesize that the reason we lost our ability to make the vitamin was because our ancestral diets were just so rich in it (up to ten times that of today, even as late as the Stone Age) we simply didn't need to produce it. Like exotic birds on faraway islands that lose the ability to fly when there aren't any big predators around, we lost our ability to produce it due to lack of evolutionary pressure. This mutation ties us, even today, to 'stealing' an essential vitamin from the plant kingdom by eating lots of fruit and veg on a regular basis.

Now, this same hypothesis has been used by some scientists to explain at least one of the apparent effects of a group of non-essential (but still beneficial) compounds also found in plants: phytonutrients. These are a huge group of up to 5,000 compounds that have so far been discovered in the botanical world and whose potential health effects are only just being uncovered. Part of the way they may work is by the aforementioned antioxidant effect (see page 14) that may shield our delicate cells from damage caused by free radicals, which can build up over time and lead to degenerative conditions like heart disease and cancer as we age. Plants create phytonutrients to protect their own cells from damage, but it often appears that when we eat them, their protective effect can be conferred to our own cells.

OK, unlike with vitamin C, our bodies do have the ability to produce their own antioxidants to defend against free radical damage, but this system is far from failsafe. In fact, it has been argued that our ancestral diet was so rich in such a broad range of other antioxidant compounds, it could well be that our bodies did not need to be quite as effective at producing them. We are talking up to 70 per cent more folate, three times the carotenes and a whopping six times the vitamin E than we currently eat, according to researchers at Hong Kong Polytechnic University. These scientists hypothesize that, much like vitamin C, as we have come to rely on these plant-derived compounds, our own defence system now gives us insufficient protection. The only way to keep these defences topped up, according to this theory, is with a constant dietary supply of fruit and veg. You might call it your daily dietary defence system.

DETOX SUPPORT

I am forever seeing recipes for 'detox' teas, pills and diet plans online. Yet the fact of the matter is that if you are in possession of a fully functioning liver and pair of kidneys, you have all you need to tackle the build-up of toxins in your body. This is the biological function of these organs, and they do it all day, every day, without you having to give it a second thought.

However, there is a growing body of research that suggests certain compounds in plants may play a role in supporting the body's own detox system, potentially boosting the production of the natural enzymes our bodies manufacture to tackle toxins. As far back as the 1990s, studies started to reveal, for example, that eating cruciferous veg such as broccoli and cauliflower can speed up the rate your liver clears the toxin caffeine from your bloodstream, to the point that you have to drink more of the stuff to get the same buzz. This has been attributed to the presence of a compound known as sulforaphane, which broccoli plants actually produce as a toxic defence against insects. Weird, right?

In a more recent (but admittedly very small) study at London's Imperial College, researchers found that this effect may last a surprisingly long period of time. The geeks at Imperial put a group of healthy adult men on a diet containing grilled meat, which naturally contains a known quantity of suspected carcinogens that form in flesh during cooking. They then introduced a hefty helping of cruciferous veg (about 3 portions of Brussels sprouts and broccoli

every day) to see what would happen. As the researchers expected, the levels of the carcinogens detectable in the men's urine when the veg was introduced dropped by about 20 per cent. However, and here's the surprising finding, 12 days after the participants had been taken off the high-veg diet, the levels of the carcinogen were *still* suppressed, despite the fact that they were continuing to chow down on the meat. An effect that supports your own detox system and may be powerful enough to carry on working for a considerable length of time.

Other compounds that might have similar effects have been found in citrus fruit, berries, tea and a range of herbs and spices. As a botanist, I find perhaps the craziest thing is that these compounds are often produced by plants to kill (or at least repel) small animals like plant-eating insects. It might just be that in our (much larger) bodies, small doses of these toxins paradoxically have the opposite effect, priming our bodies to ramp up their defences. Bonkers-sounding, I know. It may still be very early days, but that's the theory so far. I can't wait to find out what further research reveals!

> Ironically, the toxins found in plants may prime our own bodies for defence when we eat them.

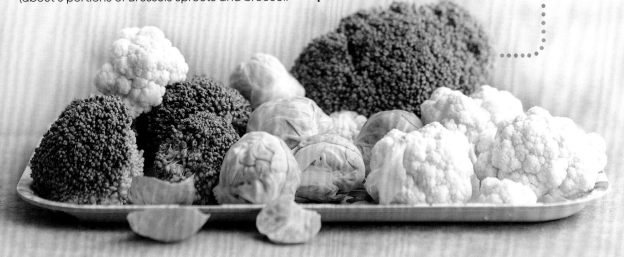

BLOOD PRESSURE & CHOLESTEROL

Potassium – a mineral found naturally in fruit and veg that is drawn up from the soil and concentrates in a plant's tissues – has consistently been shown to help reduce blood pressure across a range of studies. So much so, in fact, that it is thought to be one of the key reasons why eating a plant-based diet may reduce the risk of heart disease. Curiously, potassium works in two different ways: first, by relaxing the blood vessels, which causes them to expand and relieve internal pressure; secondly, by helping to flush out sodium (i.e. salt) in your blood, which can cause raised blood pressure. But the effect of minerals in veg on blood pressure doesn't stop there. Dietary nitrates are also drawn up through the soil by plants and are used to fuel leaf growth. When we consume these leaves, our bodies convert the dietary nitrate into a substance called nitric oxide, which studies suggest can perform a simultaneous 'health hat-trick': widening blood vessels, thinning the blood and making arteries more flexible, all at the same time. Each of these properties is associated with a reduced risk of heart disease. Get them together and you could benefit from a potential triple whammy.

The effects of potassium and dietary nitrates can kick in pretty fast, too. Scientists at the University of Exeter found that putting people on a diet containing lots of high-nitrate veg (such as chard, rocket, spinach and lettuce) for just 1 week could lower their blood pressure by approximately 4 points. This 4-point fall might not sound huge, but is relevant because every 2 point rise is thought to increase the risk of heart disease by 7 per cent and stroke by 10 per cent. In the case of potassium, an Australian research team found that a single meal containing the equivalent of the amount in two and a half bananas could temporarily improve artery function within just 2 hours of consumption. OK, it may be too early to tell if such temporary changes translate to long-term cardiovascular protection, but these studies do add to a growing stack of evidence for the apparently protective effect of potassium.

When it comes to cholesterol, research has shown that the soluble, gel-like fibres that give many fruit and veg their slippery, succulent texture can trap the cholesterol that is made naturally by our own bodies within bile, physically binding to it in the gut and blocking its reabsorption into our bloodstream. As this is thought to be an important risk factor for developing heart disease, a high-fibre diet may have a protective effect. But the benefits don't stop there. The same sticky fibrous substances can slow the absorption of sugars and fats from the food you eat, too, helping blunt their effect on your bloodstream. Pretty powerful stuff.

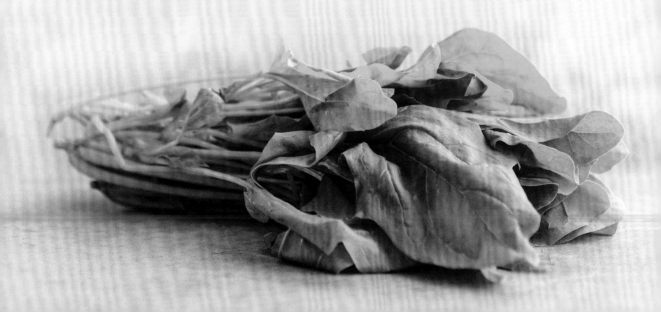

FEEDING GUT BACTERIA

In the not so distant past, it was thought that the gut's only real functions were the digestion and absorption of food; however, recent research is revealing that it (or rather the billions of friendly bacteria it is home to) plays a critical role in many other aspects of our physiology, from immunity to mental health. The indigestible fibres found in plant foods, and in particular fruit and vegetables, are what these bacteria live off, converting them into special molecules such as short-chain fatty acids, which we now know can do everything from mopping up cholesterol to boosting our mood. But here's the catch – each species of bacteria feeds off slightly different compounds, so the more diverse your diet, the more communities of bacteria your gut will be home to. Scaling up from 5-a-day to closer to 10 provides not only more food for these critters, but also a greater range of them, which may well translate into better health for both you and your little friends.

What's the evidence for this? Well, here's at least one piece. After the British government's Scientific Advisory Committee on Nutrition ran an in-depth review of all the best evidence out there, it concluded that **adults should aim to consume at least 30g (1oz) of fibre every day to ensure good health.**

What does 30g (1oz) of fibre look like in terms of a daily diet? A bunch of scientists at the British Nutrition Foundation decided to model whether this extremely high level of fibre was actually achievable given the UK's current minimum 5-a-day standard dietary recommendation for fruit and veg. They found that even if you ate loads of fibre-rich food like wholegrains and snacked on nuts and dried fruit, you would also need to eat at least 8 portions of fruit and veg a day to achieve the required 30g (1oz) of fibre. **Sticking to the minimum 5-a-day would mean missing out on more than a quarter of your daily fibre needs, yet another reason why we should aim to surpass the minimum level.** Put simply, it's basically the only way to get enough fibre!

IT'S NEARLY IMPOSSIBLE TO MEET YOUR BASIC FIBRE NEEDS JUST BY EATING 5-A-DAY.

THAT'S ONE MORE REASON TO AIM HIGHER!

'CROWD OUT' LESS HEALTHY FOOD

Here's something weird – it turns out that a significant part of the apparent benefits of fruit and veg may be about not only what they contain, but also what they don't. Take celery, for instance. You know the old claim that celery is so low in calories that our bodies burn more energy digesting it than the calories it contains? Well, scientists at Oxford Brookes University in the UK decided to put this to the test. Could it really be a 'negative calorie' food? Serving a group of female volunteers a 100g (3½oz) portion of the fresh stems, the researchers measured their calorie expenditure and found that although digesting the veg did burn more than 85 per cent as many calories as the stalks contained, there was still a small surplus, albeit of just a measly 2 calories! However, we of course don't live off celery alone. So could it be that foods that have a very high fibre and water content but are very low in calories, like celery, fill us up so much it results in us eating less of other more high-calorie foods throughout the day? Well, looking at the evidence, the answer is: 'Quite probably!'

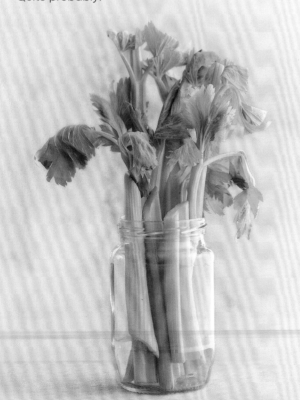

According to a study published in the *Journal of the American Dietetic Association*, for example, serving up a large side salad as a starter to a bunch of volunteers meant they tended to eat significantly less food when presented with an all-you-can-eat pasta buffet. How much less? Up to 12 per cent, even when the calories present in the salad were taken into account.

Scoff an apple before lunch and you could slash the total calories you eat in the meal by 15 per cent, knocking off an average of 187 calories. That's more than in a can of cola without you even noticing! A similar effect has been shown in a range of other foods from pears to soup, revealing that adding bulky low-calorie foods to what is served makes people so satiated they eat less of other higher-calorie foods.

This ability of foods with low-calorie density to essentially 'crowd out' other foods from our diet has revealed a curious phenomenon when it comes to our eating behaviour: we tend to eat a similar weight of food every day, irrespective of the calories it contains. This is a fascinatingly curious quirk of how our bodies regulate our appetite, which we can use to our own advantage. By simply swapping high-calorie foods for an equal weight of food lower in calories (basically any fruit and veg), studies suggest you can potentially eat significantly *more* food, feel just as satiated and still cut calories, fat and sugar from your diet. And that's before we mention the added nutrients, flavour and colour.

This is why this one dietary change seems to me to be potentially so powerful – if simply eating *more* fruit and veg also has the unintended knock-on effect of causing us to eat *less* fat and sugar and fewer calories overall, it's equivalent to making multiple, more far-reaching changes without even trying. In the concluding words of one such study by the University of Pennsylvania: 'This approach may facilitate weight loss because it emphasizes positive messages rather than negative, restrictive messages.' Amen to that!

WHAT IS A PORTION?

Pretty much any fruit and veg you can imagine counts towards your daily portions, meaning you really are spoilt for choice. Here's a quick guide to everything that counts, and an explanation for the very few exceptions to the rule.

WHAT COUNTS?

80G (2¾OZ) WHOLE FRUIT OR VEG

It doesn't have to be fresh – **frozen or canned counts**, too. Surprisingly, **80g (2¾oz) isn't even all that much**, meaning a 'portion' can be much smaller than you might think. I was certainly surprised when I got out the scales. One apple, for example, about 160g (5¾oz), is 2 portions right there. In order to get maximum benefits, enjoy as many different types of fruit and vegetables as you can. This is because different fruit and veg provide different vitamins, minerals and fibres.

OR

30G (1OZ) DRIED FRUIT OR VEG

During the drying process, water lost from fruit leads to a reduction in weight, meaning **30g (1oz) dried fruit is the equivalent of a whole portion of fresh**. Its concentrated sweetness provides a great way to replace refined sugars, syrups or honey in loads of recipes, too, while sneakily upping your daily fruit dose. Although there are fewer examples of dried veg, the same deal works: 30g (1oz) of dried mushrooms, for example, is the equivalent of 80g (2¾oz) of fresh; likewise, 30g (1oz) of tomato purée, which is made by cooking fresh tomatoes until much of the water is removed, counts as 1 portion.

To illustrate this, I've weighed a bunch of fruit and veg to show you quite how little 1 portion can be (see overleaf).

WHAT 1 PORTION LOOKS LIKE

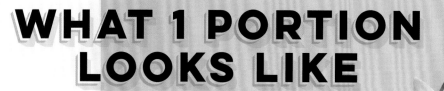

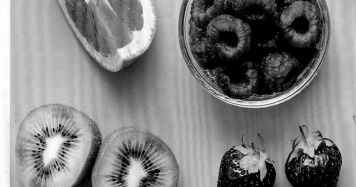

Yep. Even canned convenience foods like baked beans and vegetable soup can count. Just a measly **quarter of a can (80g/2¾oz)** is all you need!

People tend to misjudge how small an 80g (2¾oz) portion is when it comes to apples, pears, peppers, peaches and avocados. A single fruit is actually **2 portions!**

Even the dried stuff counts, whether it be snacking on sugary-sweet raisins or adding deliciously savoury dried mushrooms to a risotto.

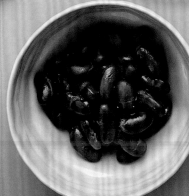

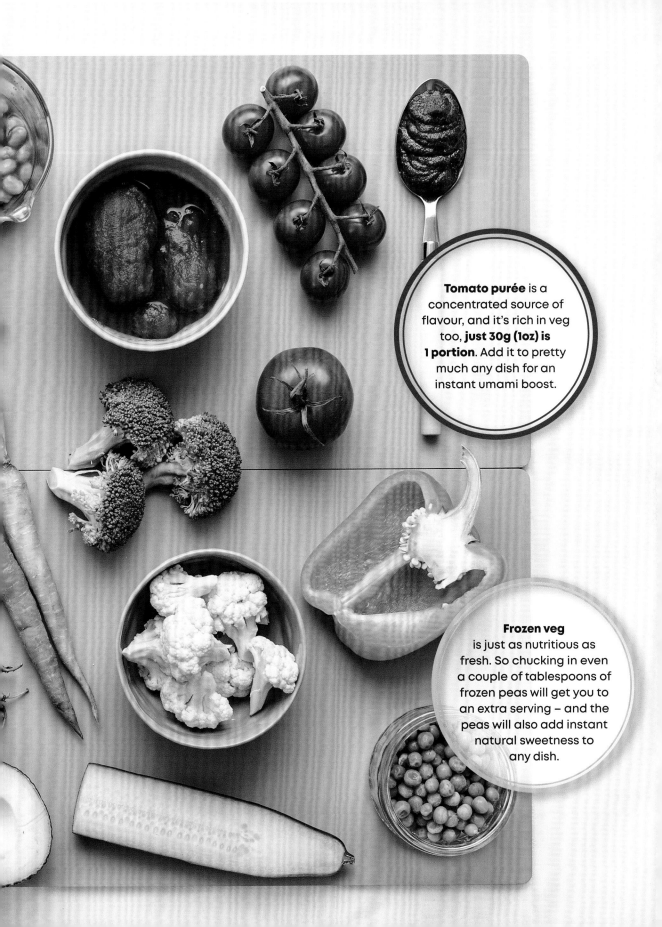

Tomato purée is a concentrated source of flavour, and it's rich in veg too, **just 30g (1oz) is 1 portion**. Add it to pretty much any dish for an instant umami boost.

Frozen veg is just as nutritious as fresh. So chucking in even a couple of tablespoons of frozen peas will get you to an extra serving – and the peas will also add instant natural sweetness to any dish.

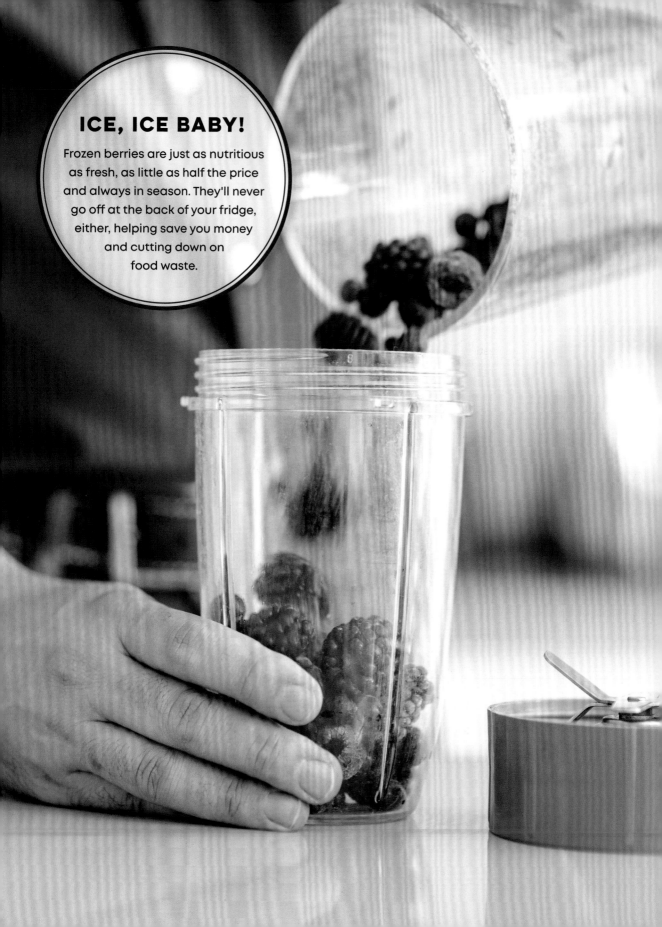

ICE, ICE BABY!

Frozen berries are just as nutritious as fresh, as little as half the price and always in season. They'll never go off at the back of your fridge, either, helping save you money and cutting down on food waste.

WHAT 'KINDA' COUNTS?

150ML (5FL OZ) JUICE OR SMOOTHIE

When fruit or veg are blitzed up into a purée, the contents trapped within their tough cell walls are released, making them far easier for your body to digest. This can be a great thing for many vitamins and minerals, for example. However, the same effect also applies to sugars, meaning these too hit your bloodstream much faster. Served in the form of a drink, it is also significantly easier to consume large amounts of these sugars very quickly, bypassing the action of chewing altogether, which triggers feelings of fullness in our brains.

This phenomenon was investigated by a team of researchers from Maastricht University in the Netherlands who found that serving a fruit salad of sliced apples, apricots and bananas along with a few glasses of water resulted in participants feeling significantly fuller than when served the exact same ingredients whacked in a blender and poured into a glass (aka, a smoothie). When it comes to juice, most of the healthful fibre is removed during the juicing process, which speeds up how quickly the sugar hits your bloodstream even further.

So, while smoothies and juices are still great sources of vitamins, minerals and other phytonutrients, only a single 150ml (5 fl oz) portion counts towards your daily target. And that's very small indeed. We are talking about half a normal juice glass. It is also recommended that juices and smoothies are consumed alongside other foods, not as a between-meal snack, because this can help protect your teeth from the sugars they contain. A useful tip.

80G (2¾OZ) BEANS OR PULSES

Beans and pulses are a great source of fibre and, unlike most other veg, are a good source of protein, too. However, as they are generally less nutrient-dense than other fruit and veg, most public health guidelines consider that they should only count towards one of your daily portions. That doesn't mean you need to limit your intake, it just means extra portions won't count towards your target.

WHAT ABOUT SOUP?

If smoothies only count in a very limited way, why do blended soups count? After all, a soup is basically just a veg smoothie served hot, with a spoon and a little added salt, right? Well, here's the weird thing. It might be all down to the *spoon*. Yes, you read that right.

Researchers at Purdue University in the USA set out to compare how eating apples affected appetite when served in a variety of ways: whole, as a smoothie and as a soup. That's kind of strange – why apple soup? Well, previous studies had shown that in contrast to smoothies, consuming soup was satiating enough that people tended to reduce their consumption of other foods later in the day. And guess what the researchers found? Volunteers who ate the apple soup reported feeling not only more full than those who drank the same mix in a smoothie, but almost as satisfied as those who ate whole fresh apples. The soup scoffers even consumed fewer overall calories for the rest of the day than those who ate whole fresh apples. A surprising finding that has turned up in a number of other trials.

This could well be explained by the fact the liquid was served in a bowl with a spoon, meaning the participants consumed it much more slowly. Other studies have shown this can also reduce calorie intake and overconsumption. The slower pace may have given the volunteers' brains time to register that they were full. Picture how long it takes to eat, say, a 200ml (7fl oz) bowl of soup. What, 10–15 minutes? Compare this to consuming the same amount of liquid served as a smoothie or juice in a glass, which people often down in less than a minute, according to the supergeeks at Wageningen University in the Netherlands, and you get the picture.

It may even be that simply the act of eating from a bowl might psychologically feel more like a 'meal' than a mere 'drink' – we know that subjective feelings of fullness are affected by how many calories people perceive a meal contains. Different serving methods can elicit different biological responses, so while smoothies don't count, soups, purées and other blitzed-up foods do. Science is nothing if not surprising!

WHAT DOESN'T COUNT?

POTATOES

Yes, I hate to be the bearer of bad news, but potatoes don't count as a fruit and veg portion. This is due to their higher calorie content and lower amounts of nutrients, when compared to other fruit and veg at least. The same also goes for other very starchy white veg like cassava, plantains and yams.

Weirdly, sweet potatoes, parsnips and swedes *do* count because, in general, the balance of nutrients to calories in these is slightly tipped in their favour. Now, as a botanist, I think this distinction can be a little arbitrary, as bananas, for example, do count, but plantains, which are very close relatives and have an extremely similar chemical composition, don't. Sweetcorn counts, but maize (which is basically fully mature sweetcorn) doesn't. Strictly speaking, white varieties of sweet potatoes that are much lower in nutrients count, whereas purple varieties of regular spuds with nutrient levels that are many times higher do not count. However, in general and pedantic plant-geekery aside, the distinction seems a pretty sound one, at least in terms of broad brushstrokes.

However, just because potatoes and other very starchy veg don't count as a vegetable, this doesn't mean we should avoid eating them. They are simply categorized together with other starches like wholegrains such as brown rice and oats, which research has shown should form the basis of a healthy diet. In fact, despite recent trendy carbophobia, based on the best available evidence, standard health guidelines still recommend that we get half of our calories from such foods. Potatoes are a great source of fibre and, gram for gram, contain as little as half the calories of bread and pasta, so don't feel you need to miss out on spuds!

PICKLES, OLIVES & CONDIMENTS

Although very high in fruit and veg content, pretty much every recipe out there for these tasty treats contains so much salt or sugar (and sometimes both) that serving up an 80g (2¾oz) portion of them would contribute excessive amounts to your diet. Take ketchup, for example. Although it is a concentrated source of tomatoes, it contains gram for gram twice as much added sugar as Coca-Cola, along with a hefty amount of salt.

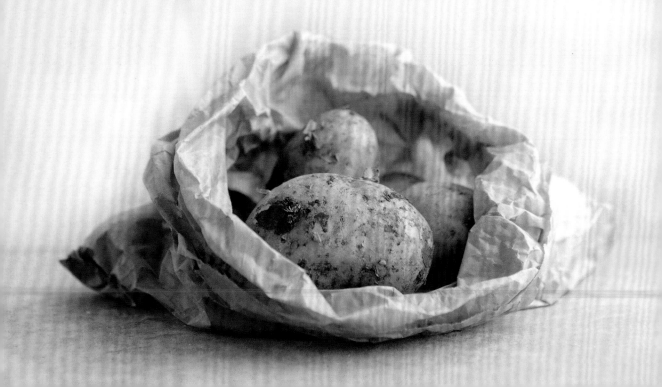

WHILE ONION RINGS AND COLESLAW DON'T COUNT, VEG THAT ARE SHALLOW-FRIED WITHOUT OIL-ABSORBING BATTER OR USE DRESSINGS WITH A MORE MODEST AMOUNT OF ADDED FAT *DO COUNT.*

YOU'LL SEE QUITE A FEW RECIPES FOR THESE DOTTED THROUGH THE BOOK, INCLUDING SWEET POTATO & PARSNIP FRIES (SEE PAGE 133).

Fortunately, however, there is a pretty easy work-around for most of these: make your own! I have been tinkering in my kitchen to find ways to make super-simple recipes for condiments from dill pickles to ketchup that are far lower in salt and sugar than the shop-bought alternative but taste just as good…if not way better! Trust me when I say they are genuinely ridiculously easy, too – as in mixing a few pre-made ingredients together in less than 2 minutes. This means that many fruit and veg favourites that would not normally count suddenly do. Check them out on pages 210–217.

JAMS & JELLIES
Although jams and jellies can contain up to 50 per cent pure fruit, as with condiments, the remainder is usually made up of an avalanche of sugar. However, if you make a no-added-sugar jam or compote (see my recipe on page 58), you really do get to have your jam and eat it.

ONION RINGS & COLESLAW
Pretty much the same deal as everything in this section I am afraid. Even though recipes for these contain a very high vegetable content, the massive amount of added fat in the batter and/or mayonnaise is considered to offset the benefits. Sadly, I don't make up the rules!

WINE
And finally. Yes, I know wine is basically gone-off grape juice. But no, it doesn't count. My mum was particularly cross about this. Don't shoot the messenger!

THE MYTHS

If foodie media stories are anything to go by, attempting to scale up your fruit and veg intake beyond 5-a-day will involve hours of chewing, ridiculous amounts of prep time and a massively prohibitive cost. And indeed, when you look at probably the biggest study to assess global governmental efforts to boost fruit and veg consumption run by the University of Sydney's food scientists, this appears to be a fair reflection of public opinion, too. But is it actually true?

Well, as with many psychological barriers, there seems to be a pretty large gap between public perception and the evidence in practice. Trust me, as someone who is notoriously lazy, tight-fisted and also likes a burger, I had genuine reservations before testing it out. So here's my break-down of the top five myths about eating more than 5-a-day, from someone who regularly does it.

MYTH 1:
IT TAKES A LOT OF TIME & EFFORT

Take a look at any clean-eating blog and you might get the impression eating healthily involves a kitchen full of fancy spiralizers, high-power blenders and multi-layered dehydrators. You'll have to spend hours soaking, grating and fermenting that stuff, too, if you want maximum benefits. Right?

Well, thankfully, no! Almost any fruit and veg in pretty much any form counts towards your daily portions – whether it's an apple as you dash out the door or a quick shop-bought fruit salad on your lunch break. Opening a can of baked beans for toast is another option and how much time does that take? Frozen mixed veg can easily be chucked into pretty much any dish, from speedy omelettes to shop-bought pasta sauce, giving an extra veggie boost.

Let's also not forget super-convenient and pre-sliced options, and yes, these can include supermarket ready meals. Food writers can be quite sniffy about these, but there is now an increasingly wide range of veggie side dishes that come without excessive amounts of fat, sugar or salt, including seemingly indulgent sweet potato wedges and store-bought hummus or guacamole, which are even better if you go for the lower fat and salt formulations. Why not dip the wedges in the hummus or guac for 2 portions in one – I kid you not.

Not only are pre-sliced options and ready meals incredibly convenient for those pushed for time or without many cooking facilities (think of the office kitchenette at lunchtime), but they can also be a total godsend for people with disabilities. A simple, pre-packed bowl of mixed fresh veg you can bung in the microwave and serve in 3 minutes is just as healthy as slicing it yourself, I promise you.

Still not sure? A study in the *British Medical Journal* that objectively analysed the composition of 100 ready meals versus 100 popular recipes from TV chefs found the ready meals contained on average less salt, sugar and fat (including saturated fat) and fewer calories as well as more fibre than the home-cooked versions. Put simply, what determines how a food affects your biology is what it contains, not whether you made it yourself. So spare yourself the guilt and eat more veg however you can.

Frankly, though, upping your portions when cooking stuff from scratch isn't as hard as you might think. If you are making spaghetti Bolognese, a stew, chilli

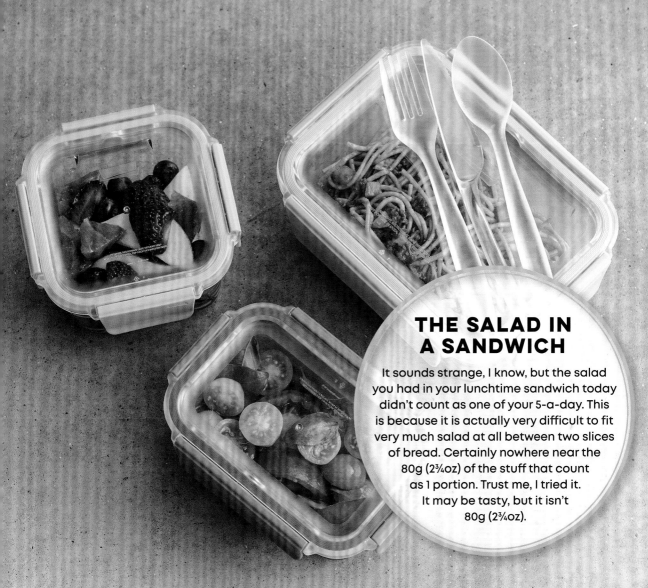

THE SALAD IN A SANDWICH

It sounds strange, I know, but the salad you had in your lunchtime sandwich today didn't count as one of your 5-a-day. This is because it is actually very difficult to fit very much salad at all between two slices of bread. Certainly nowhere near the 80g (2¾oz) of the stuff that count as 1 portion. Trust me, I tried it. It may be tasty, but it isn't 80g (2¾oz).

con carne, curry or a stir-fry, simply adding one more carrot, courgette or pepper than the recipe says will give you a couple more portions without you having to change anything else and only adds at most a few minutes to how long it takes to whip up.

If all you do is manage to sneak 1 extra portion in at each meal, given average consumption levels in somewhere like my native UK, that would *double* your daily intake from roughly 3 to 6 portions. And remember, **every extra portion you get could make a statistical difference to your risk of a range of diseases**. It really couldn't be simpler.

CONVENIENCE FOOD THAT COUNTS AS 1 PORTION

Baked beans

Baked sweet potatoes wedges

Canned pasta in tomato sauce

Canned vegetable soup

Fruit bars
(containing 30g/1oz dried fruit and no added sugar)

Fruit compote

Guacamole

Hummus

Ice lollies
(made with 100 per cent fruit juice)

Muesli
(containing 30g/1oz dried fruit and no added sugar)

Salsa

Store-bought smoothies and juice
(with no added sugar)

MYTH 2:
FRUIT & VEG ARE JUST TOO EXPENSIVE

Fruit and veg are often thought of as expensive. In an era of growing inequality and economic uncertainty, this can be a real limitation for many people, as simply getting enough calories at all can be the priority for some. But for those not on the very lowest incomes is this idea supported by the evidence? Being an unapologetic data geek, I love a good stat so I crunched the numbers and here's what I found.

Let's pick three dinner favourites at random – say, spaghetti Bolognese, Marsala chicken and fajitas. If you run their stats, in all three instances it turns out that veg are pretty much the cheapest components gram for gram. On average they clock in at roughly the same price as carbs such as pasta, bread or rice, and in some cases can be much lower, and are a fraction of the cost of cheese and meat. In fact, in some dishes the total cost of 3–4 portions of veg can still be lower than 1 portion of the meat.

Now, of course, there are exceptions. Gram for gram, lighter-weight crops like berries and salads are indeed much more expensive than most meat and carbs. However, this is offset by the fact that they tend to make up a much smaller proportion of recipes than heavier, more commonly used items like apples, onions and carrots, which can be as much as 95 per cent cheaper. This means that swapping out some of the carbs and meat for fruit and veg in all sorts of common everyday dishes, far from being more expensive, actually results in either the same or a significantly reduced cost compared to traditional recipes. Healthier, tastier recipes with a veggie boost, lower calories *and* that cost less to make – not a bad deal, really.

If you want your shopping budget to stretch even further opting for frozen and canned veg is a great way to save cash, too – frozen berries, for example, are often half the price of fresh in my local supermarket. And if these are going in homemade compotes, sauces or smoothies, truly, no one will be able to tell the difference. Likewise, canned tomatoes are far cheaper, not to mention more convenient for tipping into soups and stews, instantly eliminating the time spent slicing and dicing.

Finally, budget brands and discount supermarkets can be a great way of getting the same nutrition for a significantly reduced cost. Trust me, 'value' kidney beans in a generic white tin have pretty much the identical chemical (and therefore nutritional) composition as fancy organic brand with an Italian name and gold writing on the side, so your body won't have any idea, no matter how posh you are.

1 PORTION OF VEG CAN COST AS LITTLE AS A QUARTER THE PRICE OF 1 PORTION OF MEAT. SO, CHOOSING MORE VEG IS GOOD FOR YOUR HEALTH AND YOUR WALLET.

MYTH 3:
FRESH IS BEST

In recent years there appears to be a growing fear of 'processed' foods, and fruit and veg are no exception. According to this mind-set, fresh fruit and veg are somehow innately superior to the frozen or canned equivalents. While basing your diet on crisps and instant noodles certainly isn't a great idea, when it comes to fruit and veg, this form of foodie prejudice simply is not supported by evidence. A real shame, as it has arguably caused supermarket offerings of frozen goods, a nutritious, convenient and affordable way to consume all sorts of fruit and veg, to shrink dramatically.

This is despite research that has consistently shown that frozen fruit and vegetables are nutritionally comparable, and in some cases even superior, to the fresh kind. This is because 'fresh' is a relative term. 'Fresh' veg is still transported, packed and displayed in stores, and in some cases this time lag is enough for its nutritional value to degrade significantly. For example, researchers at the University of California found that green peas can lose up to 50 per cent of their vitamin C just a day or two after being picked, not to mention much of their natural sweetness. Freezing them within hours of picking, as is done commercially, stops the chemical reactions that degrade nutrients dead in their tracks, meaning frozen veg can, ironically, be functionally 'fresher'.

The same Californian team concluded 'Exclusive recommendations of fresh produce ignore the nutritional value of canned and frozen products and may conceal the sensitivity of fresh products to nutrient loss…The results presented here suggest that canned, frozen and fresh fruit and vegetables should all continue to be included in dietary guidelines.' Couldn't have said it better myself!

A Sheffield Hallam University study found that frozen vegetables tend to generate almost half the amount of food waste compared to fresh (anything you don't use tends to be put back in the freezer). The reduction of waste is so much less, in fact, that frozen veg can generate far lower carbon emissions, even when you count the running of the freezer.

MYTH 4:
FRUIT HAS TOO MUCH SUGAR

There is a common claim, online at least, that fruit consumption should be limited due to its sky-high sugar content. I have even seen the same theory about humble root veg like carrots and parsnips. However, when you look for the evidence, well, this just is not backed by science.

You see, the sweet stuff in whole fruit and veg is served up trapped within a matrix of plant fibres. The presence of these fibres slows not only how quickly you eat them (you have to do a lot more chewing) but also how quickly they are released into your bloodstream (as the fibres slow how quickly your gut can absorb them). Furthermore, beneficial phytonutrients they contain may also go a long way to 'offsetting' the potential adverse health effects of the sugars present. **For this reason, dietitians are clear that, although we should cut down on 'free' sugars that don't come bound up in fibre (syrups, honey and juice), the intrinsic sugars found in whole fruit and veg should not limit your consumption of them.**

But don't modern fruit varieties contain loads more sugar than they did in the past? Well, this is certainly another common claim, and there has indeed been a lot of breeding work over the centuries to make fruit taste sweeter. However, and this is a very big 'however', the reality is that increased sweetness has very rarely been achieved by upping the sugar content; instead, the amount of bitter or acid chemicals fruits contain has been reduced, causing the sweetness to come to the fore. For example, extremely tart Bramley apples contain very similar levels of sugar as well as all other nutrients to intensely sweet Jazz apples. If tasting sweeter means you are likely to eat more Jazz apples (when was the last time you scoffed a whole Bramley without an avalanche of added sugar?), then a little extra sweetness is no bad thing.

FRUIT & DIABETES

What about people with type 2 diabetes? Well, given that the positive health effects of fruit consumption have been demonstrated to outweigh the effect of the sugars they contain, most dietary guidelines for treating type 2 diabetes recommend a diet rich in high-fibre foods, including fruit.

To confirm whether this standard recommendation was indeed well supported by evidence, independent Danish scientists set up one of the first clinical trials to actually test whether restricting fruit intake might improve the health of a group of newly diagnosed type 2 diabetics. Over the course of 3 months, they found that patients who had been advised to restrict their fruit intake to less than 1 portion a day showed no greater improvement in their health than those who had

been advised to eat almost twice the amount. This led the researchers to conclude: 'We recommend that the intake of fruit should not be restricted in patients with type 2 diabetes.' A pretty clear message, but what do other trials say?

If the sugar in fruit posed a risk to health, one might imagine that if you put a group of people on an extremely fruit-rich diet and monitored their health closely, you would find some alarming results. Well, Canadian scientists decided to do just that with an admittedly very small group of volunteers, feeding them an astonishing 20 portions of fruit a day – that's 1.6kg (3lb 8oz)! What did they find? Lower body weight, blood pressure and triglycerides and a huge drop in cholesterol, with no adverse health effects. Well, there you have it.

MYTH 5:
ORGANIC IS BETTER

There are many reasons why you may choose to eat organic. Evidence has shown it is more profitable for hard-working farmers, for example, who can earn up to 35 per cent more from the same crop. It can have, according to some measures, environmental benefits such as reduced use of certain pesticides. However, being on average 18 per cent less productive, it can also mean more land is needed to generate the same amount of food, which can lead to the destruction of natural habitats as they are converted to farmland. So things are *far* from black and white in this area, no matter what social media says.

But how does the claim that organic is *healthier* for you stack up when it comes to fruit and veg? Well, this has been investigated by literally hundreds of studies and here's what they found: there is lots of evidence that suggests organic crops are indeed higher in some key nutrients. But here's the issue: there are also loads of other studies that have found either no difference or, indeed, *lower* levels of some nutrients in organic crops. Often, even in the same study, some nutrients are found to be higher, while others are found to be lower. So we have a body of evidence that is highly contradictory and from which it is really difficult, nigh on impossible, to draw any objective, meaningful and consistent conclusions. When stats geeks have gathered all the best-quality studies together and tried to sift through the numbers to find patterns, no significant difference in the levels of vitamins and minerals could be found in any study.

This is probably because making like-for-like comparisons between organic and non-organic fruit and veg is very difficult. For example, if you went to a shop and bought an organic apple and a non-organic one, it is likely that they would be different varieties, grown on different farms or even countries, with different soil types and climates, and handled and stored in different ways, all of which will affect the end results.

OK, but what about pesticides? After all, what is pretty clear from the studies we have so far is that organic crops, despite often being grown using some pesticides, do tend to contain much lower levels of pesticide residue than their non-organic counterparts. Surely this alone makes them a superior option? Well, it is important to bear in mind the amounts we are talking about when it comes to the use of the word 'residue' and, crucially, whether these residues are large enough to actually impact human health. To attempt to estimate this, an independent team of researchers from the University of Copenhagen set out to calculate the risk to the population by measuring the residues in 47 of the most common foods in the Danish market. They then established the proportions of the diet these would make up and used this to calculate the statistical risk such a diet would pose to those who consumed it. After factoring all the residues from each of these 47 foods in the total diet, the researchers concluded that the risk posed by them was 'very unlikely'. But *how* unlikely, exactly? Roughly equivalent to consuming a single glass of wine every 7 years, statistically speaking. Now that's some Danish understatement for you.

So while it is still unclear whether organic food has any nutritional benefit given the current evidence, what we *do* know is that on average organic food tends to be more expensive. So, if you can afford it and want to buy organic for whatever reason, go right ahead. I do it pretty often, and there is no reason that it will be worse for your health. However, if you feel paying a little extra for it will reward you with a proportional increase in health benefits, well, at the moment there just isn't much science to support this claim.

10 TRICKS TO MORE FRUIT & VEG

Let's face it, increasing your daily portions of fruit and veg can seem a pretty daunting task, even when you discover how surprisingly small a 'portion' really is. To help you on your way, here are 10 super-simple tips and tricks for 'botanical bolt-ons' that will easily fit in with your existing diet. A fruity dessert here, a nifty cooking tip there will dramatically increase your consumption without sacrificing anything at all. So let's get started…

DON'T BE A SLAVE TO RAW

'The *only* way to eat veg is crisp and raw, just as nature intended' is a common claim that you'll have undoubtedly seen in books, blogs and social media memes everywhere. Something we have all read so often, it simply must be true. Right?

Well here's the tricky thing with this claim: a plate of raw veg can be really hard to get through. It physically takes you a lot of time and effort to eat it, which means that the typical portion sizes of raw veg are often much smaller than their cooked equivalent. Let's take the example of spinach.

Anyone who has ever cooked the stuff will know that even a truly enormous fresh bag of leaves cooks down to just a few spoonfuls in a minute or two. This dramatic reduction in volume created by the blast of heat in a pan means that even a small portion of sautéed leaves can contain many times more grams of actual spinach than the great big handfuls in even a generous plate of the raw stuff.

Both of the plates shown below contain 1 portion of spinach. Which do you think you'd be more likely to eat?

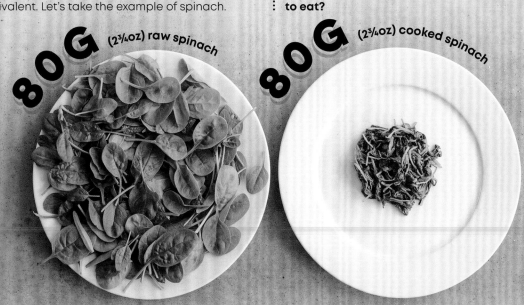

80G (2¾oz) raw spinach

80G (2¾oz) cooked spinach

But, surely, if serving food raw retains far more nutrients, do we need to eat as much of it to gain the same benefits? Well, funnily enough, eating raw food doesn't always guarantee more nutrients are retained. In fact, it can often mean quite the opposite. The cooking process breaks open the tough, indigestible cell walls of plants, releasing their contents in a liquid form that our bodies can access. You can actually see this process in action as their tissues soften and wilt after just a few minutes of heat. The net result is that many key nutrients are much more easily absorbed through cooked veg than raw.

How much more? Let's take a look at spinach again. Researchers at the University of California found that people who ate the leafy green cooked had a whopping three times more carotenes (antioxidants that can be converted to vitamin A) in their bloodstream after their meals than subjects served exactly the same amount raw. Similar findings have been noted for carrots, tomatoes and sweet potatoes. Cooking actually makes them, in effect, higher in key nutrients by making them more digestible. Combine this with the fact that cooking also means you can comfortably eat much more of them and you have a powerful double whammy.

So what's the take-away here? If you like eating veg raw, that's great! It can be a tasty way to add crunch and variety to your meal. I do it all the time, in moderation. But don't feel you need to be a martyr to the raw cause, as it is highly likely serving it cooked means you'll not only scoff more of it, you may even get more goodness gram for gram.

SO, MY NUMBER ONE TIP TO EATING MORE VEG IS SIMPLY TO SERVE IT COOKED because not only is each portion likely to contain more grams of the veg, but also it will be far easier, not to mention more enjoyable, to eat. **Simple enough, right?**

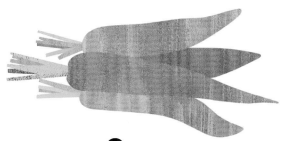

CARROTS 3X more beta carotene when cooked

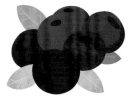

BLUEBERRIES Up to **2X** the antioxidant activity when lightly cooked

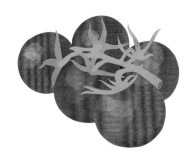

TOMATOES 2X the phytonutrient lycopene when cooked

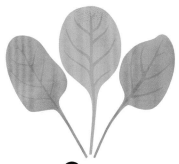

SPINACH 3X more carotenes when cooked

DON'T BE A VEGGIE BOILER

Studies looking into veg consumption across populations have consistently found that people in southern Europe tend to eat far more vegetables than those in northern Europe. In fact, the difference can be over two and a half times as much! This appears to be largely down to culture. There could well be loads of social factors at play here, but I can't help wonder if one reason is simply down to traditional methods of cooking?

Boiling vegetables, particularly those that are finely cut, also happens to be an extremely effective way of drawing water-soluble flavour chemicals, not to mention essential nutrients, from their tissues and transferring them to the cooking water. Brilliant, if you then consume that liquid along with the veg in terms of soups and stews. But if, like the home cooks of my mum's childhood in postwar Britain, you strain this off and tip it down the sink, well, that's a large chunk of the good stuff going (in a very real way) down the drain.

In terms of the taste alone, research suggests that the boiling treatment washes away about 25 per cent of their natural sugars. This significantly reduces their sweetness, which is usually the number one factor that determines how highly people rate

Compare a plate of green beans, converted to a grey mush after a good 30 minutes of boiling (as my poor mum grew up with in 1950s Wales) versus the exact same veg served tender-crisp after sautéeing in olive oil, garlic and bacon as they do in Spain. Which are you likely to eat more of?

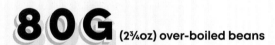

80G (2¾oz) over-boiled beans

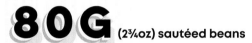

80G (2¾oz) sautéed beans

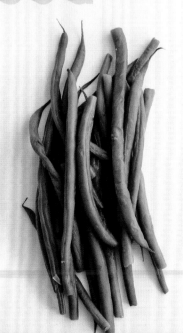

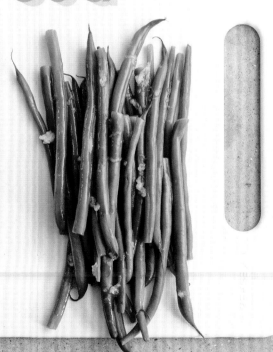

flavour in taste tests. This is important, as studies have consistently shown that of all factors influencing food preference (including flavour, texture, nutrition, cost, safety and convenience), flavour is by far the most important motivator. Along with their sweetness go a hefty chunk of their vitamin C and 20 per cent of their beta carotene – the plant precursor to vitamin A. Talk about foodie sacrilege!

The moral of the story is skip the boiling (unless it's in a soup or stew) and cook veg really any other way. Steaming and microwaving are very quick ways to get them from fridge to table with a minimum of fuss, but baking, grilling, roasting and even frying will also concentrate flavour compounds and caramelize the sugars in the crop, which can greatly enhance their flavour.

Cooking them in a small amount of oil will add to their calorie count but the addition of a little drizzle to your veg can work nutritional wonders in other ways. Some key nutrients in plants are fat soluble, which means cooking or serving them with a little oil or butter can significantly increase the amount of these nutrients your body can absorb from them. For example, Deakin University in Australia showed that cooking tomatoes in a little olive oil can increase the amount of the antioxidant lycopene (thought to help protect against certain cancers) we absorb sixfold. The same treatment works when roasting carrots (coincidentally, my favourite way of eating them), resulting in dessert-level caramelized sweetness and boosting the potentially heart-healthy carotenes we get from them by 80 per cent, according to Spanish research. Fancy a knob of butter on your sweet potatoes? Go ahead! Research has found a little fat can double the amount of beta carotene – a precursor to vitamin A – we are able to absorb from the veg.

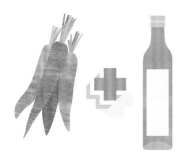

carrots + olive oil = 50% more carotenes

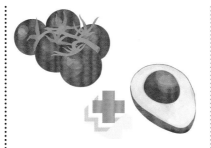

tomatoes + avocado = 4x the phytonutrient lycopene

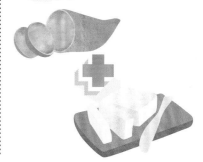

sweet potato + fats like butter = 2x the beta carotene

WHAT HAPPENS WHEN YOU COOK GREEN VEG?

Experimental 'test-tube' research suggests that compounds found in green veg can help bind the bile acids the body naturally produces during digestion. This quirky property may block the potentially harmful reabsorption of these acids, which can have the knock-on effect of reducing the risk of degenerative conditions like heart disease and cancer. Research by the United States Department of Agriculture found that, while cooking significantly improved the ability of green veg to do this (at least in test tubes), sautéeing generally was far superior to boiling for getting the best out of them. Boil kale and it can be 9 per cent more effective at binding to bile acid compared to eating it raw. Sauté it, however, and this ability jumps to 30 per cent. Serve broccoli simmered and it could be 24 per cent more effective at protecting you, but sauté it and it may become 84 per cent more effective. Well, according to this one trial, at least.

EMBRACE FLAVOUR BOOSTERS

The ability of fat to improve both the nutrition and enjoyment you get out of loads of fruit and veg is not only restricted to the cooking process. However you choose to serve them up, there are all sorts of tasty drizzles and sprinkles that can turn even the most simple plate of veg into something spectacular. From creamy dips and dressings to scatterings of grated cheese, crisp croutons, crunchy nuts, fried onions and perhaps a few shards of bacon, even quite modest amounts of these indulgent toppings can significantly increase the amount of veg you are likely to scoff, without necessarily sending the calorie count soaring.

Don't believe me? Research published in the *Journal of the American Dietetic Association* found that 12-year-olds offered helpings of carrot, celery and broccoli with a peanut butter dip for a 4-month period saw a significant increase in veg intake versus those served the same crops plain. In fact, those made to munch on straight-up veg without

the tasty peanut butter side actually saw a decrease in their consumption. Not only did the dip-eaters increase their overall intake over the semester, they were also found to eat a greater variety of veg. Why peanut butter? Because unlike other popular dips like mayonnaise, it is rich in nutrients that US dietary guidelines at the time described as being 'of concern' for adolescents, such as vitamin E, magnesium and potassium. The concern is that people tend not to get enough of these nutrients.

So as long as you don't go crazy with the oil, these tasty additions can mean you not only are likely to eat more veg, but will also get more out of each bite. Frankly, if these indulgent additions mean you are likely to eat fewer desserts and snack between meals, it's a pretty awesome trade-off.

FOOD IS ABOUT ENJOYMENT, SO DON'T BE SHY OF ADDING A FEW TASTY TOPPINGS TO YOUR VEG IF IT HELPS YOU ACHIEVE YOUR TARGET.

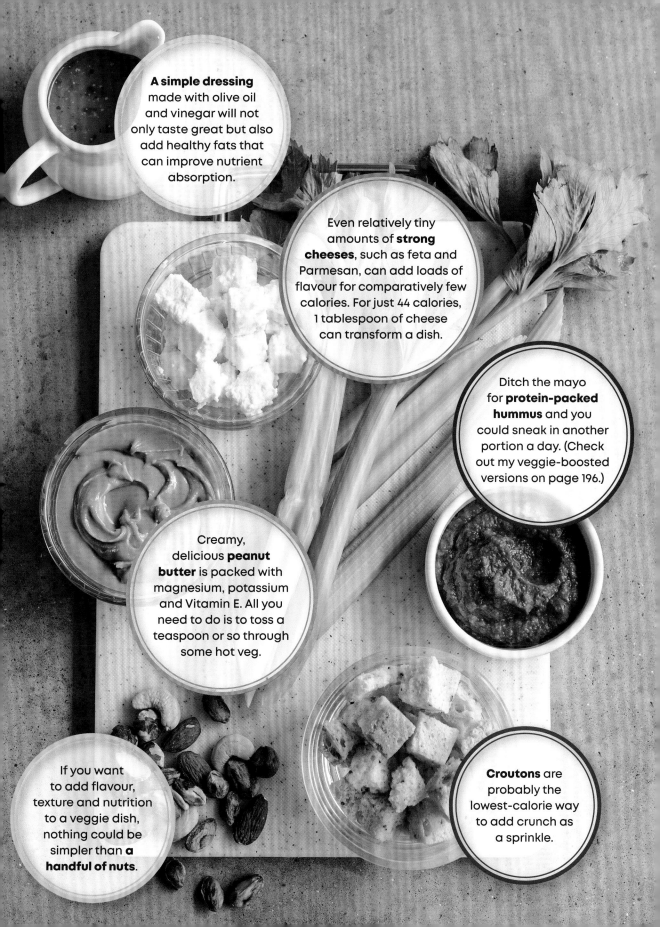

A simple dressing made with olive oil and vinegar will not only taste great but also add healthy fats that can improve nutrient absorption.

Even relatively tiny amounts of **strong cheeses**, such as feta and Parmesan, can add loads of flavour for comparatively few calories. For just 44 calories, 1 tablespoon of cheese can transform a dish.

Ditch the mayo for **protein-packed hummus** and you could sneak in another portion a day. (Check out my veggie-boosted versions on page 196.)

Creamy, delicious **peanut butter** is packed with magnesium, potassium and Vitamin E. All you need to do is to toss a teaspoon or so through some hot veg.

If you want to add flavour, texture and nutrition to a veggie dish, nothing could be simpler than **a handful of nuts**.

Croutons are probably the lowest-calorie way to add crunch as a sprinkle.

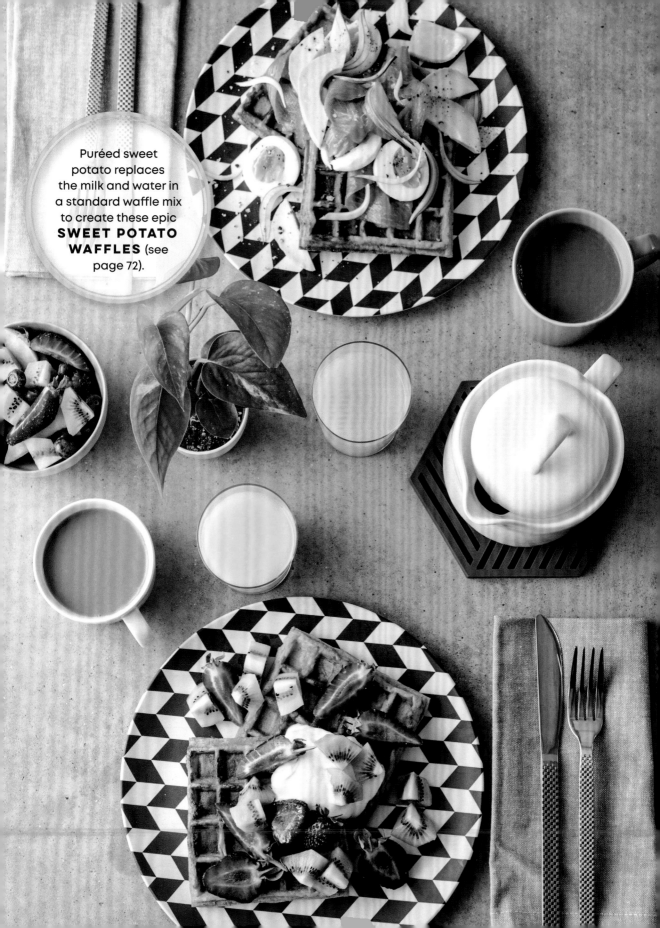

Puréed sweet potato replaces the milk and water in a standard waffle mix to create these epic **SWEET POTATO WAFFLES** (see page 72).

BLITZ 'EM UP

I was making pancakes one morning and slicing a banana into the batter, when it dawned on me: **most batters and doughs contain as much as 50 per cent water or milk by weight**. Now, as fruit and veg are usually mainly made up of water, could there be a way to replace some of the water in recipes with puréed produce? Admittedly, health benefits were far from my mind at the time. All I wanted was to make the most sweet and fruity pancakes. But lo and behold it worked!

In fact, by replacing the stock, water, milk or cream in almost any recipe, you can easily boost your fruit and veg intake, stealthily. So could this be a viable way to up our consumption without really noticing, even for ardent veg haters? Well, studies in *The American Journal of Clinical Nutrition* suggest exactly that.

Researchers at Pennsylvania State University found that the vegetable content of many of kids' favourite dishes could be quadrupled by sneakily incorporating them in the form of a purée. Folded into baking mixtures, pasta sauce and casseroles, kids reported these 'veg by stealth' dishes just as tasty as the traditional versions with less veg. The net result was a dramatic increase in veg intake, even for crops the kids normally hated! This is a useful trick, especially as (perhaps rather tellingly) the consumption of whole vegetables served as side dishes remained identical.

In their write-up, the researchers went to great lengths to point out that parents should not rely exclusively on this sort of subterfuge because 'repeated exposure' to whole veg has frequently been shown in trials to be one of the most effective ways to convince little sugar monsters that fruit and veg may not be deadly. But if puréeing veg works for you, it's worth doing – after all, puréeing veg into soups, stews and creams isn't necessarily 'subterfuge', just a traditional way of cooking that makes veg more palatable for different people's tastes. Just another trick up your sleeve!

But the Pennsylvanians did not stop there. A further study they carried out also discovered that the same technique worked just as well with adults (surprise, surprise). Not only did big kids enjoy meals such as mac and cheese and chicken rice casserole enhanced with puréed veg just as much as the regular kind, they also reported feeling equally as full afterwards. The reduced calorie density in these 'veggie-loaded' meals, however, meant that they were eating an average of 357 fewer calories a day. That's more than the number of calories in a fast-food chain cheeseburger, every single day. Quite a saving!

BY REPLACING THE STOCK, WATER, MILK OR CREAM IN ALMOST ANY RECIPE, YOU CAN EASILY BOOST YOUR FRUIT AND VEG INTAKE, STEALTHILY.

GREAT GRAIN EXTENDERS

Despite the rise of trendy carbophobia, science has consistently shown that wholegrains are one of the most nutritious foods out there. They are a great source of fibre, as well as containing essential vitamins and minerals like thiamine, magnesium and selenium. In fact, a University of Aberdeen trial found that giving patients 3 portions of wholegrains a day for 12 weeks could lower their blood pressure enough to statistically reduce their risk of coronary heart disease by as much as 15 per cent and the chances of experiencing a stroke as much as 25 per cent. What's remarkable about this is the reduction is broadly similar to that achieved by some pharmaceutical drugs, according to the number crunchers. It's perhaps no surprise then that public health advice recommends we choose higher fibre, wholegrain varieties of carbohydrates compared to refined versions. However, there is a range of ways to help bulk out the grains in your diet with extra fruit and veg, helping simultaneously to up the levels of nutrients and lower the calories in each carbolicious portion. From rice and oats to breads and pasta, here are some simple ways to get even more of the good stuff.

RICE & OATS

Adding flavourful peppers, onions, peas, carrots or sweetcorn (frankly, any veg you fancy) to rice can transform an otherwise bland side dish into something far tastier. This can be as easy as bunging your veg into the pan of rice halfway through its cooking time, or simply tossing it through leftover rice to make super-simple pilafs and fried rice.

If you pick beans and pulses as your veg of choice, you might just be in for an extra bonus. A growing body of research suggests that this traditional pairing may significantly reduce the rate at which the carbs in rice are released into your bloodstream, theoretically keeping you fuller for longer. Even when served with super-rapidly digested white rice, a generous portion of beans was found to quell its impact on blood sugar by up to 50 per cent. Perhaps surprisingly, this effect wasn't only observed after the meal itself but continued to blunt the release of carbs consumed at the next meal several hours afterwards, and even the next day. I love rice, but rice with added flavour, fibre, protein and nutrients is even better. Not to mention fewer calories.

This treatment works for porridge, too. Just pick fruit and some of the sweeter veg (I'm talking carrots, pumpkin and sweet potato) and you are good to go. Oh, and for my posher readers, it will work for couscous and quinoa, too.

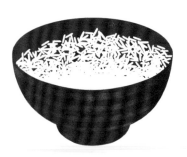

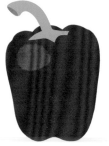
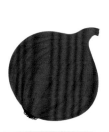
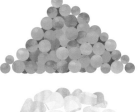

FRIED RICE made with **50%** veg = **35%** fewer calories and **2x** the fibre

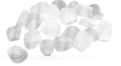

PASTA

When it comes to pasta, I have a different strategy. Instead of adding veg to the cooking water as I do with rice, I prefer to boost the number of portions of them in the sauce. This retains the flavour and nutrients of the veg better than boiling, and means there is no worry about the veg cooking at a different rate to the pasta or making either one soggy.

Oh, and if that wasn't good enough, why not switch the conventional pasta altogether for bean pasta? This is a traditional type of pasta made in Asia using bean flour instead of grain flour. The higher protein content of the beans means the pasta has a more elastic texture (similar to egg pasta) and a denser, more filling consistency.

Aside from being quicker to cook, as it is made from 100 per cent beans, 80g (2¾oz) bean pasta also conveniently counts as 1 portion of veg. A number of Western brands are increasingly making versions styled along the lines of Italian pasta, from 'fettucine' and 'spaghetti' to 'penne' and 'fusilli'. Although I am notoriously sceptical of fashionable carb alternatives (such as the abomination that is spiralized 'courgetti'), I find the bean pastas based on the most traditional recipes that use soya or mung beans really quite good. Surprisingly so, in fact. I'll never give up the wheat-based form, but these types are definitely deserving of the title 'pasta'. However, I avoid the lentil- or pea-based kinds because, no matter how many times I try them, they always end up grainy or soggy.

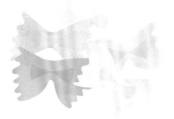

Replacing wheat-based pasta with bean-based pasta = **3X** the protein and **6X** the fibre

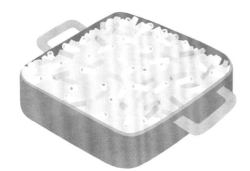

MAC AND CHEESE made with **50%** veg = **42%** fewer calories

BREAD & PANCAKES

Whether it is succulent kernels of sweetcorn dotted through buttery cornbread or the caramelized warmth of onion and peppers giving scones extra flavour, simply stirring chopped cooked veg into pretty much any batter or dough will help keep you fuller for longer using fewer calories.

In fact, by swapping grain-based flour with gram flour made from 100 per cent ground chickpeas, you can turn all sorts of breads and pancakes into a portion of veg as if by magic. This is the same stuff used to make poppadums and chapatis, and is fantastically versatile, creating deliciously satisfying pizza bases and flatbreads that have both added fibre and protein.

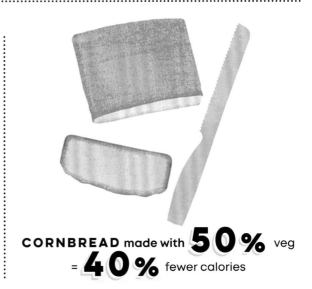

CORNBREAD made with **50%** veg = **40%** fewer calories

SPUD SWAPS & SUBSTITUTES

Potatoes might not count towards your recommended daily intake, but, fortunately for spud lovers like me, their deliciously versatile flavour pairs so well with loads of other veg, it's really easy to dramatically boost the good stuff in a whole host of traditional potato dishes. **Simply replace some of the spuds in any recipe with the veg of your choice.**

To potentially double the veg content of any meal, you could even (dare I say it?) substitute the spuds altogether with other equally comfortingly carby veg in everything from mash and fries to rösti. How far you want to go with this is up to you. Throughout the book, I'll be providing ideas for how to swap out some of the spuds without missing out on flavour.

The delicate creaminess of cannellini beans makes a surprisingly delicious substitute for mash. See my recipe on page 204.

Drizzled with oil and grilled, parsnips make amazing veggie fries. They're even more amazing when served fully loaded (see page 198).

Turned into creamy mash, sweet potatoes can help you sneak in an extra portion of veg served atop a cottage pie (see page 136).

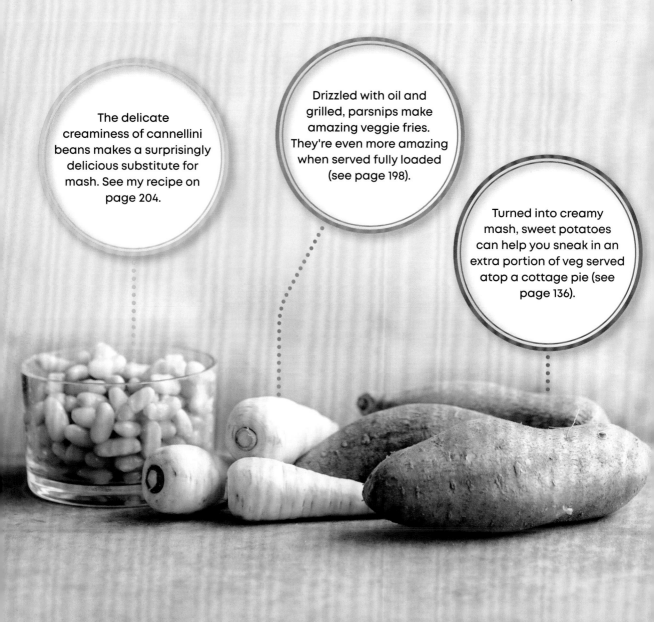

MEAT IN THE MIDDLE

Adding mushrooms, beans, lentils or any other kind of veg that takes your fancy to loads of your favourite meat recipes can be a brilliant way of upping the veg content and reducing the fat in your meal – a habit that could over time save you not only an inch or two off your waistline but also some cash off your grocery bill. We are not talking about radically changing recipes. Chucking in an extra handful of veg to your normal meat-based stews, casseroles, pasta sauces and burgers is enough to lower the ratio of meat to veg in any recipe, making the protein stretch further.

Although I am not vegetarian, I find these additions so flavourful that I will often substitute the meat entirely with veg with a meaty texture. Smoky shiitakes make great, umami-packed burgers (see page 132), without the greasy heaviness of the meaty kind. Sweet carrots and creamy peas teamed up with satisfying chickpeas to make 'meat' balls served Scandinavian-style are (to me at least) far more tasty and interesting than the pork-based type.

The same 'bulking out' approach works with eggs, too, where a veggie boost can make the same quantity of protein go further, while adding loads of great flavour. Fold leftover peppers, sweet potato, onion, mushrooms, leeks or sweetcorn into beaten eggs to make a hearty frittata or Spanish omelette in minutes.

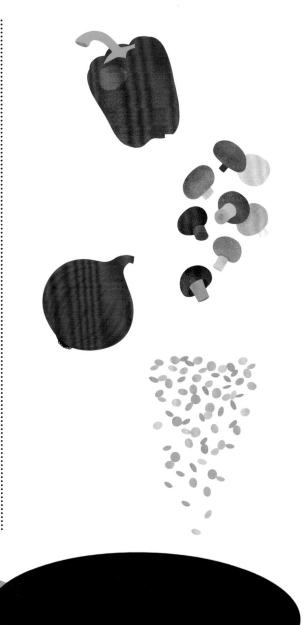

HAVE YOUR BIT ON THE SIDE

OK, I know this one isn't exactly a revolutionary idea, but simply adding a side salad is a really easy way to dramatically up your fruit and veg content in each meal without changing anything else. When I say 'salad', it doesn't necessarily have to mean the green, crisp, leafy variety. We could be talking anything from a veggie side dish like a plate of tomatoes scattered with garlic and drizzled in olive oil with your favourite pasta dish, to a fresh fruit salad or even a glass of juice with your usual breakfast cereal or toast. Even a side 'salad', and I know I am using the word loosely here, of baked sweet potato fries will make a delicious 'bolt-on' and add an extra portion of veg to any meal. (Seriously, I defy anyone to turn down the offer of some sweet potato fries!)

These culinary bolt-ons don't have to be added to your main meal. A simple soup or any other fruit- or veggie-rich starter counts, too. I am all for eating *more* in the interests of my health. Frankly, even if the only thing you did was add a small 250g (9oz) side of fruit or veg to each meal without making any other changes whatsoever, you would easily smash your daily target.

CONDIMENTS THAT COUNT

Ketchup, BBQ sauce & pickles are foods that don't normally count towards your veg intake, which is a huge shame considering their often surprisingly high fruit and veg content *and* the significant amount of these condiments you can get through in a meal without really noticing. Ever looked down at what you thought was an enormous bowl of dip and realized you have polished it off all by yourself? Well, with a few simple tweaks to bring the salt, sugar and fat content under control, these same condiments can be magically turned into vegetable portions. So dip away! Most of these recipes only take 10 minutes or less to knock together, with barely any actual cooking involved. A pretty fair deal, if you ask me.

KETCHUP

Just swap the avalanche of sugar in the shop-bought stuff with supersweet sultanas and you'll get a homemade ketchup that is pretty much 100 per cent fruit and veg with a little added cider vinegar. **See the recipe on page 210.**

MANGO CHUTNEY

Fresh, fruity and yet somehow deliciously rich, spoon on as much of this as you like on curry nights. Made using 60 per cent fruit and veg, it all goes towards your daily portions. **See the recipe on page 211.**

PICKLES

You might think you'd need all sorts of fancy canning kit and a good few hours, but all of these homemade pickles can be knocked together in minutes. I find reducing the sugar and salt actually improves their flavour, making them fresher and lighter. **See the recipes on page 216.**

AVO 'MAYO'

You can use avocados in pretty much any recipe that calls for mayonnaise, from creamy dips to sandwich fillings. I've even turned them into a foolproof 'hollandaise' that will never, ever split: blitz 1 portion of **Guac-molata (see page 193)** to a smooth sauce in a food processor with 2 tablespoons milk.

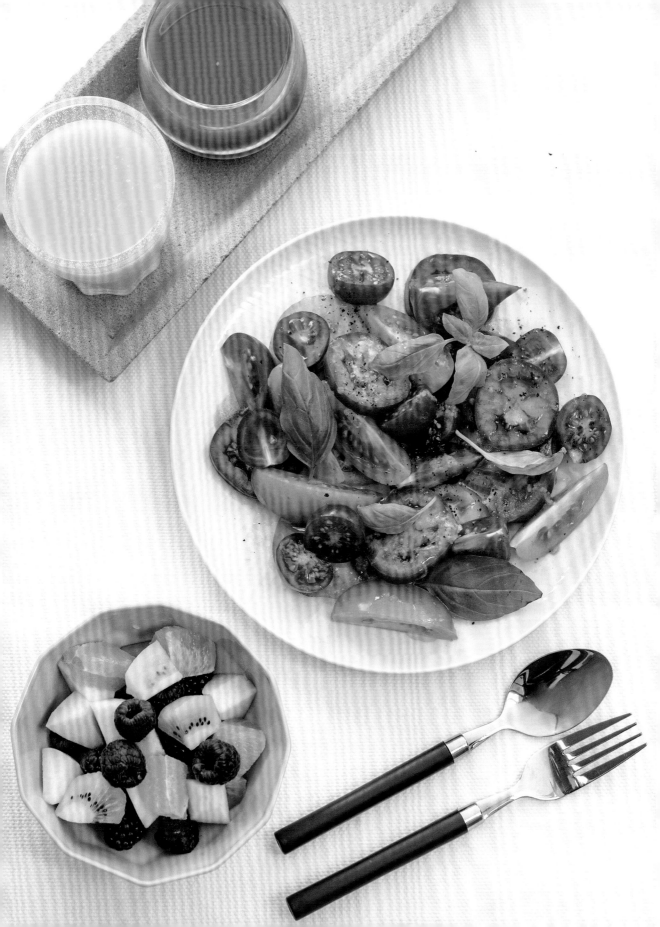

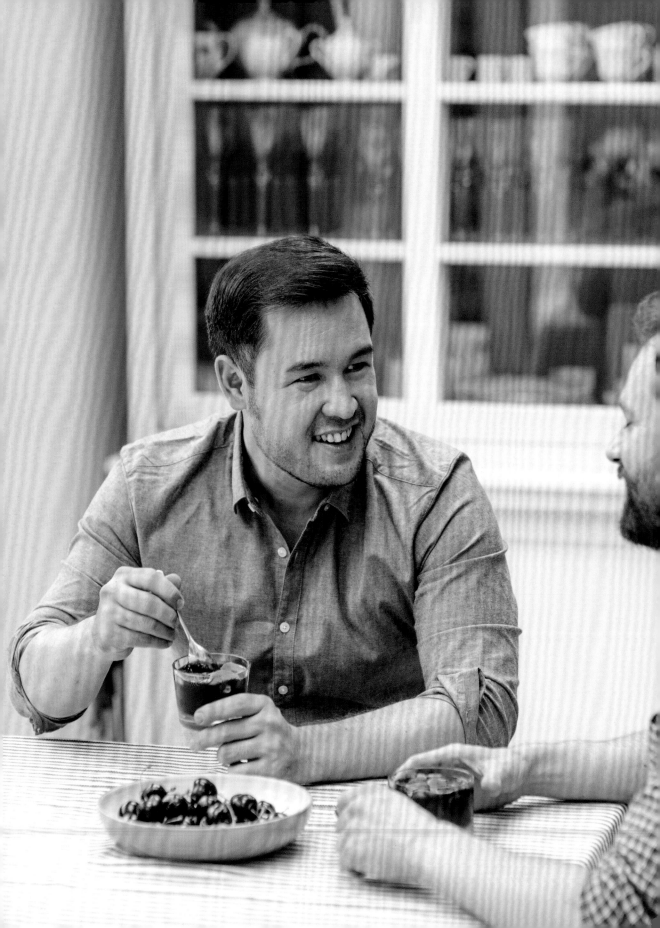

THERE'S ALWAYS ROOM FOR DESSERT

Ever notice that even after a slap-up meal, no matter how full you are feeling, there always seems to be room for dessert? Well, thankfully, you can blame biology for this one. Research suggests the miracle that is the 'dessert stomach' is all down to a phenomenon known as 'sensory-specific satiety'. When you tuck into a plate of food, the new flavour stimuli triggers feelings of pleasure, inducing you to eat more. However, the more you eat of a given dish, the less each mouthful is capable of inducing the same reaction, leading to an increased feeling of satiety. However, if you suddenly introduce new flavours and textures, your pleasure centres get fired up all over again, reigniting your hunger.

As someone afflicted with a notorious sweet tooth, I basically live my life in a permanent state of 'dessert stomach'. However, as loads of traditional desserts have a naturally high fruit content (up to 80 per cent in some cases), there is a way to turn this curse into a downright bonus. After all, what better way to cram extra portions of fruit (and veg) into your diet than in the guise of pudding?

With a few simple tips and tricks to up their fruit content even further, while keeping fat and sugar levels in check, you can truly have your pie, crumble, mousse or cake and eat it too.

FOR ME, THE EASIEST WAY TO UP YOUR INTAKE OF FRUIT AND VEG IS TO HAVE DESSERT. TAKE THIS AS YOUR OFFICIAL EXCUSE, IF YOU NEED ONE.

BREAKFASTS & BRUNCHES

TRIPLE BERRY HOTCAKES

Who can say no to a pancake breakfast? By a clever feat of culinary trickery, these bad boys pack a good 4 portions of fruit into every serving. I love it when 'health food' comes disguised as 'junk food'.

4 PORTIONS PER SERVING

Serves 2
Prep time 5 minutes
Cook time 8 minutes

4 large eggs
200g (7oz) self-raising white flour
1 tsp mixed spice
pinch of salt
300g (10½oz) strawberries (fresh or frozen and defrosted)
butter, for frying
150g (5½oz) blueberries (fresh or frozen and defrosted)

To serve
150g (5½oz) fresh mixed berries
4 tbsp Greek yogurt
½ tsp icing sugar
freeze-dried raspberries, for sprinkling

BLEND all the ingredients except the blueberries together in a food processor to form a batter.

HEAT a little butter in a large frying pan over a medium heat. Pour in 2 tablespoons of the batter per pancake, well spaced apart and swirling the pan around so each pancake spreads out to the size of a CD. Scatter 1 tablespoon of the blueberries over the still-liquid surface of the pancake.

COOK for 1 minute on each side, then remove from the pan and keep warm until you have used up all the batter to make 12 pancakes.

DIVIDE the mixed berries and yogurt among the pancakes, dust each serving with icing sugar and sprinkle with freeze-dried raspberries.

FROZEN BERRIES

are as nutritious as fresh, yet they can be less than half the price – especially in winter. And, frankly, if you are using them in this batter, no one will ever tell the difference. I do love a nutrition cheat.

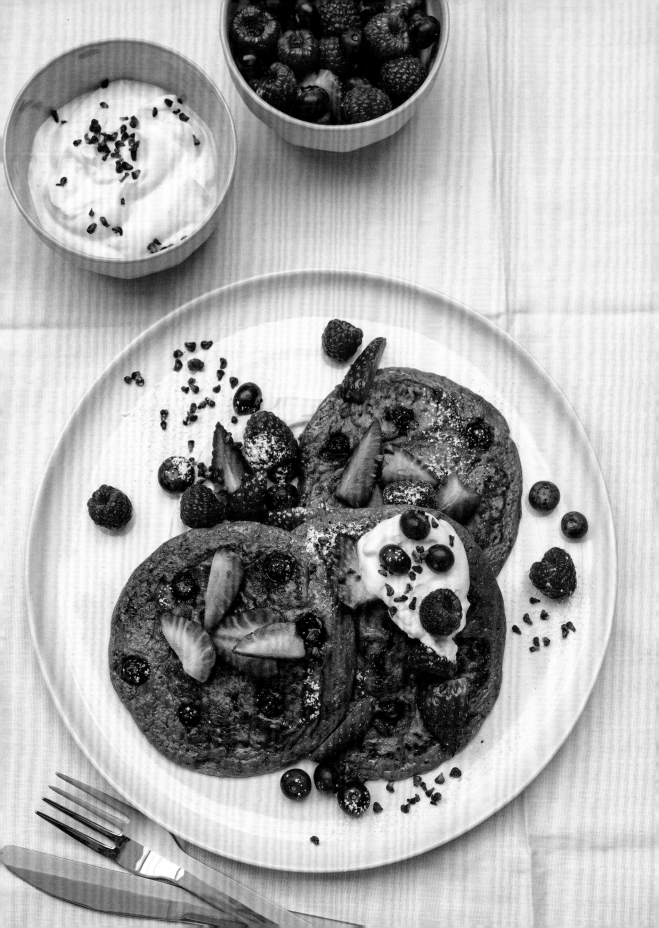

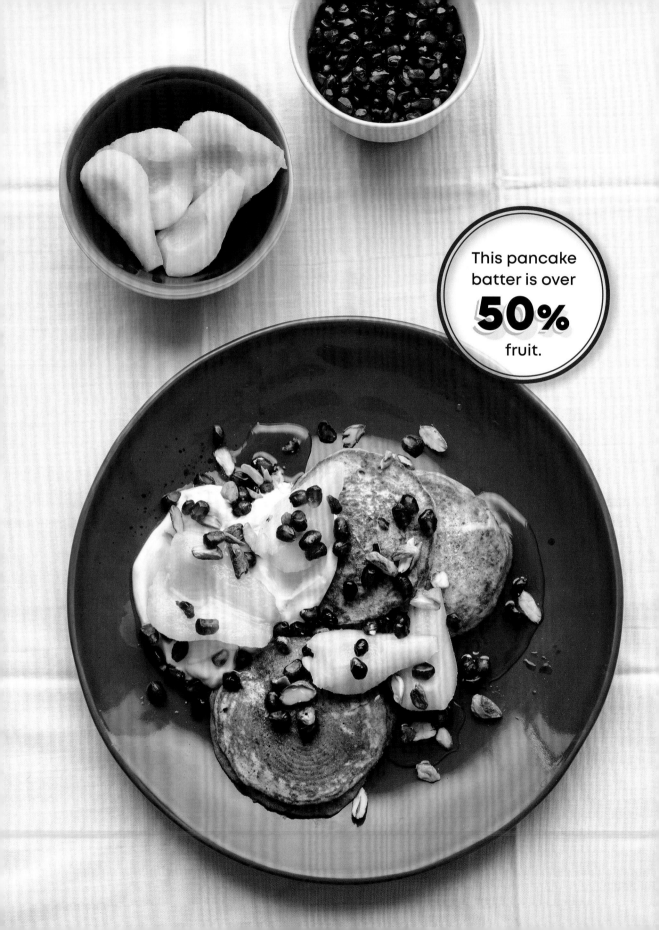

This pancake
batter is over
50%
fruit.

BANANA & PEANUT BUTTER PANCAKES

Light, fluffy pancakes that contain, as if by magic, more fruit than anything else, making up over half the batter by weight. And that's before you add the tasty, fruity toppings! Yet, perhaps surprisingly, they taste pretty much identical to the regular kind. Trust me, no one will know about your healthy cheat. Top each serving of 3 pancakes with one of the suggested toppings and it will add 2 extra portions to your daily intake.

Serves 2
Prep time 5 minutes
Cook time 8 minutes

4 bananas
1 tbsp peanut butter
4 eggs
100g (3½oz) plain wholemeal flour
1 tsp vanilla bean paste
1 tsp baking powder
large pinch of salt
1 tsp extra virgin olive oil
butter, for frying

BLEND all the ingredients together in a food processor to form a batter.

HEAT a little butter in a large frying pan over a medium heat. Pour in 2 tablespoons of the batter per pancake, well spaced apart and swirling the pan around so each pancake spreads out to the size of a CD.

COOK for 1 minute on each side, then remove from the pan and keep warm until you have used up all the batter to make 12 pancakes.

SUGGESTED TOPPINGS

① PEAR, POMEGRANATE & YOGURT

Add ½ drained 400g (14oz) can of **pears** to each serving of pancakes, then scatter with a large handful of **pomegranate seeds**. Spoon over 2 tbsp **Greek yogurt** and serve with a sprinkle of **pistachios** and a drizzle of **honey**.

② PINEAPPLE, KIWI & COCONUT

Top each serving of pancakes with 80g (2¾oz) **fresh pineapple** wedges, 1 peeled and sliced **kiwifruit** and a sprinkle of **coconut flakes**.

③ GRAPEFRUIT & ORANGE

Scatter each serving of pancakes with ½ sliced **pink grapefruit**, ½ sliced **orange** and a sprinkle of **flaked almonds**.

FRUIT CRÊPES

As you will soon be able to tell in this book, I have recently fallen in love with gram flour. Despite being made exclusively of ground-up chickpeas, if you formulate your recipe right, it tastes surprisingly similar to wholemeal wheat flour or cornmeal and can be cooked in the same way. This means that these wonderfully moreish, protein-packed crêpes are, I kid you not, pretty much 100 per cent veg. With a delicious fruit filling, that's 4 portions of fruit and veg in a super-healthy breakfast that looks more like a generous dessert.

Serves 4
Prep time 10 minutes, plus standing
Cook time 32 minutes

500ml (18fl oz) water
250g (9oz) gram flour
1 tbsp extra virgin olive oil
2 tbsp orange blossom water
1 tsp fine sea salt
butter or olive oil cooking spray, for frying

To serve
8 tbsp cottage cheese
640g (1lb 6oz) peeled and sliced oranges
320g (11¼oz) peeled and sliced kiwifruit
300g (10½oz) blueberries
finely grated lime zest
honey, for drizzling

POUR the measured water into a large bowl, then add the gram flour a little at a time, whisking constantly until it resembles smooth, thin custard. Stir in the olive oil, orange blossom water and salt, then leave to stand for 15 minutes.

MELT a small knob of butter in a frying pan over a medium-high heat. (Alternatively, spray the pan lightly with olive oil.) Give the batter a stir, then pour in enough to cover the base of the pan. Cook for 2 minutes on each side, then remove from the pan and keep warm until you have used up all the batter to make 8 large crêpes.

DIVIDE the cottage cheese and fruit among the pancakes, sprinkle each serving with a pinch of lime zest and serve with a drizzle of honey.

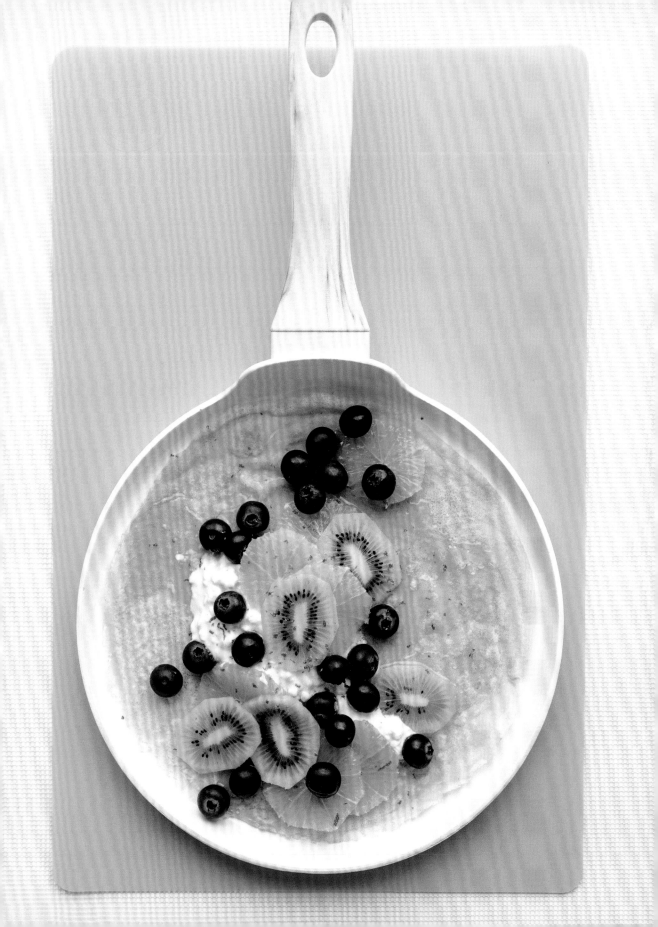

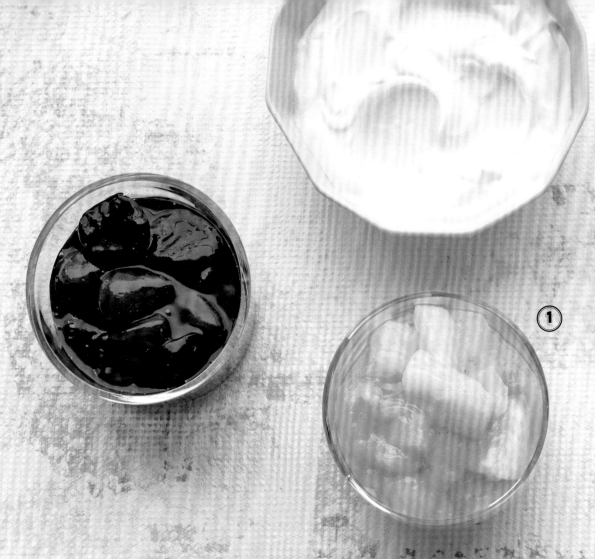

STRAWBERRY & CHERRY COMPOTE

This excellent no-added-sugar alternative to jam can be knocked together in just 5 minutes in the microwave, yet also counts as a portion of fruit. All the compotes can be made with fresh or frozen fruit.

PORTION 1 PER SERVING

Serves 4
Prep time 5 minutes
Cook time 5 minutes

200g (7oz) strawberries, chopped
200g (7oz) pitted dark cherries, halved
2 tbsp granulated stevia (baking blend)
4 tbsp lemon juice
1 tsp cinnamon
1 tbsp cornflour

COMBINE all the ingredients in a microwavable bowl and microwave for 5 minutes on full power, stopping halfway through to mash the fruit with a fork, and then mash them again at the end.

LEAVE to cool slightly before serving. The cooled compote can be stored in an airtight plastic container in the fridge for up to 1 week.

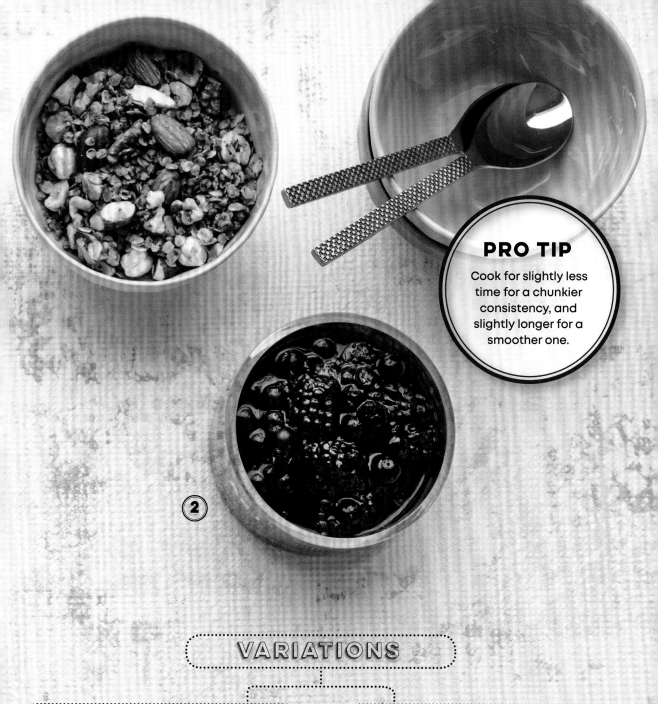

PRO TIP

Cook for slightly less time for a chunkier consistency, and slightly longer for a smoother one.

②

VARIATIONS

① MANGO & PINEAPPLE COMPOTE

Make the compote as opposite, replacing the strawberries and cherries with 200g (7oz) **mango** chunks and 200g (7oz) **pineapple** chunks, the lemon juice with 2 tbsp **lime juice** and the cinnamon with 1 tsp **ground ginger**.

② DARK BERRY COMPOTE

Make the compote as opposite, replacing the strawberries and cherries with 200g (7oz) **blackcurrants** and 200g (7oz) chopped **blackberries**, the lemon juice with 2 tsp **vanilla bean paste** and the cinnamon with 1 tsp **ground allspice**.

MANGO & GINGER PORRIDGE

Oats are one of the most nutritious, convenient and affordable of all store-cupboard staples. Pair them up with a good old helping of fruit (and potentially even veg) and you have a pretty powerful combo. I have swapped some of the water in a standard porridge recipe with tasty fruit and veg (which are, after all, made up of over 80 per cent moisture) to sneakily up the flavour, colour and portions of the good stuff to the maximum.

 PORTIONS PER SERVING 3

Serves 4
Prep time 5 minutes
Cook time 5 minutes

160g (5¾oz) jumbo rolled oats
400g (14oz) canned mango purée
200ml (7fl oz) milk
1 tsp ground ginger
100g (3½oz) goji berries
300g (10½oz) fresh pineapple wedges, chopped

PLACE everything except the pineapple in a medium saucepan and stir well.

BRING to the boil over a medium heat, then reduce the heat and simmer gently for 3–5 minutes, stirring occasionally, until thickened.

SERVE with the pineapple wedges.

VARIATIONS

1 SPICED PUMPKIN PORRIDGE

Make the porridge as above with 160g (5¾oz) **jumbo rolled oats**, 250g (9oz) **canned pumpkin purée**, 150g (5½oz) finely grated **carrots**, 100g (3½oz) **raisins**, 300ml (10fl oz) **milk**, 300ml (10fl oz) **water** and 1 tbsp **mixed spice**. Omit the pineapple and serve with 2 sliced **apples** and 12 **fresh cherries**.

2 GRAPE & APRICOT PORRIDGE

Make the porridge as above with 160g (5¾oz) **jumbo rolled oats**, 400ml (14fl oz) **purple grape juice**, 200ml (7fl oz) **soya**, **almond** or any other **non-dairy milk** and 200g (7oz) stoned and chopped **fresh apricots**. Omit the pineapple and serve topped with 300g (10½oz) **fresh blackberries** and 4 halved **fresh strawberries**.

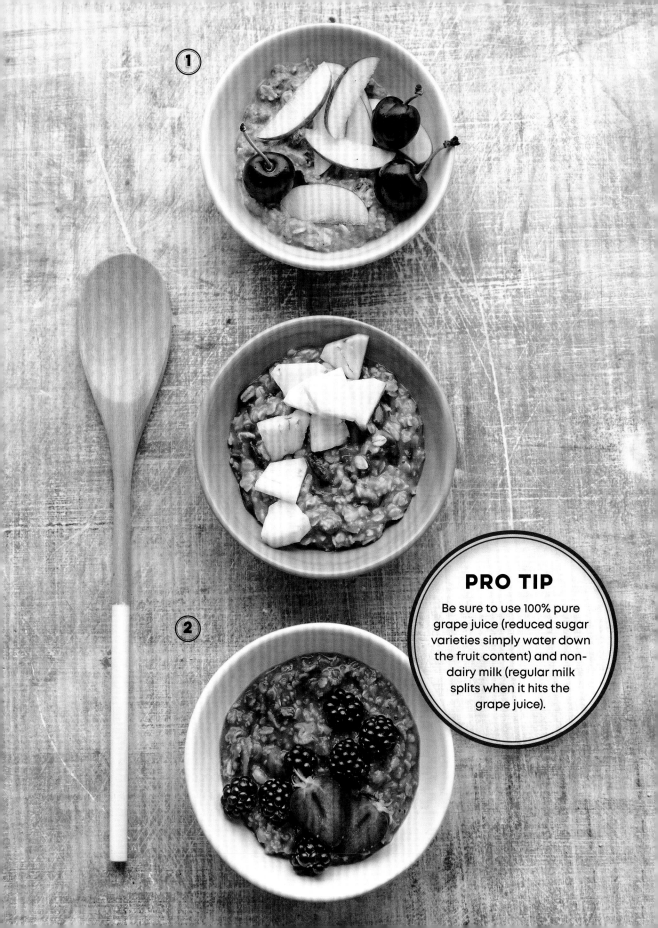

①

②

PRO TIP

Be sure to use 100% pure grape juice (reduced sugar varieties simply water down the fruit content) and non-dairy milk (regular milk splits when it hits the grape juice).

GREEN EGGS & HAM

Am I the only kid that had a Dr. Seuss obsession? Here's my breakfast tribute to the childhood classic. It's basically an Eggs Benedict with a whole lot of good stuff (4 portions to be exact), and without the stress of the hollandaise splitting. Hurray!

Serves 2

Prep time 10 minutes

Cook time 12–16 minutes

4 large eggs

1 tsp butter

150g (5½oz) asparagus spears

100g (3½oz) frozen peas

100g (3½oz) sugar snap peas

150g (5½oz) watercress

1 large avocado, stoned, peeled and cubed

salt and pepper

To serve

2 wholemeal English muffins, halved and toasted

4 slices of ham

1 x quantity Guac-molata (see page 193), blitzed to a smooth sauce in a food processor with 2 tbsp milk

BRING a saucepan of water to a gentle simmer, then stir with a large spoon to create a swirl. Carefully break an egg into the water and cook for 3–4 minutes. Remove with a slotted spoon and keep warm. Repeat with the remaining eggs.

MEANWHILE, melt the butter in a frying pan over a high heat, add the asparagus, peas and sugar snaps and cook for 2–3 minutes until just tender. Season with a little salt and pepper. Take the pan off the heat and add the watercress and cubed avocado, stirring constantly until the watercress starts to wilt.

TOP the toasted muffins with the ham and poached eggs, then add the hot vegetables. Drizzle the Guac-molata generously over the poached eggs and get eating.

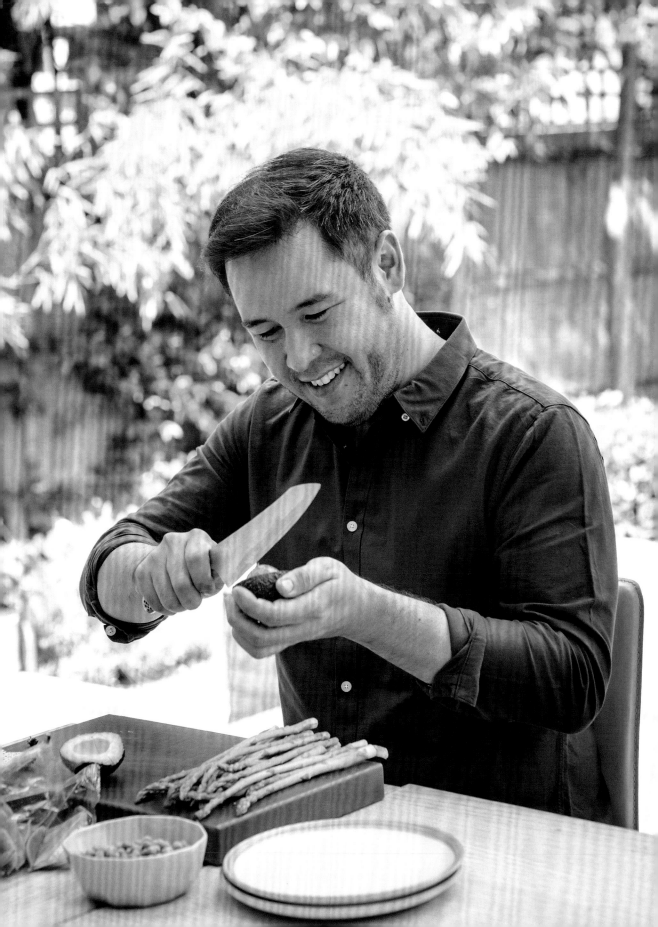

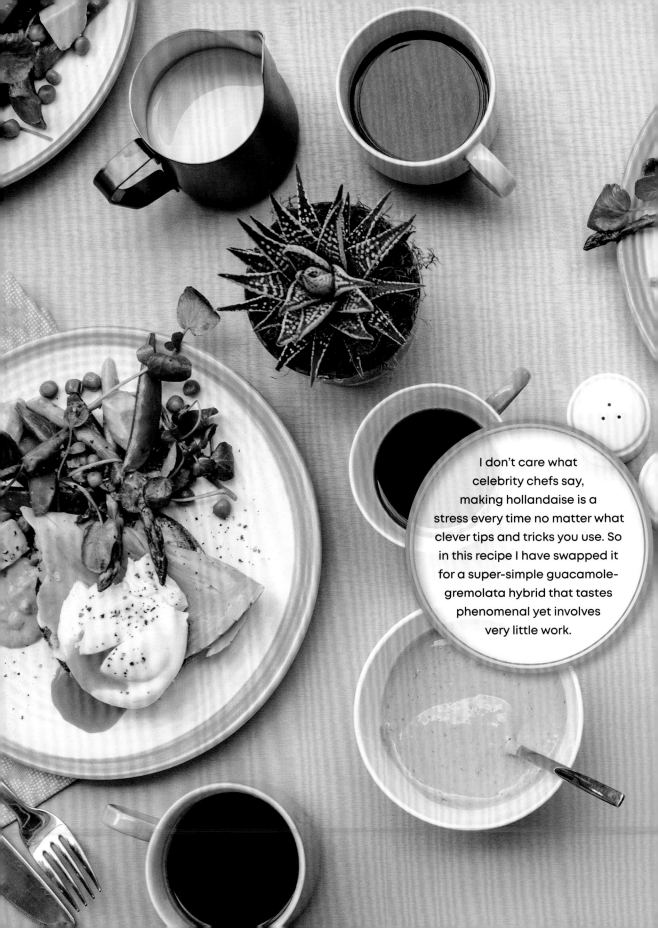

I don't care what celebrity chefs say, making hollandaise is a stress every time no matter what clever tips and tricks you use. So in this recipe I have swapped it for a super-simple guacamole-gremolata hybrid that tastes phenomenal yet involves very little work.

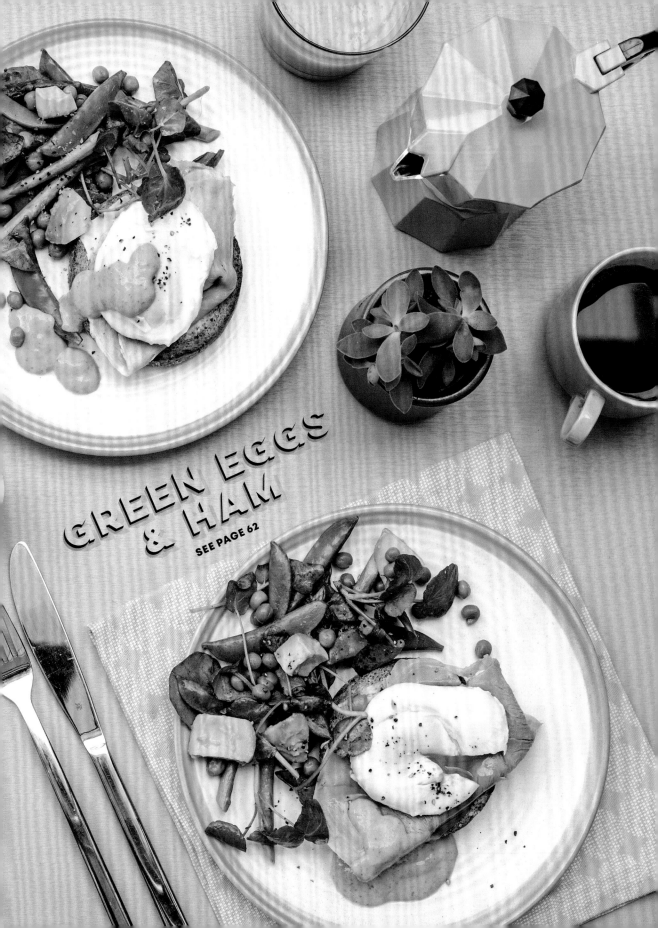

GREEN EGGS
& HAM
SEE PAGE 62

EGGS IN PURGATORY

The ultimate quick weekend breakfast that can be knocked together to restore you to feeling human, even if your head might happen to be a little fuzzy from the night before. Especially good with lots of hot, buttered wholegrain toast for dunking. Packing 3½ portions in each tasty serving, console yourself by knowing at least you have done something healthy this week.

Serves 4

Prep time 15 minutes

Cook time 40 minutes

1 tbsp extra virgin olive oil

300g (10½oz) white onions, thinly sliced

300g (10½oz) cored and deseeded mixed peppers (ideally, green and yellow), sliced lengthways

400g (14oz) can chopped tomatoes

4 garlic cloves, minced

2 tsp smoked paprika

2 large fresh bay leaves

4 large eggs

pepper

To serve

1 tbsp chopped parsley

1 red chilli, finely sliced

finely grated zest of 1 lemon

½ x quantity Guac-molata (see page 193)

toasted and buttered rye bread

PREHEAT the oven to 200°C (400°F), Gas Mark 6.

HEAT the olive oil in a large, deep frying pan over a medium heat, add the onions and peppers and fry for 20 minutes until softened and reduced by half.

TIP in the chopped tomatoes, garlic and paprika. Tear the edge of the bay leaves in several places (this helps release their flavour) and add to the pan. Mix together well, then cook for 5 minutes. Remove the bay leaves.

TRANSFER the piping hot mixture to a 2-litre (3½-pint) baking dish. Make a well for each egg, then crack them into the indentations. Season the eggs with a little pepper.

BAKE for about 15 minutes, or until the eggs are cooked to your liking.

SPRINKLE with the parsley, chilli and lemon zest and serve with the Guac-molata and toasted and buttered rye bread.

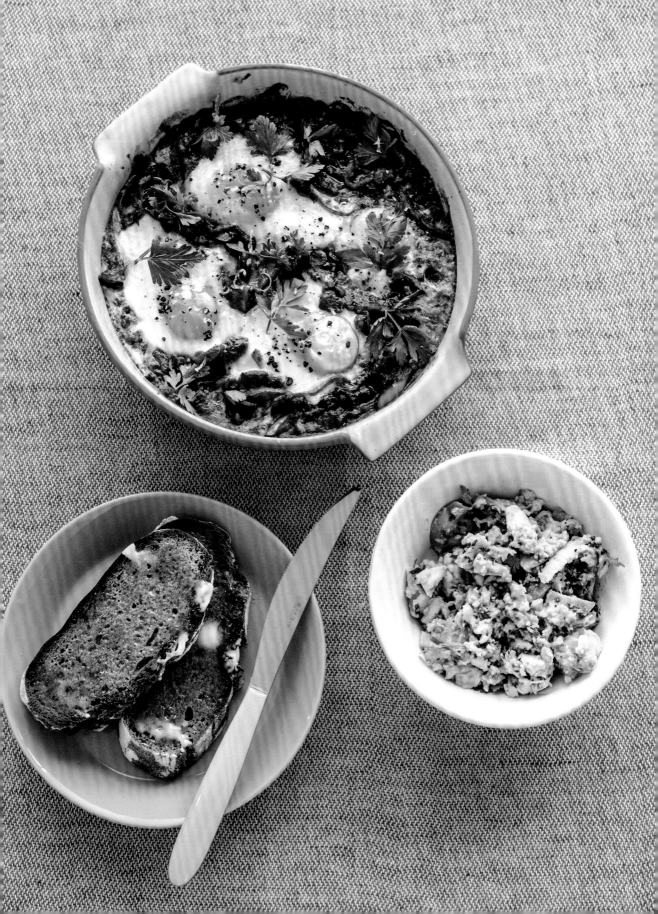

FULL MEXICAN

In my 20s, I lived with two lovely Mexican ladies who always made earth-shatteringly good food, including some of the richest, fieriest breakfasts known to man, that were somehow super fruit- and veg-packed, too. Tuck into slices of golden, buttered cornbread with smoky beans, runny eggs and creamy avocado and you will wonder why you ever went Full English.

Serves 4
Prep time 10 minutes
Cook time 25–30 minutes

8 eggs

1 x quantity Cheesy Jalapeño Cornbread (see opposite), sliced and buttered

2 large avocados, stoned, peeled and sliced lengthways

14 baby plum tomatoes, halved

Smoky beans

2 tsp extra virgin olive oil

300g (10½oz) diced onions

2 garlic cloves, minced

400g (14oz) can black beans, rinsed and drained

1 tbsp Worcestershire sauce

400g (14oz) can chopped tomatoes

1 tbsp smoked paprika

1 tsp chipotle chilli flakes

pinch of salt

BRING a saucepan of water to a gentle simmer, then stir with a large spoon to create a swirl. Carefully break an egg into the water and cook for 3–4 minutes. Remove with a slotted spoon and keep warm. Repeat with the remaining eggs.

MEANWHILE, for the Smoky Beans, heat the olive oil in a large frying pan over a medium heat, add the onions and fry until starting to brown, then add the garlic, beans and Worcestershire sauce and cook for 2–3 minutes, stirring occasionally. Add all the remaining ingredients, bring to a simmer and cook gently for 5 minutes. Keep warm.

PLACE 2 or 3 slices of buttered cornbread on each plate and top with the poached eggs. Divide the Smoky Beans, avocado slices and tomatoes among the plates and serve.

CHEESY JALAPEÑO CORNBREAD

Who knew that cheesy cornbread could be made so healthy? Containing roughly 50 per cent pure veg in every slice, it will help you to pack in portions of veg effortlessly. It is best eaten on the day it is baked, but is still good toasted the next day.

1 PORTION PER SERVING

Serves 4
Prep time 10 minutes
Cook time 25–30 minutes

300g (10½oz) drained canned sweetcorn

2 large eggs

½ tsp sea salt

1 tbsp olive oil, plus extra for greasing

1 tbsp clear honey

200g (7oz) coarse cornmeal or polenta

2 tsp baking powder

30g (1oz) fresh jalapeño chillies, halved and thinly sliced

20g (¾oz) strong Cheddar, crumbled

PREHEAT the oven to 220°C (425°F), Gas Mark 7. Grease and line a 900g (2lb) loaf tin with nonstick baking paper.

BLITZ together the sweetcorn, eggs, salt, olive oil and honey in a blender until the batter is thick and lumpy.

COMBINE the remaining ingredients in a large mixing bowl. Tip the sweetcorn mixture into the bowl and stir well to combine.

POUR the batter into the prepared tin and bake for 25–30 minutes until deep golden. Leave to cool in the tin for 10 minutes before transferring the bread to a wire rack.

SERVE warm or cold. The cornbread can be stored in an airtight plastic container in the fridge for up to 1 week.

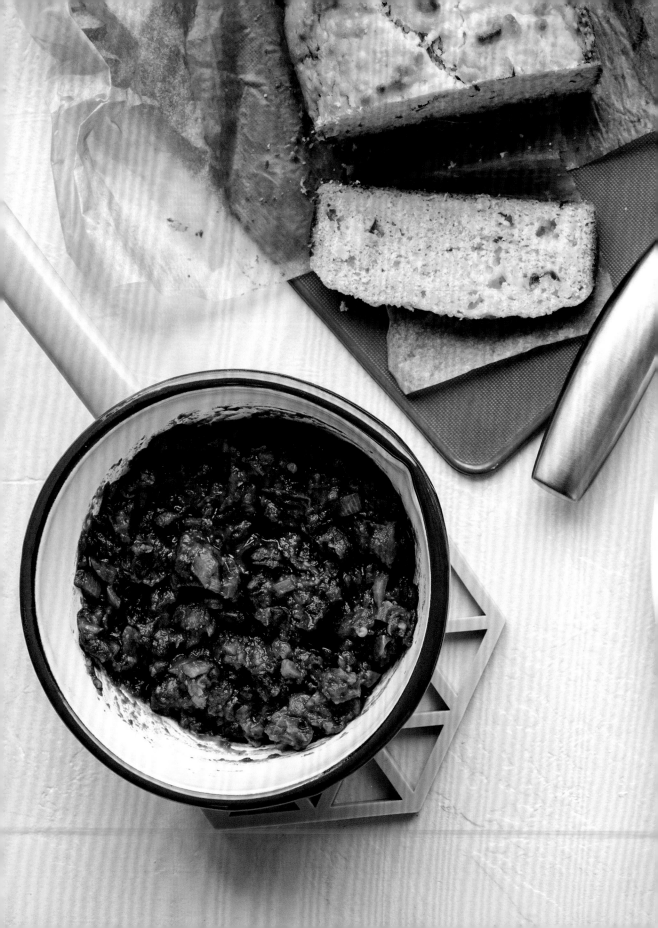

FULL MEXICAN SEE PAGES 68–69

SWEET POTATO WAFFLES

My trick for achieving a proper crisp texture with these veg-packed waffles, not to mention a wonderful rich, biscuity flavour, is to use custard powder instead of flour. This just happens to make them gluten-free, too. These guys are super-versatile and work just as well with sweet or savoury toppings – a tasty way to up the fruit and veg content even further. A couple of waffles with one of the suggested toppings will give you 3.5 portions of fruit and veg.

Serves 2
Prep time 5 minutes
Cook time 8 minutes

olive oil, for greasing
250g (9oz) cooked sweet potato
150g (5½oz) custard powder
100ml (3½fl oz) milk
2 eggs
1 tsp mixed spice
½ tsp finely grated orange zest
large pinch of salt
150g (5½oz) finely grated carrots

GREASE and preheat a waffle iron.

BLITZ together all the ingredients except the carrots in a food processor until smooth.

TRANSFER the mixture to a bowl and gently fold in the finely grated carrots.

SPOON the batter into the waffle iron to make 4 waffles. Cook over a high heat for 4 minutes on each side if using an old-school iron. If you are using a fancy electric one, these timings may vary.

SUGGESTED TOPPINGS

① APPLE, PEANUT BUTTER & BLUEBERRY

Spread 2 waffles with 1 tbsp **peanut butter**, then top with ½ cored and sliced **apple** and 80g (2¾oz) **blueberries.** Dust with ¼ tsp **cinnamon**.

② SALMON, AVOCADO & BOILED EGG

Top 2 waffles with ½ peeled, stoned and sliced **avocado**, 2 slices of **smoked salmon**, 2 halved boiled **eggs** and ⅛ sliced **red onion**.

③ KIWI, MIXED BERRIES & YOGURT

Spread 2 waffles with a dollop of **yogurt**, then top with ½ peeled and sliced **kiwifruit** and a handful of **mixed berries**.

④ BACON, BANANA & MAPLE SYRUP

Cook 4 **bacon rashers**, then divide between 2 waffles with 1 sliced **banana**. Drizzle with **maple syrup**.

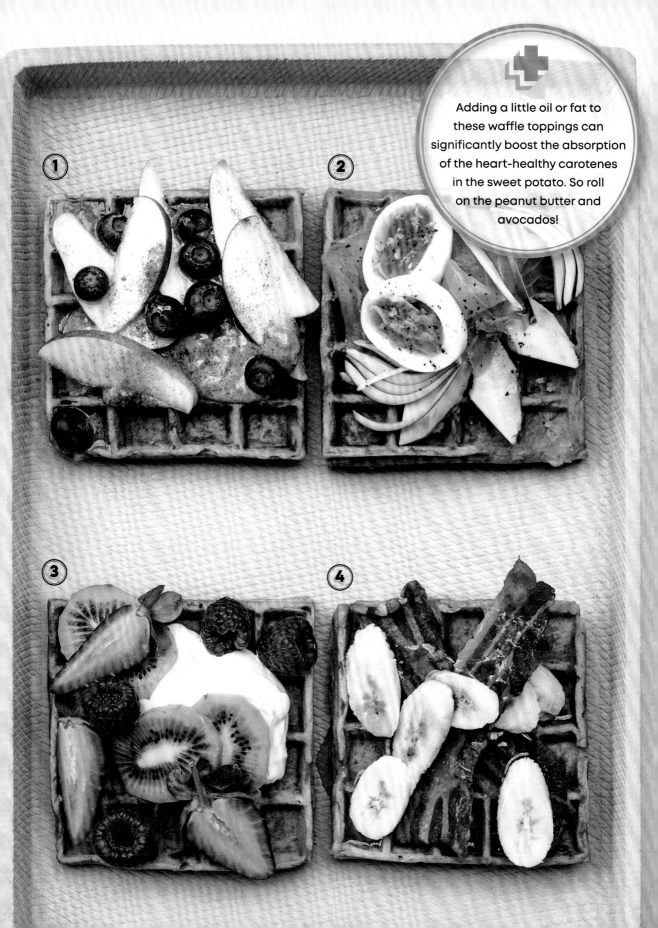

1

2

Adding a little oil or fat to these waffle toppings can significantly boost the absorption of the heart-healthy carotenes in the sweet potato. So roll on the peanut butter and avocados!

3

4

STICKY-SWEET BANANA BREAD

As a life-long lover of cake, banana bread is probably my absolute favourite. So I didn't take tinkering with this classic lightly. But after a good year of trial and error I think I have well and truly cracked it! This is a deliciously sticky, sweet banana bread that swaps loads of oil and refined sugar for a ton of hidden fruit and veg, yet is still more than worthy of the name. Delicious as a snack with a cup of tea, or toast a couple of slices and serve with fruit compote for an extra few portions.

Serves 4
Prep time 15 minutes
Cook time 1 hour

350g (12oz) ripe peeled bananas (about 3)
100g (3½oz) finely grated parsnip
150g (5½oz) chopped dates
2 large eggs
2 tbsp extra virgin olive oil
1 tsp vanilla bean paste
250g (9oz) self-raising wholemeal flour
¼ tsp salt
1 tsp bicarbonate of soda
1 tsp cinnamon
50g (1¾oz) walnuts, chopped

PRO TIP

Chopped dates, which can be picked up in the baking aisle of most good supermarkets, will save you *loads* of time and faff because you won't need to stone and slice the sticky things by hand.

PREHEAT the oven to 200°C (400°F), Gas Mark 6 and line a 20 x 10cm (8 x 4in), 6.5cm (2½in) deep loaf tin with nonstick baking paper.

PLACE 2 of the bananas in a mixing bowl and mash together, then whisk in the parsnip, dates, eggs, olive oil and vanilla.

COMBINE the dry ingredients except the walnuts in a separate large mixing bowl, giving it a good stir to thoroughly incorporate the bicarbonate of soda, then tip in the banana mixture and nuts and mix together just until the last bits of powdery flour disappear (don't overmix it as this will result in a denser, chewier texture).

POUR into the prepared tin. Slice the remaining banana lengthways, then press it into the top of the mixture. Cover the tin with foil, crimping the edges around the sides to form a loose seal. (This is important to ensure the bread cooks evenly and avoid a hard, cracked crust.)

BAKE for 1 hour, or until a skewer inserted into the centre comes out clean. Leave to cool in the tin for 10 minutes before transferring to a wire rack.

SERVE warm or cold. The banana bread can be stored in an airtight plastic container in the fridge for up to 1 week.

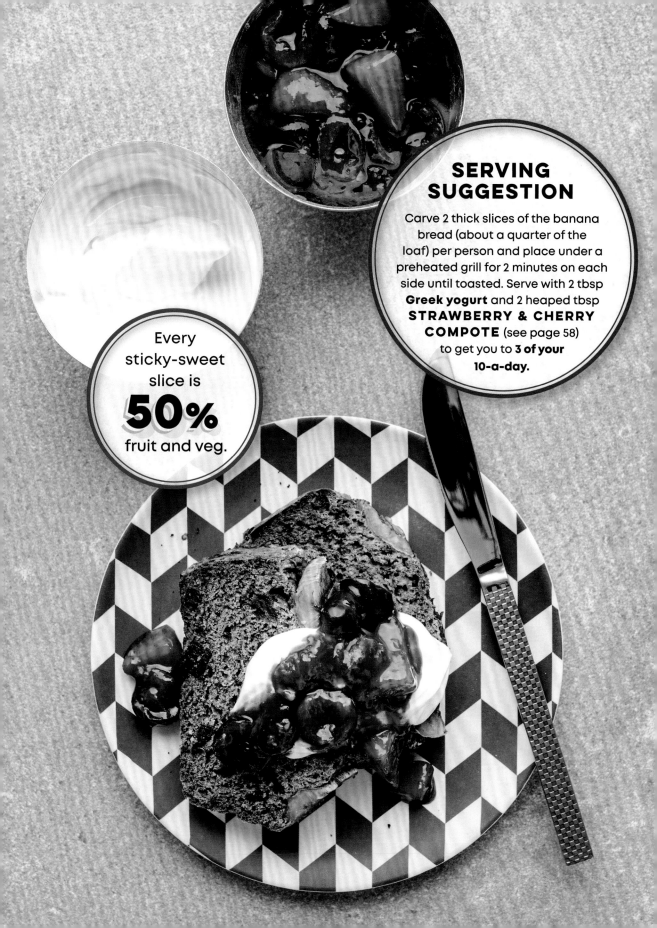

Every sticky-sweet slice is 50% fruit and veg.

SERVING SUGGESTION

Carve 2 thick slices of the banana bread (about a quarter of the loaf) per person and place under a preheated grill for 2 minutes on each side until toasted. Serve with 2 tbsp **Greek yogurt** and 2 heaped tbsp **STRAWBERRY & CHERRY COMPOTE** (see page 58) to get you to **3 of your 10-a-day.**

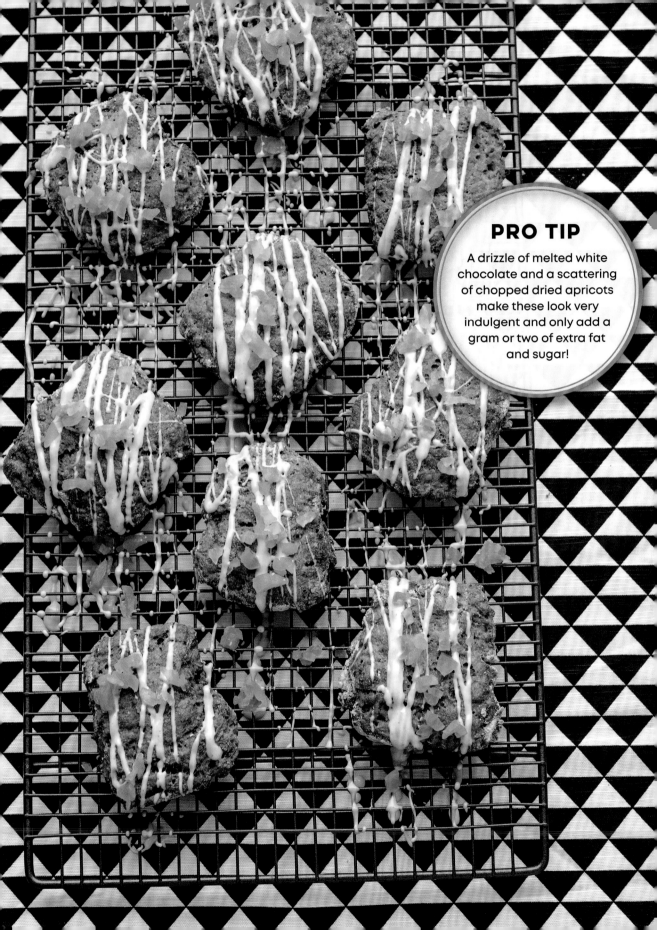

PRO TIP

A drizzle of melted white chocolate and a scattering of chopped dried apricots make these look very indulgent and only add a gram or two of extra fat and sugar!

CARROT CAKE BAKES

OK, it's not exactly a cool foodie thing to admit, but I love those fruit-studded 'breakfast scones' you get at chain coffee shops. Sometimes it's all I get to grab as I run for a train. Haven't we all been there? So I wondered if I could make my own fruit- and veg-packed version, without all the added sugar and – after more than ten versions and hours of kitchen experiments – here we have it! Soft, sweet and chewy bakes (not exactly scones) made with almost 60 per cent fruit and veg, plus a healthy dose of wholegrains. Two of these delicious bakes will give you 1 portion of your recommended daily intake.

Makes 10
Prep time 15 minutes
Cook time 25 minutes

200g (7oz) finely grated carrots
1 tbsp extra virgin olive oil
1 tsp mixed spice
1 tsp vanilla bean paste
50g (1¾oz) dried apricots, chopped
250g (9oz) plain wholemeal flour, plus extra for dusting
1 tbsp baking powder
large pinch of salt
¼ tsp turmeric
finely grated zest and juice of 1 orange (about 200ml/7fl oz)
100g (3½oz) mashed banana
milk, for brushing

PREHEAT the oven to 200°C (400°F), Gas Mark 6 and line a baking sheet with nonstick baking paper.

COMBINE all the ingredients together in a mixing bowl until they form a rough, wet dough.

TURN the dough out on to a floured chopping board and shape into a flat rectangle about 1.5cm (⅝in) deep. It might seem implausibly wet at this point, but keep the faith!

CUT into 10 equal-sized squares, then place on the prepared baking sheet and brush the tops with a little milk. Bake for 25 minutes, or until golden.

TRANSFER to a wire rack and leave to cool completely. They can be stored in an airtight container for a few days.

Grab 2 of these, along with an apple and glass of juice and that's **4 portions** of your recommended daily intake right there.

LUNCHES

PHILLY CHEESESTEAK SANDWICH

Forget this vegetable-munching malarkey, sometimes only a good old steak will do. Pair it up with melted cheese, cram it into a baguette and you are on to something so good you might not believe it can help towards your recommended daily intake. Each packed with 3.5 portions of flavourful veg, these guys help crowd out excessive amounts of meat or cheese in this US classic, without compromising on flavour. Don't believe me? Make it and tweet me your verdict.

Serves 2

Prep time 20 minutes

Cook time 25 minutes

2 demi baguettes

1 tsp olive oil, plus extra for drizzling

200g (7oz) sliced onions

200g (7oz) cored, deseeded and sliced green pepper

180g (6¼oz) minute steak, finely sliced

butter, for spreading

4 mature Cheddar cheese square slices, cut in half

pepper

Mushroom peppercorn spread

1 tsp extra virgin olive oil

160g (5¾oz) fresh shiitake mushrooms, finely diced

1 tsp white wine vinegar

1 tsp coarsely ground black peppercorns

2 tbsp Greek yogurt

FIRST, make the mushroom peppercorn spread. Heat the olive oil in a frying pan over a medium heat, add the mushrooms and fry for 5 minutes until softened, then tip in the vinegar and continue to cook until the liquid has just evaporated. Combine the cooked mushrooms with the remaining ingredients in a small bowl and set aside.

SLICE the baguettes in half horizontally, without cutting them all the way through. Open them out, then cook under a preheated grill for a few minutes until toasted. Set aside.

HEAT the olive oil in a frying pan, add the onions and green pepper and cook over a medium heat for 10 minutes until softened, stirring occasionally.

PLACE the steak in a bowl, add a light drizzle of olive oil and a generous sprinkling of pepper and toss together. Clear a space in the centre of the pan and add the beef. Fry for 1 minute, or to your liking, then take off the heat.

SPREAD the mushroom mixture over the base of each baguette, then butter the top halves. Place 2 half-slices of cheese on top of the mushroom spread, then divide the steak and veg mixture between the sandwiches. Top with the remaining cheese and close the sandwiches. Wrap each sandwich in kitchen foil, then place under a preheated grill for 5 minutes, or until the cheese has melted.

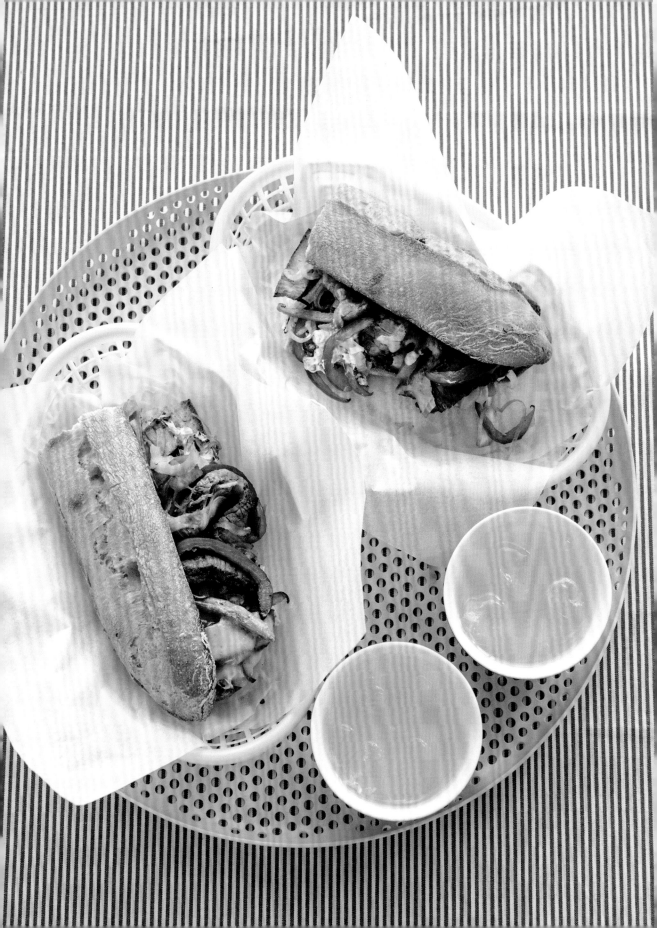

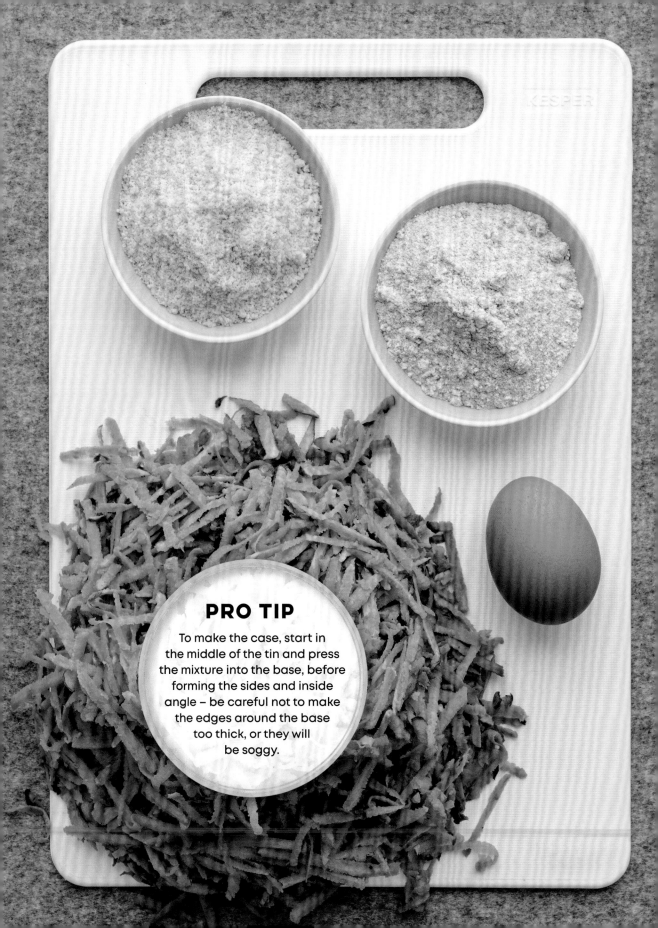

PRO TIP

To make the case, start in the middle of the tin and press the mixture into the base, before forming the sides and inside angle – be careful not to make the edges around the base too thick, or they will be soggy.

CHEESE & DOUBLE VEG QUICHES

Vegetable quiche where even the 'pastry' case itself is made from veggies sounds like it couldn't possibly work. Right? Well, it took a few tries, but I think we have cracked it! Plus, the super-simple sweet potato and cornmeal flan case is far quicker and easier than faffing with homemade pastry. These quiches provide at least 3 portions of veg crammed into every serving, without sacrificing on the creamy, cheesy filling.

SWEET POTATO & CORNMEAL FLAN CASE

Swapping fat- and flour-based pastry for a flan case made with shredded sweet potatoes and cornmeal gives you a golden, crisp base with an extra dose of veg snuck in. Plus, no laborious rolling, chilling and trimming to get you there.

PORTION 1 PER SERVING

Serves 4
Prep time 15 minutes
Cook time 40 minutes

olive oil, for greasing

350g (12oz) grated sweet potatoes (no need to peel)

1 large egg

50g (1¾oz) coarse cornmeal or polenta

50g (1¾oz) cornflour

pinch of salt

4 twists of black pepper

PREHEAT the oven to 200°C (400°F), Gas Mark 6 and grease a 25cm (10in) flan dish with a little olive oil.

WRAP the grated sweet potatoes in a muslin cloth or clean tea towel and squeeze out the excess liquid over the sink. Transfer to a large bowl, then add the remaining ingredients and mix together. The best way to do this is to get in there and use your fingers.

PRESS the mixture firmly and evenly into the prepared dish to form the case. Pinch off any little bits that stick above the rim to prevent them burning during cooking, then cover with foil.

BAKE for 20 minutes. Remove from the oven, then gently press the now-softened sweet potato against the dish with the back of a fork to give it a more compressed shape. Return to the oven, uncovered, and cook for another 20 minutes, or until the base is dry to the touch. Remove from the oven and leave to cool completely.

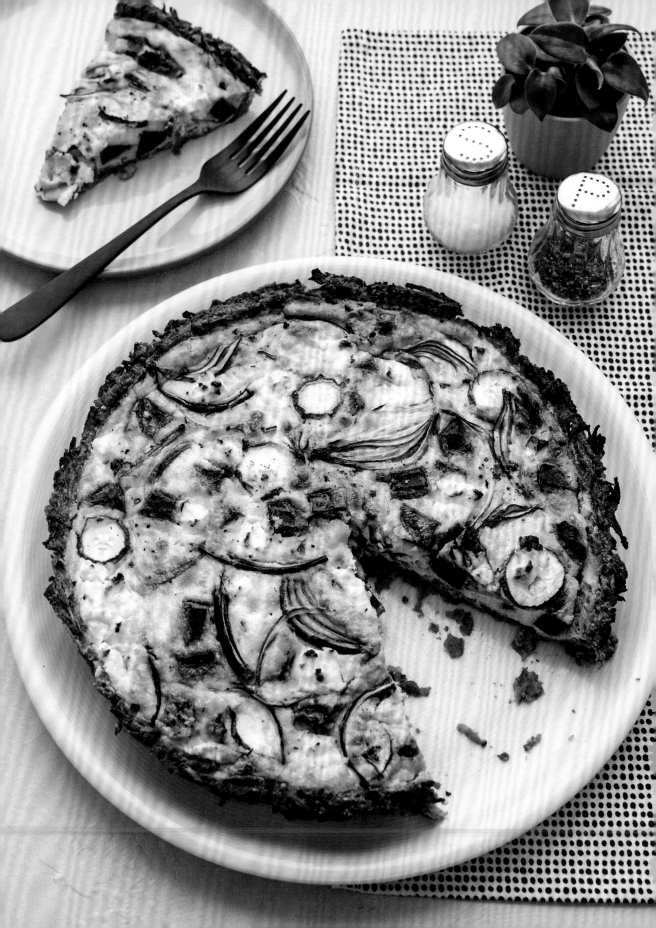

BEETROOT, COURGETTE, RED ONION & GOATS' CHEESE QUICHE

Fresh, light and packed full of veg. A perfect weekday lunch al desko.

Serves 4

Prep time 15 minutes

Cook time 25–30 minutes

200g (7oz) ready-cooked beetroot, cut into 3mm- (⅛in-) thick slices

1 Sweet Potato & Cornmeal Flan Case (see page 83)

200g (7oz) finely sliced red onions

200g (7oz) trimmed courgette, cut into 2–3mm- (⅛in-) thick slices

60g (2¼oz) soft white goats' cheese, such as Chavroux, sliced into rounds

Cream filling

400g (14oz) crème fraîche

3 large eggs

½ tsp freshly grated nutmeg

pinch of salt

8 twists of black pepper

PREHEAT the oven to 220°C (425°F), Gas Mark 7.

WHISK all the cream filling ingredients together in a bowl, then set aside.

ARRANGE the beetroot in the baked sweet potato case, reserving 3 slices. Pour over half of the cream filling, tilting the dish to ensure even distribution.

SCATTER over three-quarters of the onions, then add a layer of courgette, reserving 8 slices. Pour over the remaining cream mixture and smooth out with a spoon. Top with the reserved veg and remaining onions, and the goats' cheese.

PLACE the quiche on the middle shelf of the oven and bake for 25–30 minutes until set. Leave to cool in the tin for 10 minutes before serving.

SPINACH, PEAR, ASPARAGUS & BLUE CHEESE QUICHE

Who knew sweet pears and dates would work so well with bitter spinach and tangy blue cheese? Don't believe me? Give it a go!

Serves 4

Prep time 20 minutes

Cook time 30 minutes

350g (12oz) frozen chopped spinach, defrosted

4 large eggs

100ml (3½fl oz) crème fraîche

pinch of salt

8 twists of black pepper

½ tsp dried garlic granules

125g (4½oz) asparagus spears

2 firm dessert pears, about 100g (3½oz) each when cored

1 Sweet Potato & Cornmeal Flan Case (see page 83)

60g (2¼oz) pitted dates, sliced lengthways

finely grated zest of 1 lemon

40–50g (1½–1¾oz) Roquefort cheese

PREHEAT the oven to 220°C (425°F), Gas Mark 7.

SQUEEZE out as much liquid from the defrosted spinach as you can, then set to one side.

BEAT together the eggs, crème fraîche, salt and pepper in a jug, then stir in the squeezed spinach and the garlic granules.

CUT 7.5cm (3in) from the top of the asparagus spears to separate the tips. Set aside, then cut the remaining stalks into 4mm- (¼in-) thick slices. Dice 1 pear and cut the other into 16 wedges.

SCATTER the asparagus stalks and diced pear over the baked sweet potato case, then add half the sliced dates and the lemon zest. Pour over the spinach cream mixture and spread out evenly.

ARRANGE the asparagus tips and pear wedges on top of the filling, adding the remaining dates between them and pushing everything into the liquid. Finally, crumble over the cheese.

PLACE the quiche on the middle shelf of the oven and bake for 20 minutes until the cheese begins to brown. Cover loosely with foil and cook for another 10 minutes until set. Leave to cool completely before serving.

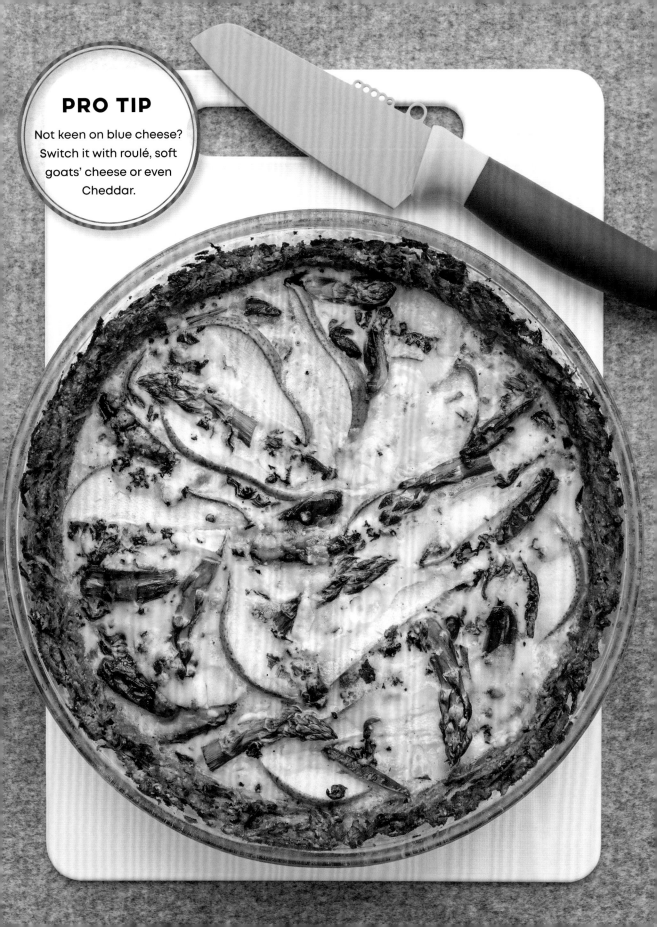

SAUSAGES IN TOMATO GRAVY WITH SWEETCORN & PUMPKIN POLENTA MASH

I love this poshed-up take on sausage and mash, and my favourite part has to be the super-simple, veg-filled 'cornbread' mash that takes less than a quarter of the time to make (I'm a geek, I timed it) yet hasn't lost any of the comforting creaminess.

Serves 4

Prep time 10 minutes

Cook time 25 minutes

1 tbsp olive oil

200g (7oz) sliced red onions

200g (7oz) cored, deseeded and finely sliced red pepper

4–6 low-fat sausages

50g (1¾oz) tomato purée

1 tbsp cornflour

1 chicken stock cube, crumbled

350ml (12fl oz) boiling water

pepper

200g (7oz) steamed French beans, to serve

Polenta mash

400g (14oz) canned pumpkin purée

200g (7oz) frozen sweetcorn

300ml (10fl oz) milk

1 tbsp butter

¼ tsp sea salt

150g (5½oz) instant polenta

HEAT the olive oil in a large frying pan over a medium heat, add the onions and red pepper and cook for 5 minutes until the veg start to soften. Add the sausages and cook for another 15 minutes, or until cooked through, turning occasionally.

MEANWHILE, put all the mash ingredients except the polenta in a large saucepan and bring to the boil. Reduce the heat to low, then gradually sprinkle in the polenta, stirring constantly until fully combined. Continue to cook for 10 minutes, stirring occasionally.

WHILE the sausages and mash are cooking, put the tomato purée, cornflour and stock cube in a measuring jug and add the measured water, a little at a time, mixing as you go to prevent lumps forming.

REMOVE the cooked sausages from the pan and set aside, leaving in the onions and peppers. Add the gravy mixture, stirring to deglaze the pan. Cook for a few minutes, then season with a little pepper.

DIVIDE the sausages and mash among 4 plates. Pour over the gravy and serve with a side of steamed French beans.

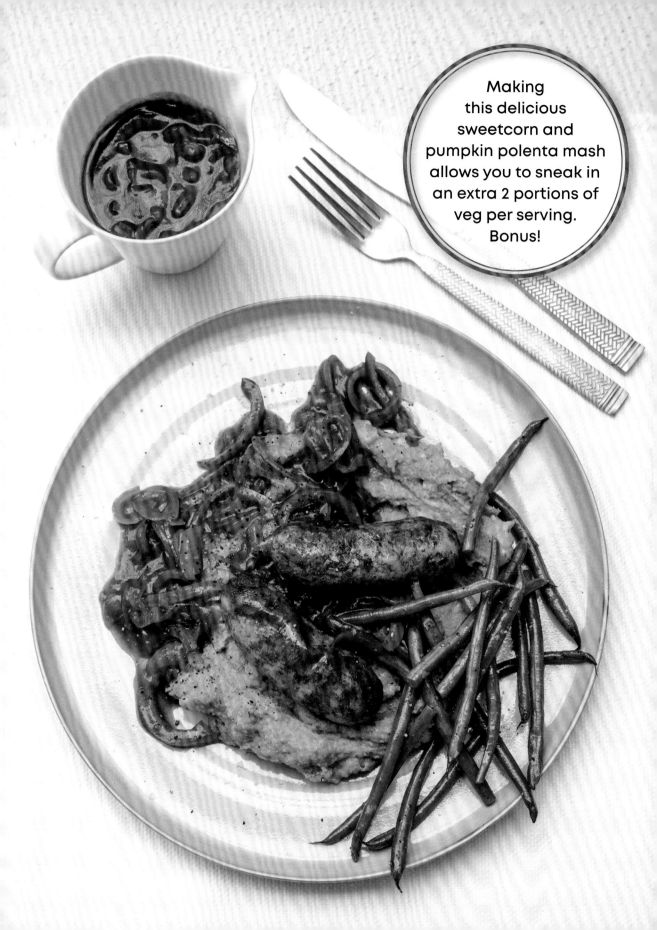

Making this delicious sweetcorn and pumpkin polenta mash allows you to sneak in an extra 2 portions of veg per serving. Bonus!

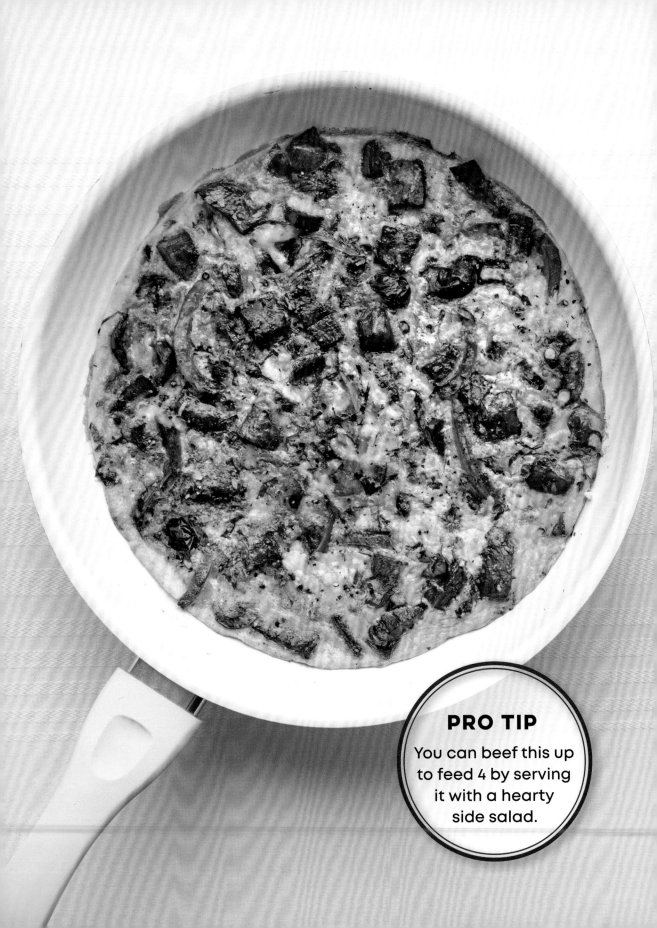

PRO TIP

You can beef this up
to feed 4 by serving
it with a hearty
side salad.

FRITTATAS

I love a good frittata, the ultimate healthy fast food that can be knocked together in minutes with whatever you have left in the fridge. Make that loads of veg and a generous dusting of Parmesan and you are on to a pretty delicious thing! These recipes can easily be scaled up or down to create a sharing size or individual portions by halving or doubling them. Serve with buttered wholegrain bread for the working lunch of champions.

BACON & SWEET POTATO FRITTATA

Bacon and sweet potatoes are a flavour match made in heaven. Add them to a frittata and you have the ultimate fast-food dish.

 PORTIONS PER SERVING 3

Serves 2
Prep time 10 minutes, plus cooling
Cook time 20 minutes

200g (7oz) whole purple sweet potato
6 large eggs
1 tsp extra virgin olive oil
100g (3½oz) lardons or diced unsmoked bacon
160g (5¾oz) cored, deseeded and thinly sliced yellow pepper
160g (5¾oz) cherry tomatoes, halved
small handful of parsley, chopped
10g (¼oz) Cheddar cheese, grated
salt and pepper

PRICK the potato all over with a fork, then microwave on full power for 5 minutes, or until softened. Leave until cool enough to handle, then peel and cut the flesh into chunks. Set aside.

BEAT the eggs in a bowl with a little salt and pepper and set aside.

HEAT the olive oil in a large flameproof frying pan over a medium-high heat, add the lardons or bacon and fry for 5 minutes. Add the yellow pepper and tomatoes to the pan and fry for another 5 minutes until softened.

TIP in the cooked sweet potato, then spread the veg out evenly in the pan. Pour in the beaten egg, tilting the pan to distribute it evenly. Sprinkle in the parsley and cheese.

COOK for 4 minutes, or until the egg is just set and you can slide a spatula around the side.

PLACE the pan under a preheated hot grill for a few minutes until the top of the frittata has set and the cheese is golden.

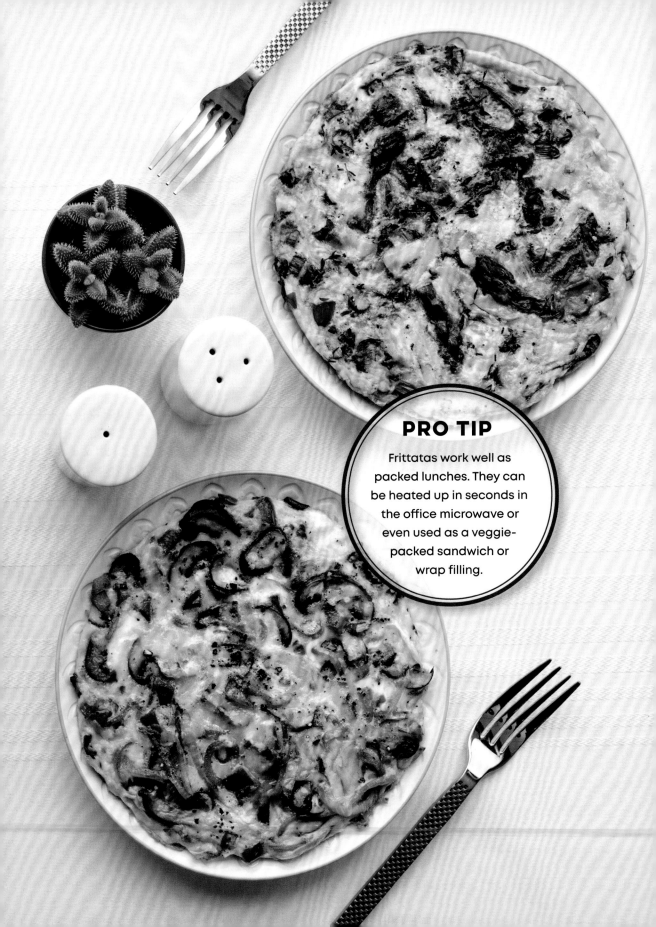

PRO TIP

Frittatas work well as packed lunches. They can be heated up in seconds in the office microwave or even used as a veggie-packed sandwich or wrap filling.

LEMONY SPINACH, RED PEPPER & ASPARAGUS FRITTATA

This combination is one of my 'go-tos' for a super-quick working lunch.

Serves 1
Prep time 10 minutes
Cook time 10 minutes

100g (3½oz) frozen chopped spinach, defrosted

3 large eggs

1 tsp extra virgin olive oil

80g (2¾oz) trimmed asparagus, finely chopped

1 garlic clove, finely chopped

1 tbsp lemon juice

a few thyme sprigs, leaves picked

80g (2¾oz) cored and deseeded red pepper, cut into chunks

10g (¼oz) Cheddar cheese, grated

salt and pepper

SQUEEZE out as much liquid from the defrosted spinach as you can, then set to one side.

BREAK the eggs into a bowl and beat together with a little salt and pepper. Set aside.

HEAT the olive oil in a small flameproof frying pan, add the asparagus and garlic and fry for 2 minutes. Stir in the lemon juice and thyme leaves and fry for another 1 minute. Add the red pepper and spinach and cook for 3 minutes.

SPREAD the veg out evenly in the pan, then pour in the beaten egg, tilting the pan to distribute it evenly. Sprinkle in the cheese and cook for 3 minutes, or until the egg is just set and you can slide a spatula around the side.

PLACE the pan under a preheated hot grill for a few minutes until the top of the frittata has set and the cheese is golden.

MUSHROOM & GREEN PEPPER FRITTATA

Cheese, mushrooms and peppers are one of my all-time favourite combinations.

Serves 1
Prep time 10 minutes
Cook time 15 minutes

3 large eggs

1 tsp extra virgin olive oil

100g (3½oz) sliced onion

80g (2¾oz) chestnut mushrooms, sliced

80g (2¾oz) cored and deseeded green pepper, cut into chunks

10g (¼oz) Cheddar cheese, grated

salt and pepper

BREAK the eggs into a bowl and beat together with a little salt and pepper. Set aside.

HEAT the olive oil in a small flameproof frying pan over a medium-high heat, add the onion, mushrooms and green pepper and fry for 10 minutes, stirring occasionally, or until the veg has reduced by nearly half.

SPREAD the veg out evenly in the pan, then pour in the beaten egg, tilting the pan to distribute it evenly. Sprinkle in the cheese and cook for 3 minutes, or until the egg is just set and you can slide a spatula around the side.

PLACE the pan under a preheated hot grill for a few minutes until the top of the frittata has set and the cheese is golden.

PUMPKIN & AMARETTO SOUP

I am forever fascinated by cultural differences when it comes to food. In the West, soups are almost always made by first laboriously sweating veg in butter or oil before adding stock in a complex, multi-stage process, while in Asia people simply chuck everything in a saucepan in one go. So would this lazy, all-in-one technique work in a Western-style, puréed soup? Well, I tried it and the answer is yes! And in my experience, and comparing both techniques in a side-by-side taste test (I *am* a geek after all), there is zero difference in flavour. So here goes: my recipe for a super-easy soup – the mix of golden autumn veg makes an incredible, warming soup and there's no need for slow sweating or multiple steps. Just tip everything in and get cooking. The best bit? 3.5 portions of veg per serving in this light lunch.

PORTIONS PER SERVING

Serves 4

Prep time 15 minutes

Cook time 18 minutes

300g (10½oz) trimmed, cleaned and chopped leeks

300g (10½oz) peeled, deseeded and chopped winter squash

300g (10½oz) cored, deseeded and chopped red peppers

300g (10½oz) chopped sweet potato (no need to peel)

800ml (1⅓ pints) vegetable or chicken stock

800ml (1⅓ pints) milk

1 tsp mixed spice

2 tbsp olive oil

2 tbsp Amaretto liqueur

4 tbsp double cream

handful of parsley, chopped

PLACE the vegetables, stock, milk and mixed spice in a large saucepan and bring to the boil, then cover, reduce the heat to medium and simmer for 15 minutes, or until the veg are tender.

REMOVE the pan from the heat and blitz the soup with a stick blender until smooth, then stir in the olive oil and Amaretto.

LADLE into bowls and add 1 tablespoon of cream to each. Serve scattered with the parsley.

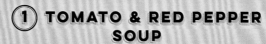

VARIATIONS

① TOMATO & RED PEPPER SOUP

Make the soup as opposite, replacing the veg with 300g (10½oz) halved **cherry tomatoes**, 300g (10½oz) diced **onions**, 120g (4¼oz) **tomato purée** and 300g (10½oz) cored, deseeded and diced **red peppers**. Omit the Amaretto.

② WATERCRESS, ASPARAGUS & PEA SOUP

Make the soup as opposite, replacing the veg with 300g (10½oz) diced **onions**, 300g (10½oz) **frozen peas**, 200g (7oz) trimmed and diced **asparagus**, 200g (7oz) diced **parsnips** and 100g (3½oz) **watercress**. Omit the Amaretto and cook the veg at a simmer for only 4 minutes.

③ SWEETCORN & YELLOW PEPPER SOUP

Make the soup as opposite, replacing the veg with 300g (10½oz) **frozen sweetcorn**, 300g (10½oz) diced **onions**, 300g (10½oz) diced **sweet potato** and 300g (10½oz) cored, deseeded and diced **yellow peppers**, and the Amaretto with ¼ tsp **turmeric**.

④ PURPLE SWEET POTATO SOUP

Make the soup as opposite, replacing the veg with 300g (10½oz) diced **onions**, 600g (1lb 5oz) finely diced **purple sweet potatoes** and 300g (10½oz) diced **cauliflower**. Omit the Amaretto.

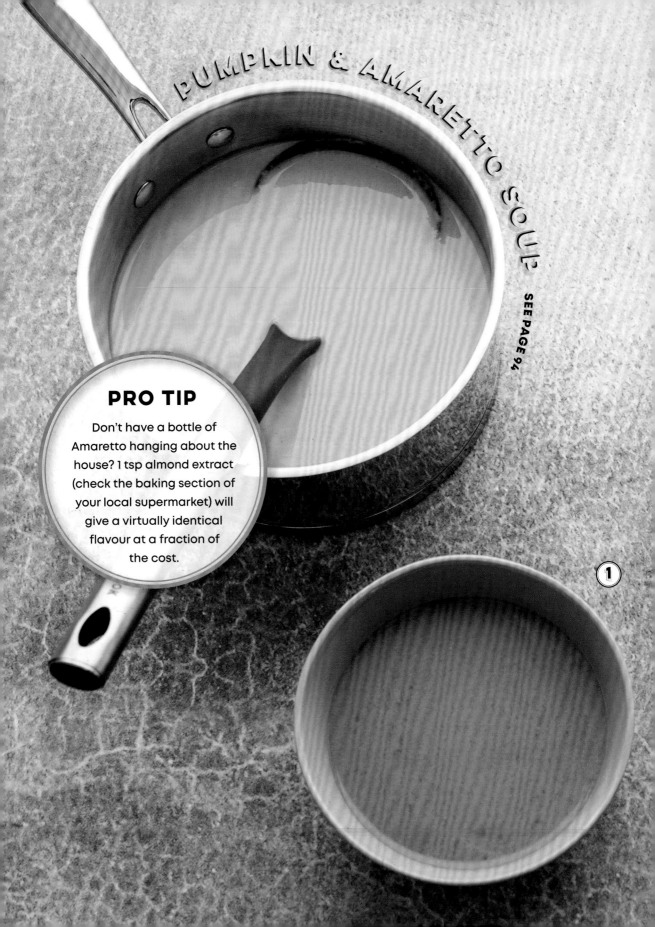

SEE PAGE 94

PRO TIP

Don't have a bottle of Amaretto hanging about the house? 1 tsp almond extract (check the baking section of your local supermarket) will give a virtually identical flavour at a fraction of the cost.

1

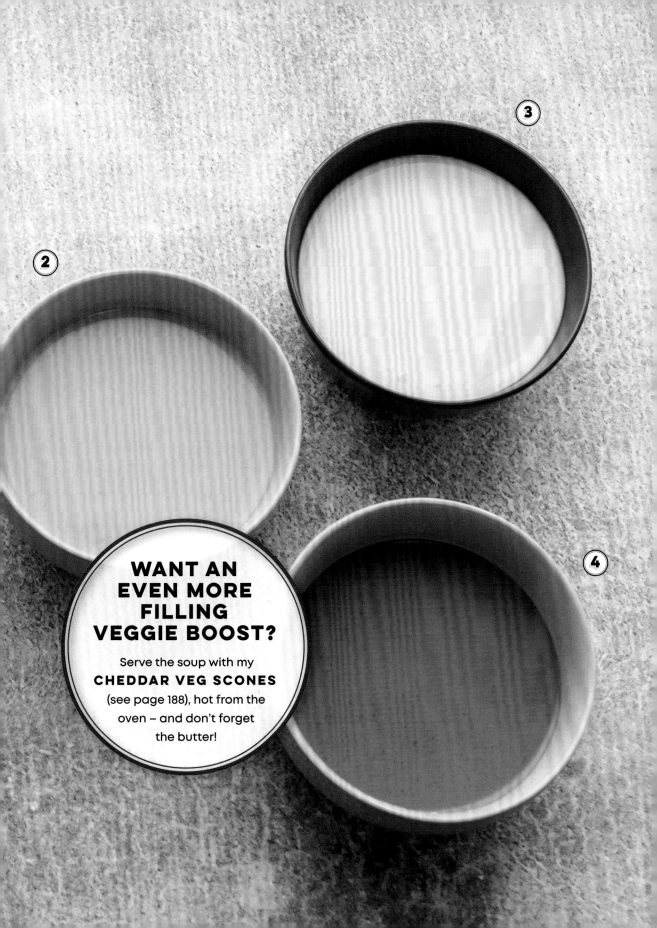

WANT AN EVEN MORE FILLING VEGGIE BOOST?

Serve the soup with my **CHEDDAR VEG SCONES** (see page 188), hot from the oven – and don't forget the butter!

10-MINUTE RAVIOLI SOUP

I really wish I was one of those people who had the time to make their own ravioli from scratch. But, sadly, my life is just way too busy. Hence why I am such a huge fan of shop-bought ravioli, which can go from fridge to plate in a grand total of 3 minutes. And what if you could make these super-convenient dumplings of deliciousness even easier by, say, ditching the need to heat up a sauce and not even bothering to strain the pasta?

Well, with ravioli soup you can do exactly this. Toss in a few super-quick-cooking veg and you have a hearty soup with 3 veg portions made in a jiffy and for absolute minimal effort.

 PORTIONS **3** PER SERVING

Serves 4
Prep time 5 minutes
Cook time 10 minutes

2 litres (3½ pints) chicken stock

600g (1lb 5oz) frozen mixed vegetables, such as carrot, peas, sweetcorn and beans

300g (10½oz) finely sliced onions

2 x 400g (14oz) packs fresh ravioli or tortellini pasta (any flavour will work)

2 garlic cloves, crushed

50ml (2fl oz) sherry

To serve

2 tbsp chopped fresh herbs (I like dill, parsley and mint)

2 tbsp grated Parmesan cheese

1 tbsp extra virgin olive oil

BRING the stock to the boil in a very large saucepan, then add the remaining soup ingredients. Bring back to the boil (this will take about 5 minutes due to the frozen veg), then reduce the heat to a simmer and cook for 3 minutes until the pasta is tender.

SERVE scattered with the herbs and Parmesan, with a little drizzle of olive oil.

VARIATION

ASIAN-STYLE RAVIOLI SOUP

Make the soup as above, using 2 x 400g (14oz) packs ham or chicken-filled pasta (anything without cheese) and replacing the frozen veg with 300g (10½oz) finely sliced **fresh shiitake mushrooms** and 300g (10½oz) **Tenderstem broccoli**, broken into thin florets. Serve scattered with 1 sliced **red chilli** and 2 finely sliced **spring onions**, and drizzled with 1 tbsp **sesame oil**.

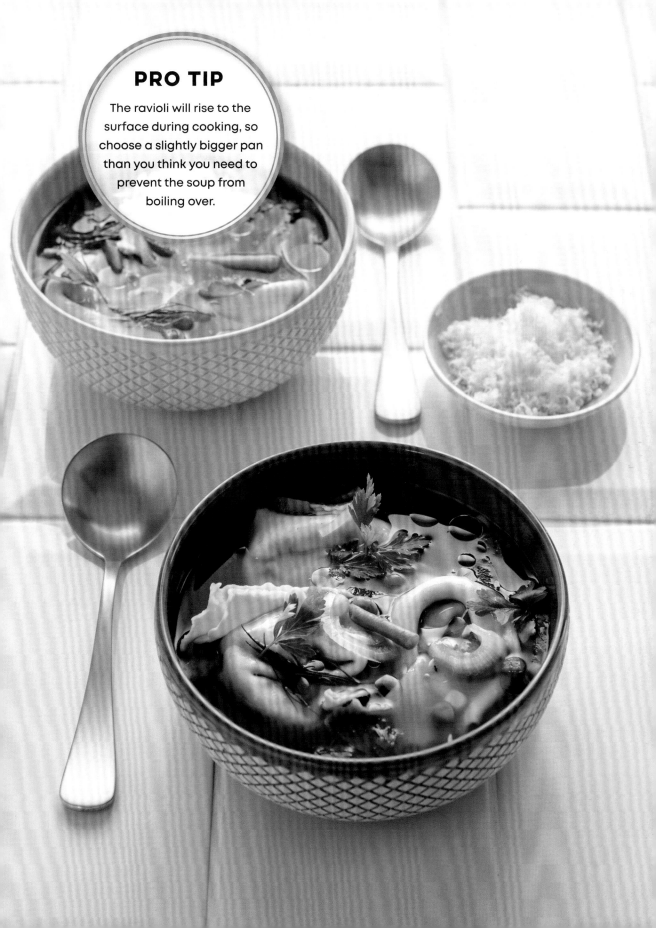

PRO TIP

The ravioli will rise to the surface during cooking, so choose a slightly bigger pan than you think you need to prevent the soup from boiling over.

SAVOURY PROTEIN CRÊPES

Looking at this picture, you might not imagine that each serving of these indulgent filled crêpes contains 3.5 veg portions. But how? Where? Well, I'll let you in on my secret. It's all about the batter. I have swapped wheat flour for gram flour, which counts as a portion of veg, giving you a dose of healthy protein as a bonus. Don't like the sound of chickpea flour? Well, if you like poppadums or pakoras, that's what they are made out of, so you're going to love these!

Serves 4

Prep time 10 minutes, plus standing

Cook time 32 minutes

250ml (9fl oz) water

250ml (9fl oz) milk

250g (9oz) gram flour

1 tbsp olive oil, plus extra for frying

1 tsp fine sea salt

POUR the measured water and milk into a large bowl, then add the gram flour a little at a time, whisking constantly until it resembles a smooth, thin custard. Stir in the olive oil and salt, then leave to stand for 30 minutes.

HEAT a little olive oil in a large 30cm (12in) frying pan over a medium-high heat. Pour in enough batter to cover the base of the pan, then fry for 2 minutes on each side until golden. Remove from the pan and keep warm until all the batter is used to make 8 crêpes.

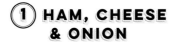

① HAM, CHEESE & ONION

Fry 400g (14oz) roughly chopped **onions** in 2 tsp **extra virgin olive oil** over a medium-high heat for 5–7 minutes, or until browned. Divide 160g (5¾oz) **tomato purée** among the crêpes, spreading it out thinly. Top with 400g (14oz) sliced **ham**, then add a line of the fried onions down the middle of each. Scatter 80g (2¾oz) grated **Cheddar cheese** over the crêpes. Fold the lower side of each crêpe into the centre to form a cone. Microwave each crêpe on full power for about 1 minute until the cheese starts to melt. Enjoy warm!

② CHICKEN & AVOCADO CRUNCH

Slice 400g (14oz) **carrots** into thin ribbons using a vegetable peeler and set aside. Mash 2 large stoned and peeled **avocados**, about 400g (14oz) flesh, with 2 tsp **cider vinegar** and 2 pinches of **salt**, then spread over the crêpes. Arrange the carrot ribbons over the avocado mix, then sprinkle with a handful of chopped **curly parsley** and the grated zest of 2 **lemons**. Divide 600g (1lb 5oz) **cooked chicken breast pieces** among the crêpes, adding it in a line down the middle of each one, then season with **pepper**. Fold the lower sides of the crêpes into the centre to form cones.

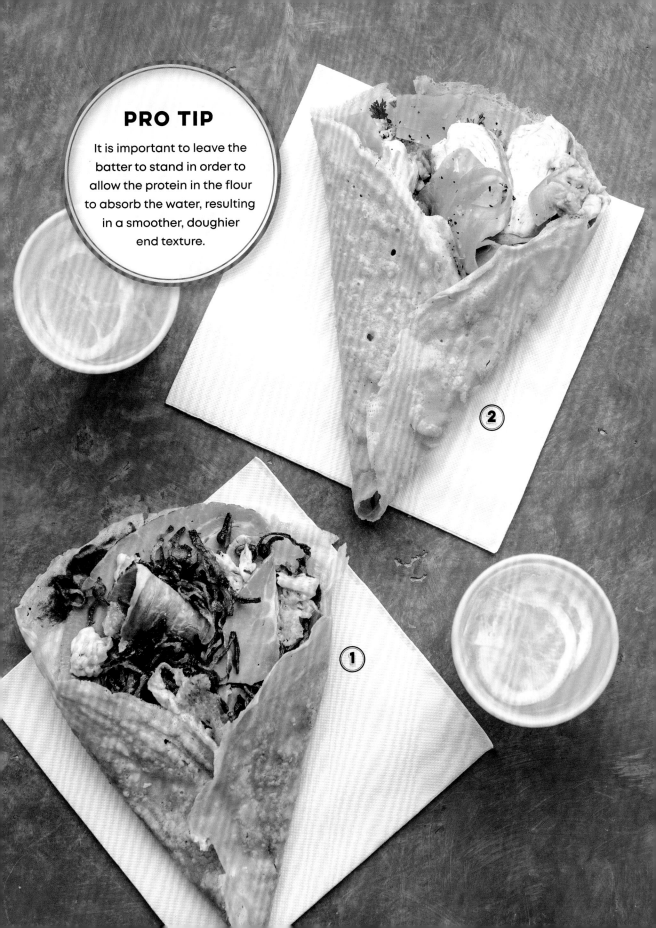

PRO TIP

It is important to leave the batter to stand in order to allow the protein in the flour to absorb the water, resulting in a smoother, doughier end texture.

①

②

FIG & GOATS' CHEESE FARINATA PIZZA

Pizza and beer are two things that make life worth living. And despite often being snobbishly labelled 'junk food' (gosh, I hate that term), pizza really can be the epitome of a balanced meal, combining protein, carbs and a potentially hefty dose of veg. It all depends what you choose to put on it! While I love the classic type, this twist of mine manages to up the veg content even further by sneaking it into the dough itself. Based on the Genovese flatbread 'farinata', which is made using gram flour, the base is given its beautiful golden hue and subtle sweetness with canned pumpkin, creating a dough that contains 2 veg portions in one serving.

Serves 4
Prep time 15 minutes, plus standing
Cook time 20–22 minutes

Base
250ml (9fl oz) water
250g (9oz) gram flour
1 tbsp cornflour
250g (9oz) canned pumpkin purée
1 tsp sea salt
1 tbsp extra virgin olive oil, plus 2 tsp

Topping
120g (4¼oz) tomato purée
160g (5¾oz) red onion, cut into 5–7mm (¼–⅜in) strips
160g (5¾oz) fresh figs, cut into thin wedges
80g (2¾oz) goats' cheese
2 tsp clear honey
60g (2¼oz) pomegranate seeds

POUR the measured water into a large bowl, then add the gram flour a little at a time, whisking constantly until smooth. Transfer a little of the gram flour mixture to a separate small bowl, add the cornflour and combine to form a smooth paste. Stir the paste back into the remaining gram flour mixture, then mix in the pumpkin purée, salt and the 1 tablespoon olive oil to form a surprisingly thin batter. Leave to stand for 30 minutes.

PREHEAT the oven to 220°C (425°F), Gas Mark 7. Line 2 x 27cm (10¾in) diameter Pyrex dishes with baking paper and grease with the remaining oil. Place the dishes in the oven for 3–5 minutes to heat up.

DIVIDE the batter between 2 bowls (there should be about 350g/12oz batter per bowl), then pour the batter from each bowl into a heated Pyrex dish and spread out evenly with a spatula. Return to the oven on the top and middle shelves and bake for 10 minutes, swapping the positions of the dishes halfway through to ensure even cooking.

REMOVE the dishes from the oven and spread the tomato purée evenly over the pizza bases. Scatter over the onion strips, then add the figs, spacing the wedges out evenly across the top. Crumble over the goats' cheese.

POP the pizzas back in the oven for 10–12 minutes, or until the cheese turns slightly golden and the edge crisps up. Serve drizzled with the honey and scattered with the pomegranate seeds.

VARIATIONS

① PAPAYAN FARINATA PIZZA

Make the pizza bases, spread with the tomato purée and scatter with the red onion as opposite. Omit the remaining topping ingredients. Cut 160g (5¾oz) **papaya** (nectarine and mango make good substitutes) into wedges, then add evenly over the bases and sprinkle with 80g (2¾oz) grated **mature Cheddar cheese**. Continue to bake as opposite, then serve topped with a few slices of **jamón Ibérico**, the pulp of 2 small **passion fruit** and a handful of **curly parsley** leaves, chopped.

② MUSHROOM & ASPARAGUS FARINATA PIZZA

Make the pizza bases and spread with the tomato purée as opposite. Omit the remaining topping ingredients. Cut 160g (5¾oz) **asparagus spears** in half lengthways, then widthways, and 160g (5¾oz) **chestnut mushrooms** into 5–7mm- (¼–⅜in-) thick slices. Toss the vegetables with 2 tsp **extra virgin olive oil**, 2 tsp finely grated **lemon zest**, 2 tsp **dried oregano** and a little **salt** and **pepper**. Scatter the veg mixture over the bases, then sprinkle with 50g (1¾oz) grated **pecorino cheese**. Continue to bake as opposite, then serve scattered with a small handful of **rocket leaves**.

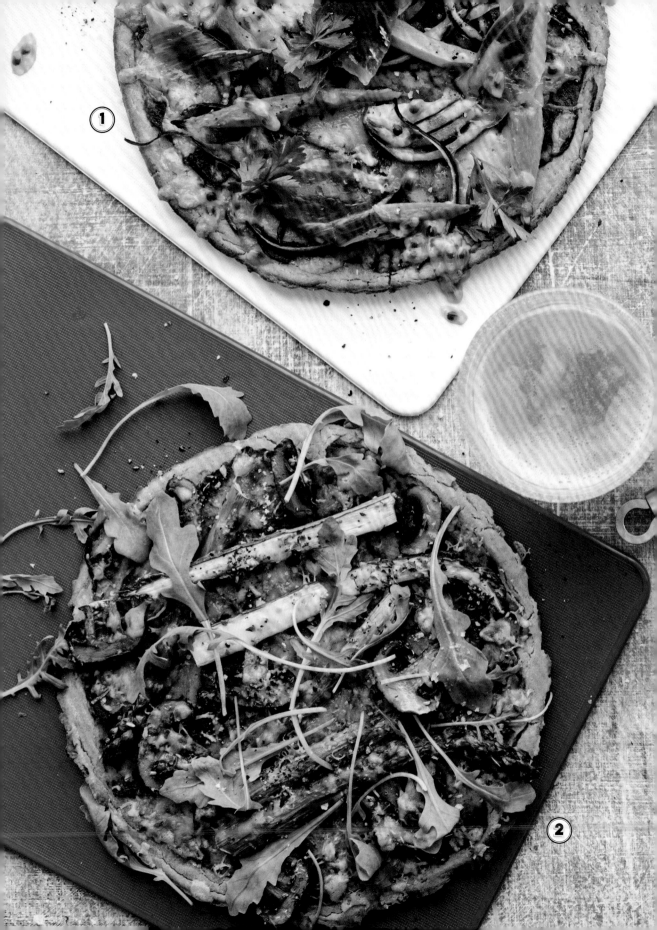

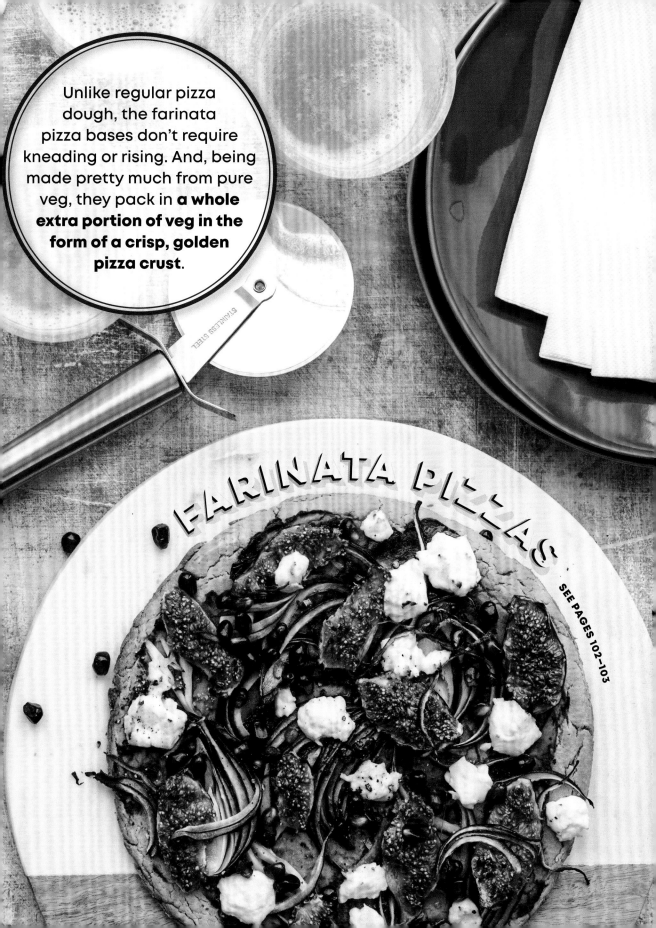

Unlike regular pizza dough, the farinata pizza bases don't require kneading or rising. And, being made pretty much from pure veg, they pack in **a whole extra portion of veg in the form of a crisp, golden pizza crust**.

FARINATA PIZZAS

SEE PAGES 102–103

VEG TAGINE

There is just something about veg from the Med. Perhaps it's the umami from the tomatoes or maybe the creamy savoury-ness of the chickpeas that makes them seem somehow more hearty than green veg? So I decided to combine a whole bunch of them in a dish to put veg squarely at the heart of a meal, instead of being a mere culinary sidekick.

Serves 4

Prep time 15 minutes

Cook time 5 minutes

1 x quantity Tomacado Salsa (see page 209)

320g (11¼oz) couscous

60g (2¼oz) raisins

60g (2¼oz) dried apricots, diced

2 chicken stock cubes

420ml (14½fl oz) boiling water

1 tbsp extra virgin olive oil

200g (7oz) finely sliced onions

400g (14oz) can chickpeas, rinsed and drained

a few mint leaves, finely sliced

a few curly parsley sprigs, finely chopped

pepper

To serve

lemon wedges

soy sauce

WHILE the Tomacado Salsa is marinating, tip the couscous into a large, wide heatproof bowl or large saucepan, add the dried fruits, crumble in the stock cubes and mix well. Pour over the measured water and give it a quick, thorough stir, then cover with a plate or saucepan lid and set aside.

HEAT the olive oil in a medium frying pan over a medium-high heat. Add the onions and fry for about 5 minutes, stirring frequently, or until browned to your liking.

REMOVE the cover from the couscous and fluff it up with a fork. Stir in the onions, the salsa (including its marinade), the chickpeas, chopped herbs and a few twists of pepper.

SERVE with the lemon wedges and a drizzle of soy sauce.

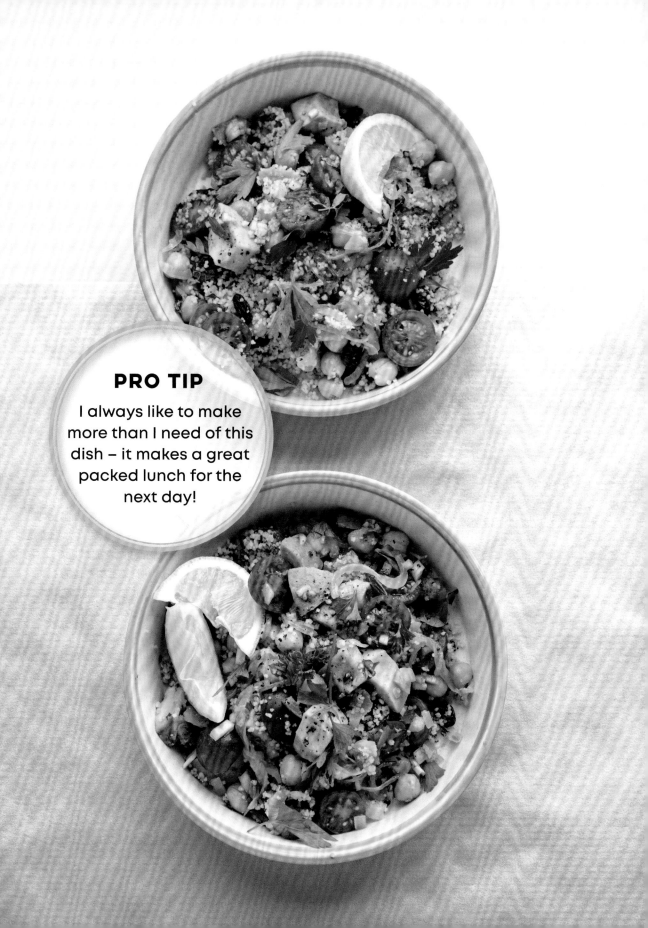

PRO TIP

I always like to make more than I need of this dish – it makes a great packed lunch for the next day!

PRAWN 'TACO' SALAD

One of my favourite packed lunches, inspired by my two lovely Mexican housemates, both *phenomenal* cooks, who I lived with in my 20s. Sorry *chicas*, for the shameless gringo-fication!

Serves 4
Prep time 25 minutes
Cook time 2 minutes

Pink pickled onions

300g (10½oz) finely sliced red onions

1 tsp sugar

¼ tsp salt

100ml (3½fl oz) cider vinegar

'Taco' prawns

250g (9oz) raw peeled king prawns

finely grated zest and juice of 1 lime

1 tsp smoked paprika

2 garlic cloves, crushed

1 tsp oregano

1 tsp olive oil, for frying

Salad

300g (10½oz) drained canned sweetcorn

300g (10½oz) rinsed and drained canned black-eyed, kidney or butter beans

300g (10½oz) cherry tomatoes, halved

90g (3¼oz) sliced green jalapeño chillies from a jar

1 large avocado, stoned, peeled and cubed

150g (5½oz) feta cheese, crumbled

small handful of curly parsley, finely chopped

1 x 30g (1oz) packet corn tortilla chips

1 lime, quartered

2 tbsp extra virgin olive oil

salt and pepper

PLACE all the pink pickled onion ingredients in a non-reactive bowl and toss together, then set aside for about 20 minutes – the reaction is pretty fast so by the time you have finished making the rest of the salad they will be ready.

COMBINE all the 'taco' prawns ingredients except the olive oil in a separate non-reactive dish and set aside while you assemble the salad.

DIVIDE all the salad ingredients except the extra virgin olive oil and seasoning among 4 bowls. Drizzle over the extra virgin olive oil and season with salt and pepper.

HEAT the olive oil in a frying pan over high heat. Add the 'taco' prawn ingredients and fry for 2 minutes, or until the prawns turn pink and are cooked through. Divide among the bowls, top with the pickled onions and dig in!

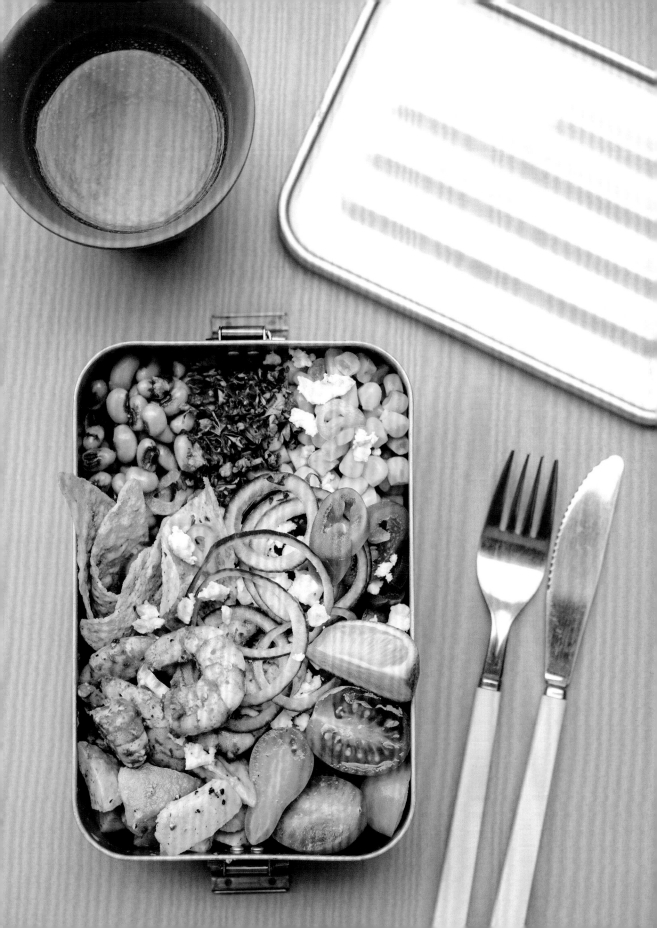

TZATZIKI CHICKEN SALAD

I have a lifelong love of tzatziki. Creamy Greek yogurt and warm garlic tag-teaming with fresh cucumber and cooling mint is to me one of the all-time great flavour combinations. The problem is I usually eat it as a dip with a giant pile of crisps and, sadly, those have yet to count as a portion of veg. So here's my deconstructed take on it, based on all the same flavours, but with loads of veg and lean protein for a perfect weekday lunch. And if you fancy some crisps on the side, go ahead! Life is too short to cut them out.

Serves 2

Prep time 20 minutes

30g (1oz) rocket leaves

1 tsp extra virgin olive oil

40g (1½oz) feta cheese, cut into different-sized cubes

finely grated zest and juice of ½ lemon

½ cucumber (about 200g/7oz)

200g (7oz) stoned and peeled avocado (about 1 large avo), sliced lengthways

300g (10½oz) ready-cooked or leftover cooked chicken breast pieces

160g (5¾oz) fresh blackberries

pepper

a few mint sprigs, to garnish

Dip

200g (7oz) Greek yogurt

½ tsp minced garlic

1 tsp extra virgin olive oil

1 tsp finely chopped dill

1 tsp finely chopped parsley

1 tsp finely chopped mint

1 tsp lemon juice

pinch of salt

MIX all of the dip ingredients together in a small bowl and set aside while you assemble the salad.

PLACE the rocket on a serving plate, toss with the olive oil and season with a little pepper. Top with the cubed feta and a sprinkle of lemon zest.

SHRED the cucumber into long, thin ribbons using a vegetable peeler, then taking a few strips at a time, fold into 'S' shapes and add to the plate.

ARRANGE the avocado slices on the plate, then drizzle with a little lemon juice. Top with the chicken pieces and blackberries, garnish with a few sprigs of mint and serve with the dip.

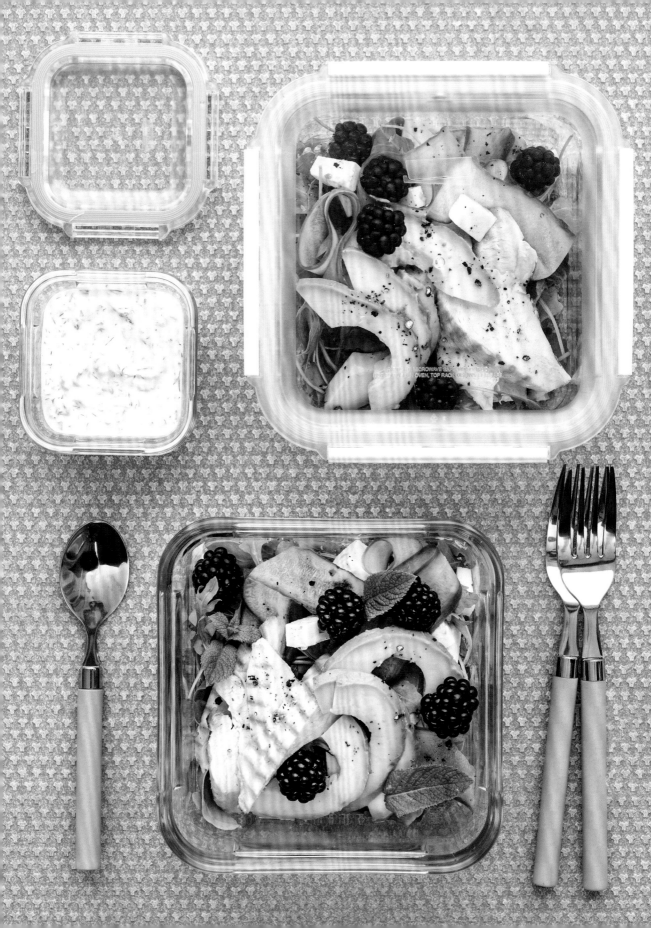

ONE-PAN RISOTTOS

I do love the comforting creaminess of homemade risotto. However, if you go too low on the veg, it can become a bit of a stodge-fest. The good news is by making two simple tweaks to an old-school recipe – bumping up the amount of veg a little and swapping the white rice for brown – not only do you get way more flavour and a far more satisfying 'bite' with this dish, but a whole lot more potential health benefits. How much more? Well, each serving of brown rice contains a whopping six times more fibre than the same amount of white according to the United States Department of Agriculture, with up to double the levels of many other vitamins and minerals. Just as well that brown short-grain rice is now becoming increasingly widely available, and can be picked up easily and inexpensively at health food stores and online.

MUSHROOM, PEA & ASPARAGUS RISOTTO

Rich, smoky mushrooms meet the sweetness of peas and asparagus.
An elegant dinner party dish, which can be knocked together in minutes.

Serves 4
Prep time 10 minutes
Cook time 1 hour

400g (14oz) fresh shiitake mushrooms, finely sliced

300g (10½oz) finely sliced onions

200g (7oz) brown short-grain rice, rinsed well

500ml (18fl oz) milk

500ml (18fl oz) water

2 chicken stock cubes, crumbled

1 garlic clove, minced

50ml (2fl oz) sherry

200g (7oz) frozen peas

100g (3½oz) asparagus, sliced at an angle

salt and pepper

To serve

2 tbsp grated Parmesan cheese

1 tbsp olive oil

small handful of parsley, chopped

COMBINE the mushrooms, onions, rice, milk, measured water and stock cubes in a large, shallow saucepan.

BRING to the boil, then reduce the heat and simmer, uncovered, for 50 minutes until the rice is tender, but still retains a little bite.

STIR in the garlic, sherry, peas and asparagus and simmer for another 2 minutes until the vegetables are tender, stirring occasionally. Season to taste and serve topped with the cheese, olive oil and parsley.

Serves 4

Prep time 10 minutes

Cook time 1 hour

....

400g (14oz) can chopped tomatoes

300g (10½oz) cored, deseeded and diced red peppers

300g (10½oz) diced onions

200g (7oz) brown short-grain rice, rinsed well

750ml (1⅓ pints) milk

2 chicken stock cubes, crumbled

50ml (2fl oz) sherry

1 garlic clove, minced

finely grated zest of 1 lemon

salt and pepper

To serve

2 tbsp grated Parmesan cheese

1 tbsp olive oil

small handful of basil leaves

TOMATO & RED PEPPER RISOTTO

This tasty risotto swaps out loads of white carbs and fat for wholegrains and veg.

....

COMBINE the tomatoes, red peppers, onions, rice, milk and stock cubes in a large, shallow saucepan.

BRING to the boil, then reduce the heat and simmer, uncovered, for 50 minutes until the rice is tender, but still retains a little bite.

STIR in the sherry, garlic and lemon zest and simmer for another 2 minutes, stirring occasionally. Season to taste and serve topped with the cheese, olive oil and basil.

Serves 4

Prep time 10 minutes

Cook time 1 hour

....

300g (10½oz) finely diced carrots

300g (10½oz) peeled, deseeded and finely diced butternut squash

400g (14oz) diced onions

200g (7oz) brown short-grain rice, rinsed well

large pinch of saffron threads

500ml (18fl oz) milk

500ml (18fl oz) water

2 chicken stock cubes, crumbled

1 garlic clove, minced

50ml (2fl oz) sherry

salt and pepper

To serve

2 tbsp grated Parmesan cheese

1 tbsp olive oil

small handful of dill, chopped

BUTTERNUT SQUASH & CARROT RISOTTO

The sweet, warming deliciousness of this dish is my fail-safe antidote to the autumn blues.

....

COMBINE the carrots, squash, onions, rice, saffron, milk, measured water and stock cubes in a large, shallow saucepan.

BRING to the boil, then reduce the heat and simmer, uncovered, for 50 minutes until the rice and vegetables are tender, but the rice retains a little bite.

STIR in the garlic and sherry, then simmer for another 2 minutes, stirring occasionally. Season to taste and serve topped with the cheese, olive oil and dill.

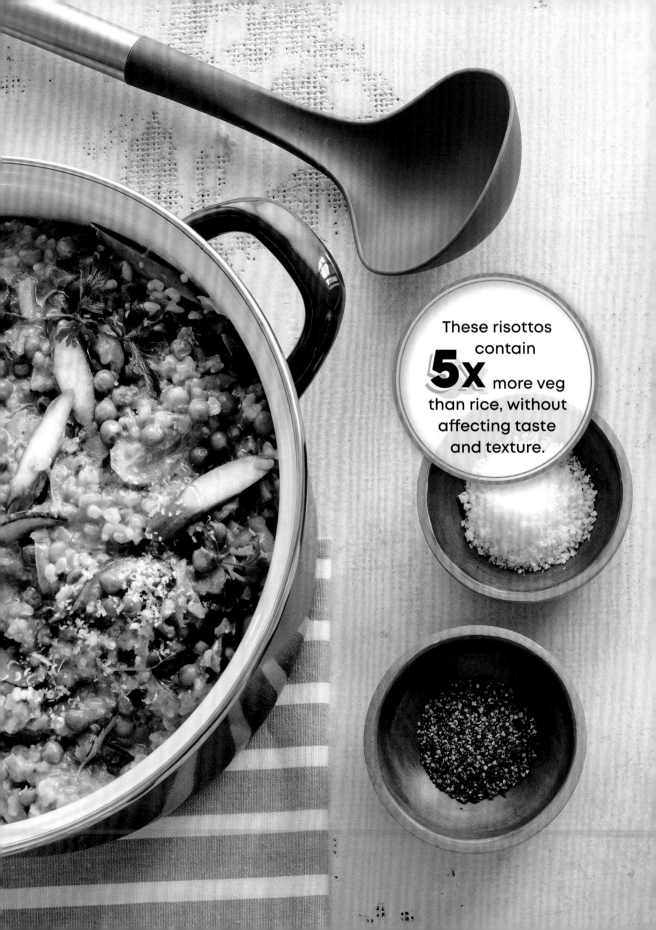

These risottos contain **5x** more veg than rice, without affecting taste and texture.

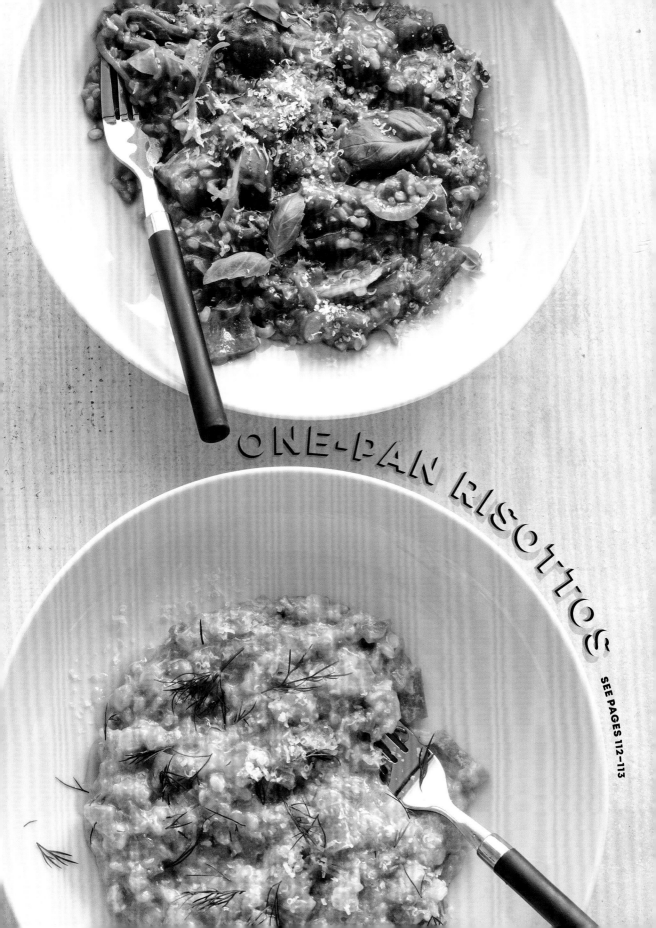

ONE-PAN RISOTTOS

SEE PAGES 112–113

MAC & CHEESE

The comforting, rich gooeyness that is mac and cheese is always popular. However, as most of the other traditional ingredients (basically flour, milk and a bit of butter) are pretty bland, it does require an awful lot of cheese for its flavour. However, by sneaking in 3 portions of golden, caramelized veg per serving, this recipe has so much depth and warmth you can slash the quantity of cheese by up to a whopping 75 per cent without missing it one bit. An astonishing saving of nearly 1,000 calories! And trust me, this is coming from a bit of a cheese fiend. You can always add more cheese at the table if I'm wrong!

Serves 4

Prep time 20 minutes

Cook time 50 minutes

1 tbsp extra virgin olive oil

300g (10½oz) cored, deseeded and finely diced red peppers

300g (10½oz) finely diced sweet potato (no need to peel)

300g (10½oz) finely diced onions

300g (10½oz) dried macaroni

2 tbsp sherry

1 chicken stock cube, crumbled

400ml (14fl oz) milk

½ tsp dried garlic granules

75g (2¾oz) mature Cheddar cheese, grated

3 tbsp cornflour, mixed with a little water to form a thin paste

4 spring onions, finely sliced

2 tbsp panko breadcrumbs

2 tbsp smoked lardons or diced bacon

salt and pepper

HEAT the olive oil in a large, shallow saucepan over a low heat, add the peppers, sweet potato and onions and cook for about 30 minutes, stirring occasionally, until completely softened and golden brown.

MEANWHILE, cook the macaroni in a saucepan of boiling water for 2 minutes less than the packet instructions, then drain the pasta.

PREHEAT the oven to 200°C (400°F), Gas Mark 6.

ADD the sherry, stock cube, milk and garlic granules to the softened veg and give it a good stir to deglaze the pan. Cook for another minute or two, then take off the heat and blitz together using a stick blender until you have a smooth sauce.

STIR in the cheese, drained macaroni and cornflour paste and season well, then pour the mixture into a large baking dish (about 30 x 20cm/12 x 8in and 10cm/4in deep), or 4 smaller individual ones.

SCATTER over the spring onions, breadcrumbs and lardons or diced bacon, then bake for 20 minutes until golden and bubbling. Leave to stand for 10 minutes before serving.

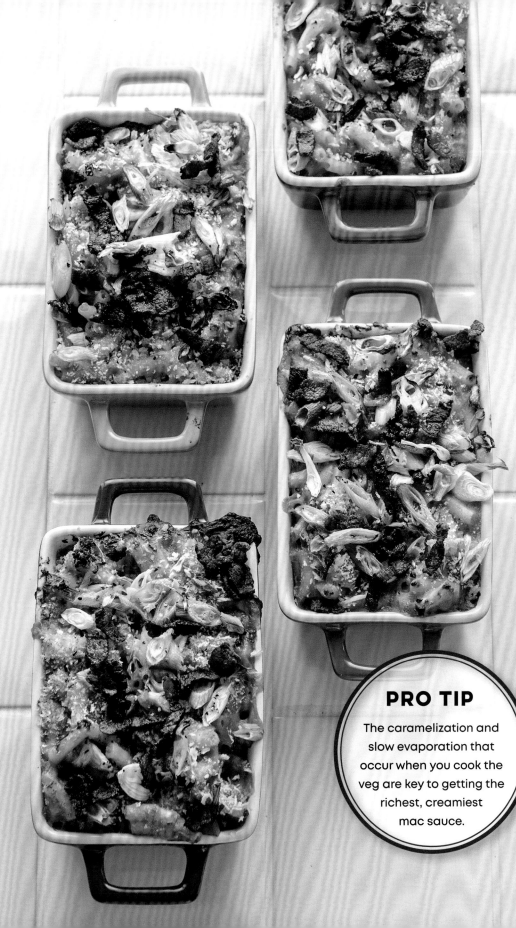

PRO TIP

The caramelization and slow evaporation that occur when you cook the veg are key to getting the richest, creamiest mac sauce.

DINNERS

MARSALA CHICKEN

Warm, comforting, delicious Italian food, quick enough to be knocked together in under 30 minutes for a weekday supper. How many chicken dishes can you think of that'll give you 2 portions of veg before you even reach for the mash or veggie side?

Serves 4
Prep time 10 minutes
Cook time 25–30 minutes

2 tbsp extra virgin olive oil

4 large boneless, skinless chicken breasts, about 150g (5½oz) each

300g (10½oz) thinly sliced onions

300g (10½oz) cored, deseeded and thinly sliced red peppers

200g (7oz) fresh shiitake mushrooms, thinly sliced

200g (7oz) button mushrooms, thinly sliced

1 tbsp plain flour

150ml (5fl oz) Marsala wine

150ml (5fl oz) milk

1 chicken stock cube, crumbled

2 garlic cloves, minced

1 tbsp chopped parsley

HEAT 1 tablespoon of the olive oil in a large, shallow saucepan over a medium heat, add the chicken breasts and fry for about 4 minutes on each side, or until cooked through and golden brown. Remove from the pan with a slotted spoon and set aside, but do not clean the pan.

ADD the remaining olive oil to the pan and fry the onions, red peppers and all the mushrooms over a medium heat until they soften and any excess water from the mushrooms has evaporated. This will take about 10–15 minutes.

SPRINKLE the flour evenly over the cooked veg and stir well to combine. Stir in the Marsala, milk, crumbled stock cube and garlic, then cook for another 2–3 minutes, stirring constantly, until the sauce thickens slightly.

RETURN the chicken to the pan to coat and heat through. Sprinkle over the parsley and serve.

PRO TIP

You can use all plain old button mushrooms if you can't find shiitake, but for me, they're totally worth it for that extra umami hit.

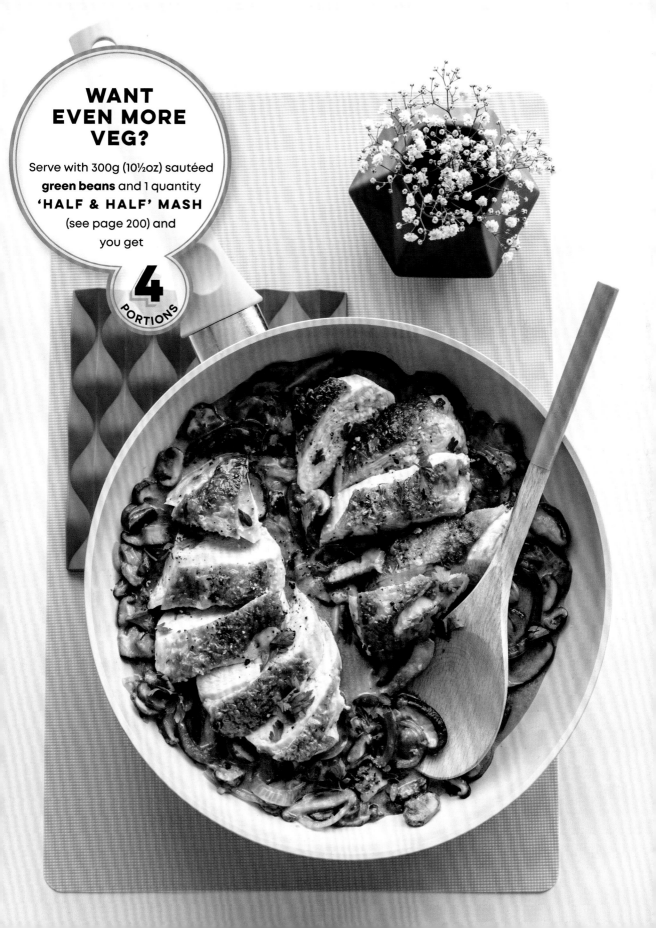

WANT EVEN MORE VEG?

Serve with 300g (10½oz) sautéed **green beans** and 1 quantity **'HALF & HALF' MASH** (see page 200) and you get

4 PORTIONS

FISH PIE

A brightly coloured take on an old favourite that's as simple to put together as it is tasty. Did I mention the 4 portions a day in each slice?

Serves 4

Prep time 20 minutes

Cook time 25 minutes

400g (14oz) red cabbage (about ¼ large head), grated or finely chopped

1 tbsp sea salt flakes

35g (1¼oz) butter, plus extra for greasing

400g (14oz) trimmed and cleaned leeks, halved lengthways and cut into 5mm- (¼in-) thick strips

500g (1lb 2 oz) frozen white fish fillets, such as haddock, cod or pollock

320g (11¼oz) sweet potatoes, cut into chunks (no need to peel)

320g (11¼oz) cubed swede

1½ tbsp finely chopped dill, plus extra to garnish

finely grated zest of 1 lemon

salt and pepper

PLACE the red cabbage in a large mixing bowl and sprinkle over the salt flakes, then using your fingers, massage the salt into the cabbage for a good 2 minutes, squeezing as you go. Leave to stand while you cook the leeks and fish, then rinse thoroughly in a colander to wash off the salt.

MELT 25g (1oz) of the butter in a large, deep frying pan over a medium heat. Add the leeks and fry for 5 minutes until softened, stirring occasionally. Add the frozen fish, cover and cook for 5 minutes, then flip the fish over and give the mixture a stir. Re-cover and cook for another 5 minutes, or until you can break the fish apart with a wooden spoon. Break the fish up, re-cover and cook for 5 minutes until the fish is just cooked through. Stir the rinsed cabbage into the fish mixture, then continue to cook for 5 minutes, uncovered. Take off the heat and drain away any remaining liquid. Cover and set aside.

MEANWHILE, simmer the sweet potatoes in a separate large saucepan of boiling water for 5 minutes, then add the swede and cook for another 5 minutes, or until the veg are soft. Drain and return to the pan. Add the remaining butter, the dill, lemon zest (reserving a little to garnish) and salt and pepper to taste, then mash together and keep warm.

WHILE the fish and cabbage are cooking, remove the base from a 7.5cm (3in) deep, 24cm (9½in) diameter springform cake tin, then lightly grease the ring with the spring clip closed. Place upside down on a serving plate.

TIP the fish mixture into the ring and press flat. Spread the mash on top and garnish with a few sprigs of dill, the reserved lemon zest and some pepper. Slide off the cake ring and serve.

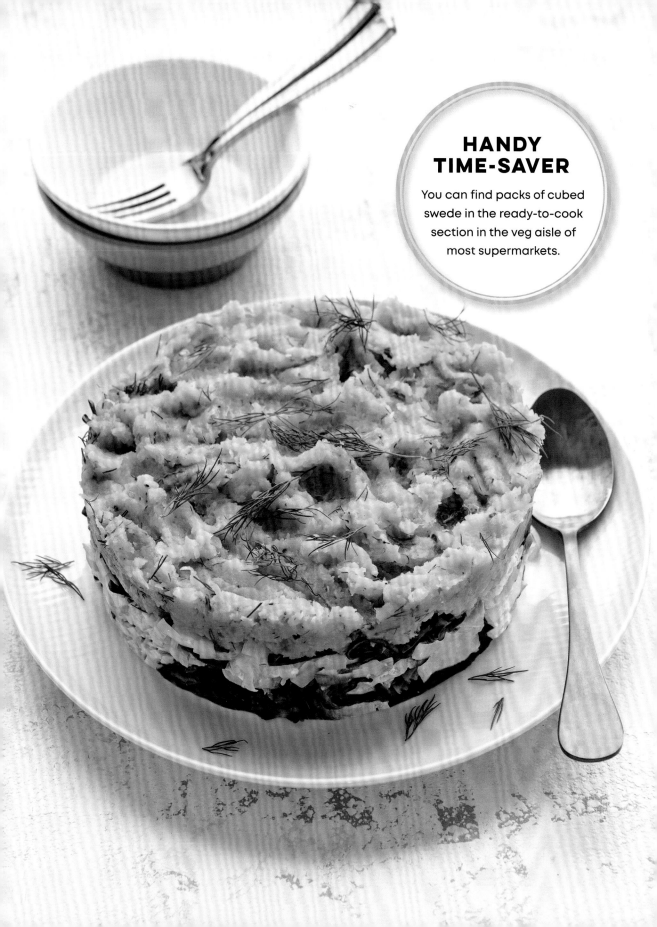

HANDY TIME-SAVER

You can find packs of cubed swede in the ready-to-cook section in the veg aisle of most supermarkets.

CHINESE FAKEAWAY

Eating healthy doesn't need to mean salads and smoothie bowls. Here's my take on a Friday night treat that's as healthy as it it gets.

BEET & SOUR CHICKEN

Sweet and sour chicken is one of the first recipes I made in home economics class at school in Singapore back in the 1990s. (Yes, some cultural stereotypes are true!) What surprised me, even then, was quite how much fruit and veg was crammed into the recipe, the avalanche of added sugar and lurid-red food colouring aside. So here you go, guys. My 21st-century revise that swaps refined sugar with the natural sweetness of fruit and is coloured only by the dazzling pigment of beetroot.

Serves 4
Prep time 10 minutes
Cook time 15 minutes

2 tsp extra virgin olive oil

320g (11¼oz) chicken breast strips

cornflour, for dusting

1 tbsp rapeseed oil

400g (14oz) onions, cut into 2cm (¾in) chunks

200g (7oz) carrots, cut into 7mm (⅜in) cubes

160g (5¾oz) cored and deseeded red pepper, cut into 3cm (1¼in) chunks

160g (5¾oz) canned pineapple chunks in juice, drained

pepper

Bacon & Egg Fried Rice (see page 127), to serve

Sauce

160g (5¾oz) canned pineapple in juice, drained and 160ml (5½fl oz) juice reserved

160g (5¾oz) cooked beetroot, roughly chopped

60g (2¼oz) tomato purée

40ml (1¼fl oz) soy sauce

60ml (2¼oz) rice wine vinegar

2 tbsp rapeseed oil

1 tsp dried garlic granules

HEAT the olive oil in a large frying pan over a medium-high heat. Dust the chicken strips in cornflour and a good amount of pepper until well coated. Add to the pan and fry for 4–5 minutes on each side, or until cooked through, adding extra pepper when you turn the strips over. Remove from the pan and set aside.

BLITZ all of the sauce ingredients including the reserved pineapple juice together in a food processor, then set aside.

HEAT the rapeseed oil in the pan over a high heat. Add the onions and stir-fry for 3 minutes until browned and softened. Add the carrots, red pepper and pineapple chunks and continue to stir-fry for 1 minute.

POUR in the sauce and cook for another minute, then add the cooked chicken and heat through for 1 minute.

SERVE immediately with Bacon & Egg Fried Rice.

BEEF IN BLACK BEAN SAUCE

When I was growing up, my Malaysian grandma always made the best super-fast food by padding out expensive ingredients like meat with loads of veg. Compare these old-school recipes with the meat-dominated modern versions and, well, there is just no contest not only in the flavour stakes, but also the cost and nutrition. Here's my attempt to piece together how she made this Chinese-Malaysian dish from hazy childhood memories.

Serves 4
Prep time 15 minutes
Cook time about 30 minutes

2 sirloin steaks, about 300g (10½oz) in total

1 tbsp olive oil, plus 1 tsp

400g (14oz) onions, roughly chopped into 2cm (¾in) chunks

320g (11¼oz) carrots, halved lengthways and cut into 2mm- (⅛in-) thick pieces

2 red bird's-eye chillies, sliced diagonally into thin rings

160g (5¾oz) cored and deseeded green pepper, cut into 2cm (¾in) chunks

160g (5¾oz) cored and deseeded orange pepper, cut into 1cm (½in) strips

Bacon & Egg Fried Rice (see page 127), to serve

Black bean paste (makes 1 small jar)

2 tbsp extra virgin olive oil

50g (1¾oz) salted black beans, rinsed and mashed with a fork

25g (1oz) fresh root ginger, peeled and minced

25g (1oz) garlic, minced

50g (1¾oz) spring onions, thinly sliced diagonally

100ml (3½fl oz) chicken stock

2 tbsp sherry

2 tsp rice vinegar

juice of ½ lime

1 tsp honey

1 tbsp cornflour, mixed with 1 tbsp water to form a thin paste

1 tsp coarsely ground black pepper

FIRST, make the black bean paste. Heat the olive oil in a small frying pan over a medium heat. Add the beans, ginger and garlic and cook for 3 minutes, stirring occasionally. Stir in the spring onions and cook for another 3 minutes. Pour in the stock, sherry, vinegar, lime juice and honey, stir well and simmer for 10–12 minutes until thickened. Stir in the cornflour paste and pepper, then cook for 1 minute. Take off the heat and leave to cool.

RUB the steaks with the 1 teaspoon olive oil, then fry in a large frying pan over a high heat for 2 minutes on each side, or to your liking. Remove from the pan and set aside.

HEAT the remaining olive oil in the same pan over a high heat. Add the onions and fry for 3 minutes until they start to brown and soften. Add the carrots, chillies and peppers and stir-fry for a further 3 minutes.

STIR in half the black bean paste (store the rest in an airtight jar – it'll keep in the fridge for up to 2 weeks) and cook for 1 minute. Slice the cooked beef diagonally into thin strips, then stir into the mixture, heating it through for 1 minute.

SERVE immediately with Bacon & Egg Fried Rice.

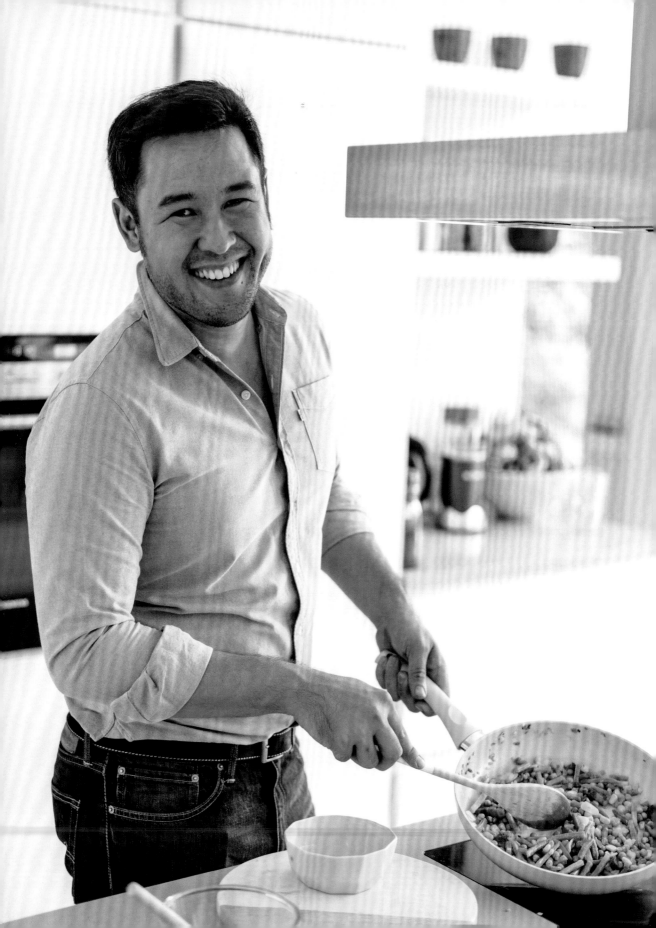

BACON & EGG FRIED RICE

My lovely mum used to make me a hot packed lunch, like many of the other kids in my Singapore state school, by packing food in a Thermos lunch box. She even wanted to make me the same kind of food my classmates had, so I wouldn't feel left out. However, being from a small village in Wales, her versions of Singaporean dishes were always, shall we say, a little bit British…and with some delicious consequences! Fusion, before fusion.

Serves 2
Prep time 5 minutes
Cook time 15–20 minutes

1 tsp olive oil

50g (1¾oz) lardons or 4 bacon rashers, diced

250g (9oz) diced onions

250g (9oz) frozen mixed vegetables

2 tbsp dry sherry

2 large eggs, lightly beaten

2 garlic cloves, minced

250g (9oz) cold leftover brown rice

1 tbsp soy sauce

¼ tsp black pepper

HEAT the olive oil in a large frying pan over a medium heat, add the lardons or bacon rashers and onions and fry until the onions soften and turn golden and the bacon starts to crisp up, about 5–10 minutes. Add the frozen vegetables and sherry and stir well, then cook for another 5 minutes.

STIR in the eggs and garlic and continue to cook until the eggs start to set, then break them up into pieces with a spatula.

ADD the rice, soy sauce and pepper and cook for a further few minutes until the rice starts to catch on the bottom of the pan and everything is piping hot. Serve immediately.

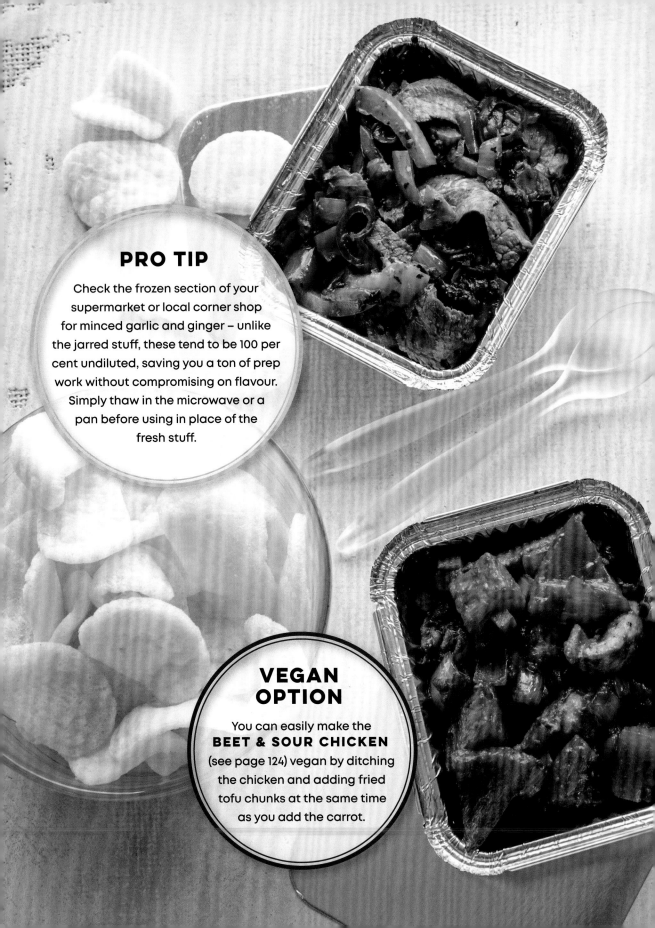

PRO TIP

Check the frozen section of your supermarket or local corner shop for minced garlic and ginger – unlike the jarred stuff, these tend to be 100 per cent undiluted, saving you a ton of prep work without compromising on flavour. Simply thaw in the microwave or a pan before using in place of the fresh stuff.

VEGAN OPTION

You can easily make the **BEET & SOUR CHICKEN** (see page 124) vegan by ditching the chicken and adding fried tofu chunks at the same time as you add the carrot.

SEE PAGES 124–127

CHINESE FAKEAWAY

AUBERGINE PARMIGIANA

This is basically a lasagne that has swapped pasta sheets for deliciously rich, breaded aubergine slices, which dramatically ups the amount of veg per serving in this ultimate Italian comfort-food dish. I experimented with the traditional method of frying these slices, but frankly, baking them involved far less time, effort and mess *and* simultaneously slashed the fat and calorie content without any real noticeable effect on flavour.

Serves 4

Prep time 25 minutes

Cook time 1 hour 20 minutes

2 large eggs

1 tbsp milk

120g (4¼oz) panko breadcrumbs

30g (1oz) Parmesan cheese, grated

1kg (2lb 4oz) aubergines, thickly sliced

500g (1lb 2oz) shop-bought tomato pasta sauce

300g (10½oz) reduced-fat mozzarella cheese, sliced

pepper

Spinach & ricotta filling

100g (3½oz) frozen spinach, defrosted

2 eggs

30g (1oz) Parmesan cheese

400g (14oz) ricotta cheese

¼ tsp freshly grated nutmeg

1 tsp dried garlic granules

handful of basil, torn, plus extra to garnish

PREHEAT the oven to 190°C (375°F), Gas Mark 5.

BEAT the eggs and milk together in a bowl. In a separate bowl, combine the breadcrumbs and Parmesan and season very generously with pepper. Dip the aubergine slices first in the egg mixture, then in the breadcrumbs to coat them evenly. Transfer the coated slices to 2 large baking sheets.

BAKE the aubergines for 30 minutes until the slices are golden, turning them once halfway through cooking.

MEANWHILE, prepare the spinach and ricotta filling. Squeeze out as much liquid from the defrosted spinach as you can, then place with all the remaining filling ingredients in a bowl and combine.

REMOVE the baked aubergines from the oven, leaving it on. Arrange a single layer of the aubergines in a large baking dish (about 30 x 20cm/12 x 8in and 7cm/2¾in deep), top with some of the filling and a few spoonfuls of the tomato pasta sauce. Repeat the layers until all the ingredients except the mozzarella are used up.

TOP with the mozzarella, cover the dish with foil and bake for 40 minutes. Remove the foil and continue to bake for 10 minutes, or until the cheese topping has melted and turned golden. Serve garnished with basil leaves.

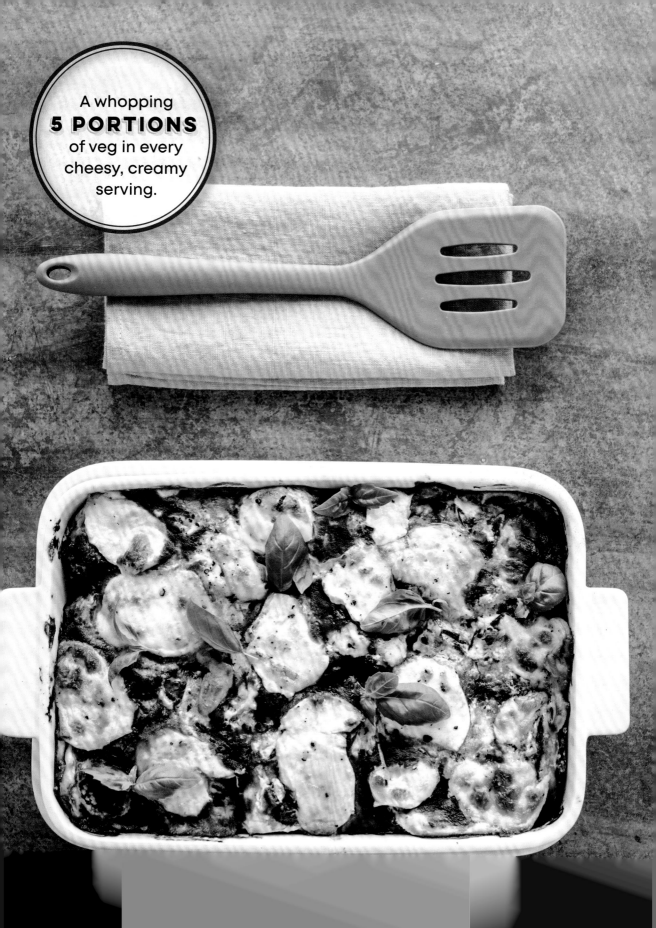

A whopping
5 PORTIONS
of veg in every
cheesy, creamy
serving.

SHIITAKE BURGERS

As I may have mentioned once or twice before, I do love a good burger. And being no vegetarian, a meat-free twist has to be pretty darn good to be worthy of the name. Fortunately, after 12 different attempts at this with my awesome recipe tester Chris, I think we have finally cracked it.

Serves 4

Prep time 20 minutes, plus soaking and chilling

Cook time 30–35 minutes

100g (3½oz) dried shiitake mushrooms

2 tbsp olive oil, plus extra for frying the patties

400g (14oz) sliced red onions

1 tsp coarsely ground black pepper

1 mushroom stock cube, crumbled

1 tsp finely chopped sage

50g (1¾oz) wholemeal plain flour, plus extra for dusting

To serve

4 burger buns, halved

8 thick tomato slices

½ red onion, sliced

8 lettuce leaves

4 slices of Cheddar cheese

1 large avocado, stoned, peeled and sliced

PLACE the shiitake mushrooms in a heatproof bowl, pour over freshly boiled water and leave to soak for 10 minutes until rehydrated. Drain and squeeze out the excess water, then finely slice.

HEAT the olive oil in a frying pan, add the sliced mushrooms, the onions, pepper, stock cube and sage and cook over a medium heat for about 10–15 minutes until the onions soften and become translucent. If the veg mixture starts sticking, add a splash or two of water and cook until all of the liquid has evaporated. Take off the heat.

MIX the mushroom mixture with the flour, then tip into a food processor and blitz until it forms a loose dough. Dust your hands with a little flour, then form the mixture into 4 patties. Chill for at least 1 hour.

FRY the patties, in batches if necessary, in a little olive oil over a medium-high heat for 5 minutes on each side. Serve in the burger buns with the tomato, onion, lettuce, cheese and avocado.

PRO TIP

Leave out the cheese to make this an all-vegan, umami-packed dream.

SWEET POTATO & PARSNIP FRIES

Hey, I'm not ashamed to admit it, chips are one of my favourite foods, especially when doused with salt and vinegar and eaten on Brighton seafront. However, sweet potato fries, dare I say it, might even be a slight improvement on the familiar potato version. They have all the same golden, crisp deliciousness, but with a caramel sweetness to boot. By tag-teaming sweet potatoes and parsnips, this simple recipe magically takes chips and turns them into one of your daily portions of veg, without adding a sky-high amount of fat or salt. Ta dah!

Serves 4
Prep time 10 minutes, plus standing
Cook time 20 minutes

200g (7oz) unpeeled sweet potato, sliced into thin strips

200g (7oz) unpeeled parsnips, sliced into thin strips

4 tbsp salt

Seasoning mix
1 tsp cayenne pepper
1 tsp dried garlic granules
1 tbsp olive oil

PREHEAT the oven to 220°C (425°F), Gas Mark 7.

THROW the veg together in a large mixing bowl with the salt. Leave to stand for 30 minutes for the salt to draw out a lot of the water (this will give you a much firmer, crispier end result). Drain off the liquid, then rinse thoroughly and pat dry with kitchen paper.

PUT the seasoning mix ingredients in a small bowl and mix well.

TOSS the prepared veg with the seasoning on a baking sheet, then bake for 20 minutes until tender and golden brown. Leave to cool for 5–10 minutes before serving.

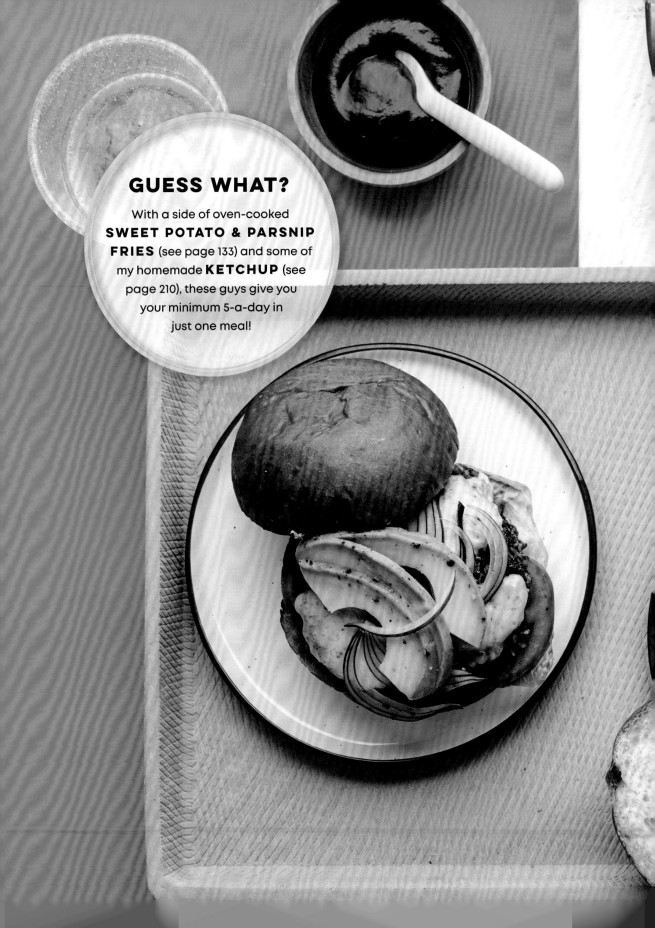

GUESS WHAT?

With a side of oven-cooked **SWEET POTATO & PARSNIP FRIES** (see page 133) and some of my homemade **KETCHUP** (see page 210), these guys give you your minimum 5-a-day in just one meal!

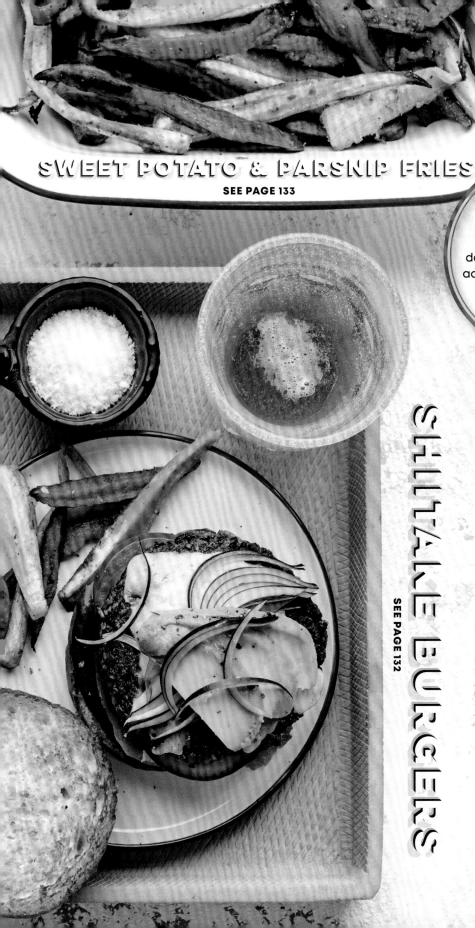

SWEET POTATO & PARSNIP FRIES
SEE PAGE 133

PRO TIP

For extra-spicy fries, double the **cayenne** and add 1 tsp coarsely ground **black pepper**. Watch out, they're hot!

SHIITAKE BURGERS
SEE PAGE 132

MED VEG COTTAGE PIE

Take my mum's resolutely 1980s recipe, add a couple of Med veg and swap the spuds with sweet potatoes and, hey presto, you have a childhood favourite with an astonishing 4 portions in each serving. Adding so much veg means a 250g (9oz) pack of mince stretches to feed 4, without you even noticing the healthy cheat.

Serves 4
Prep time 15 minutes
Cook time 40 minutes

1 tbsp extra virgin olive oil

200g (7oz) diced onions

250g (9oz) minced beef (5% fat)

2 large fresh bay leaves, torn along the edges in several places

200g (7oz) diced aubergine

200g (7oz) diced carrots

2 tbsp Worcestershire sauce

3 tbsp red wine

200ml (7fl oz) hot vegetable stock

4 tbsp tomato purée

120g (4¼oz) rinsed and drained canned chickpeas

80g (2¾oz) cored, deseeded and roughly chopped red pepper

½ tsp cayenne pepper

30g (1oz) Red Leicester cheese

Mash

400g (14oz) unpeeled sweet potatoes, cut into chunks

2 heaped tbsp half-fat crème fraîche

¼ tsp freshly grated nutmeg

HEAT the olive oil in a large, deep frying pan over a medium heat. Add the onions and fry for 5 minutes until softened. Add the mince and continue to fry for 5 minutes, stirring occasionally and breaking it up with a wooden spoon, until the meat has browned all over.

ADD the bay leaves, aubergine and carrots to the pan and cook for a further 5 minutes. Stir in the Worcestershire sauce, wine, stock and tomato purée and season with a little salt and pepper. Cover and simmer for 10 minutes. Add the chickpeas, red pepper and cayenne and continue to simmer for 3 minutes, uncovered.

WHILE the meat sauce is cooking, cook the sweet potatoes in a large saucepan of boiling water for 8–10 minutes, or until soft. Drain and set aside.

TIP the meat and veg mixture into a medium baking dish (about 25 x 20cm/10 x 8in and 7cm/2¾in deep). Mash the cooked sweet potato with the crème fraîche and nutmeg, then spread over the vegetable mixture and smooth out with a spatula. Crumble over the cheese.

PLACE under a preheated medium grill for 10 minutes, or until bubbling up at the sides and golden on top.

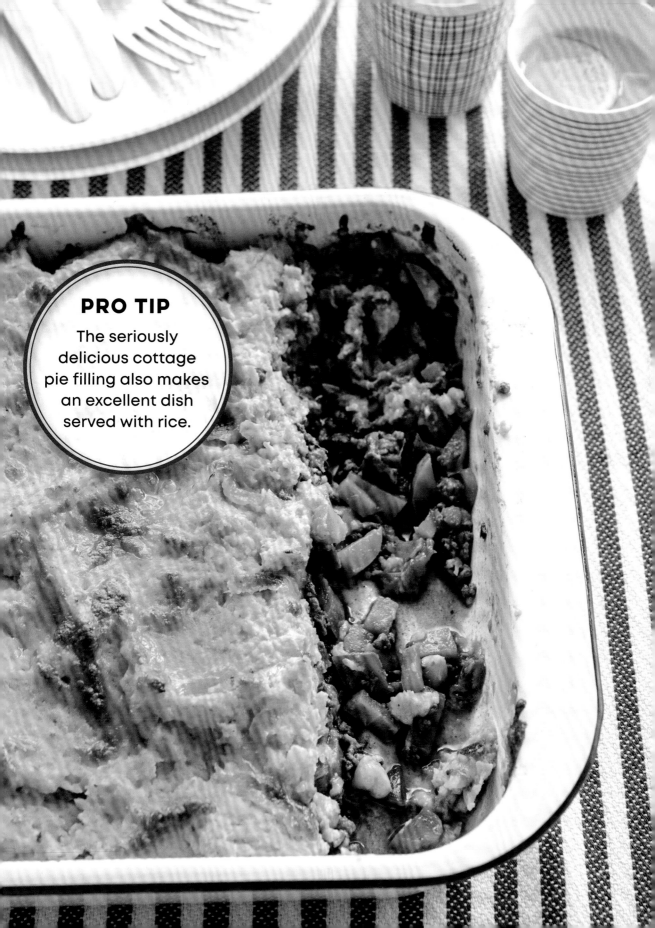

PRO TIP

The seriously delicious cottage pie filling also makes an excellent dish served with rice.

INDIAN FEAST

Curry-house favourites, these are all packed with lots of colourful and flavourful veg. Get your mates over, crack open some beers and toast your good health.

SMOKY CHICKPEA & PEPPER CURRY

Sadly, no cute 'origin story' behind this one. I was up super late recently, working away on a certain science cookbook, with no food in the fridge. I was so hungry I threw this together with the random contents found at the back of my tin cupboard and somehow I struck culinary gold. Even if I do say so myself.

Serves 4

Prep time 5 minutes

Cook time 25 minutes

1 tbsp olive oil

300g (10½oz) diced red onions

300g (10½oz) cored, deseeded and finely sliced red peppers

1 tbsp medium curry powder

1 tbsp smoked paprika

400g (14oz) can chickpeas, rinsed and drained

1 vegetable stock cube, crumbled

400g (14oz) can chopped tomatoes

400ml (14fl oz) can coconut milk

2 garlic cloves, minced

To garnish

sliced red chillies

mint leaves

HEAT the olive oil over a low heat, add the onions and peppers and fry gently for 10 minutes, or until softened.

ADD the remaining ingredients and bring to the boil, then reduce the heat and simmer, uncovered, for 15 minutes until slightly thickened.

SERVE garnished with the chillies and mint leaves.

PRO TIP

Swap the canned chickpeas with 225g (8oz) rinsed and drained chickpeas from a jar. This might sound ridiculous, but I promise you, although they might be harder to find, chickpeas from a jar are always far larger, creamier and altogether superior than canned.

GREEN HARYALI CHICKEN

Teaming up fresh herbs and leafy greens makes this the lightest, freshest and, frankly, the greenest green curry around. A bit of a left-field take for those used to traditional curry-house staples, but make this recipe once and you'll be back for more.

· ·

Serves 4
Prep time 20 minutes
Cook time about 25 minutes

20g (¾oz) butter
400g (14oz) diced onions
300g (10½oz) boneless, skinless chicken breasts, cut into chunks
160g (5¾oz) broccoli florets, halved
160g (5¾oz) cauliflower florets, quartered
400ml (14fl oz) can coconut milk
2 tbsp honey
salt and pepper

Spinach paste
400g (14oz) frozen spinach, defrosted
40g (1½oz) mint, plus extra small sprigs to garnish
40g (1½oz) curly parsley
4 green bird's-eye chillies (optional)

Spice paste
30g (1oz) garlic, minced
30g (1oz) fresh root ginger, peeled and minced
4 tbsp water

Spice mix
1 tsp turmeric
4 tsp ground cumin
4 tsp ground coriander
2 tsp ground fenugreek
½ tsp ground cardamom

SQUEEZE out as much liquid from the defrosted spinach as you can, then blend with all the remaining spinach paste ingredients in a food processor. Set aside.

MIX the spice paste ingredients together in a small bowl to form a thin paste, then set aside.

COMBINE the spice mix ingredients together in another small bowl and set aside.

MELT the butter in a large flameproof casserole dish over a medium-low heat, add the onions and sweat for 10 minutes until softened. Stir in the spice mix and cook for 2 minutes. Turn the heat up to medium, add the spice paste and stir to deglaze the pan. Add the chicken and cook for about 8–10 minutes, or until cooked through.

MEANWHILE, bring a small pan of water to the boil and blanch the broccoli and cauliflower for 3 minutes, then drain.

WHEN the chicken is cooked, add the drained veg to the casserole dish with the spinach paste, coconut milk, honey and a little salt and pepper. Stir well and simmer for 2–3 minutes, then serve garnished with a few sprigs of mint.

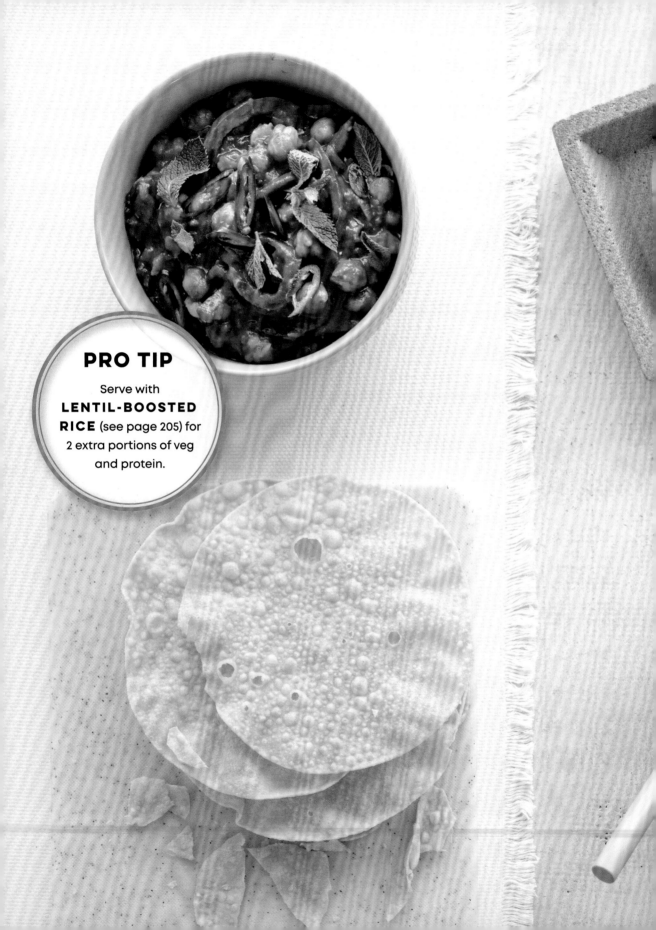

PRO TIP

Serve with **LENTIL-BOOSTED RICE** (see page 205) for 2 extra portions of veg and protein.

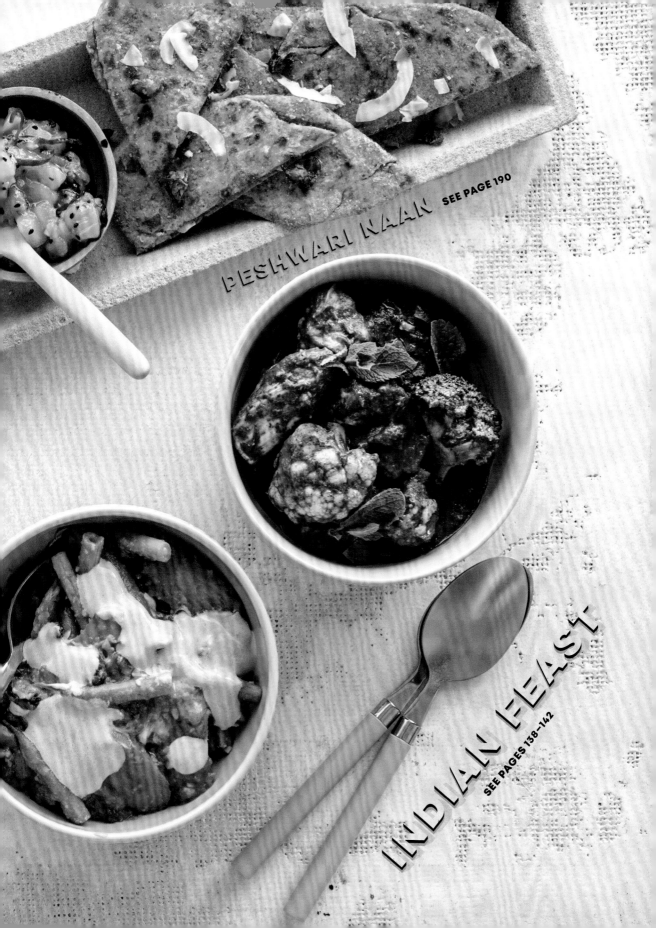

PESHWARI NAAN SEE PAGE 190

INDIAN FEAST SEE PAGES 138–142

KORMA-SPICED CHICKEN & SWEET POTATO CURRY

Creamy, coconutty curry that contains 5 fruit and veg portions in every serving.
Yes, it's possible. So have your curry and eat it.

5 PORTIONS PER SERVING

Serves 4

Prep time 25 minutes

Cook time 35 minutes

400g (14oz) unpeeled sweet potatoes, cut into 1.5cm (⅝in) cubes

1 tbsp extra virgin olive oil

400g (14oz) diced white onions

3 large fresh bay leaves, torn along the edges in several places

450g (1lb) boneless, skinless chicken breasts, cut into chunks

400ml (14fl oz) can coconut milk

400g (14oz) can chopped tomatoes

1 chicken stock cube, crumbled

160g (5¾oz) diced carrots

160g (5¾oz) trimmed green beans, halved

120g (4¼oz) raisins

Spice mix

2 tsp ground coriander

2 tsp ground cumin

1 tsp cumin seeds

½ tsp turmeric

½ tsp ground cardamom

Spice paste

15g (½oz) fresh root ginger, peeled and minced

15g (½oz) garlic, minced

2 tbsp water

To serve

4 heaped tablespoons Greek yogurt

2 tsp turmeric

1 tsp dried garlic granules

COOK the sweet potatoes in a large saucepan of simmering water for about 10 minutes until soft, then drain, tip back into the pan and leave to cool.

COMBINE all the spice mix ingredients in a small bowl, and the spice paste ingredients in another.

HEAT the olive oil in a large flameproof casserole dish over a medium heat. Add the onions and fry for 5 minutes, stirring occasionally. Stir in the dry spice mix and bay leaves and cook for another 2 minutes. Add the chicken and stir well to cover in the spices, then cook for 5 minutes, turning occasionally. Stir in the spice paste and continue to cook for 3 minutes.

MASH the sweet potatoes with the coconut milk, then add to the curry with the chopped tomatoes. Stir well, then cover and simmer for 5 minutes.

MIX the stock cube with a little of the curry liquid to form a thin paste, then stir back into the pan with the diced carrots, green beans and raisins. Re-cover and simmer for 5 minutes until the chicken is cooked through and the sauce is thickened.

MEANWHILE, whisk together the yogurt, turmeric and garlic granules in a bowl.

SPOON the curry on to plates, then drizzle over a little of the yogurt and serve.

RAINBOW TARTIFLETTE

Cheese, cream, potato and bacon: traditionally beige French tartiflette is high up the ranks of ultimate comfort food! Pair this colourful version with a sharp side salad.

Serves 4

Prep time 15 minutes

Cook time 40 minutes

400g (14oz) unpeeled purple sweet potatoes, cut into chunks

1 tbsp olive oil

400g (14oz) finely sliced onions

150g (5½oz) lardons or diced unsmoked bacon

100ml (3½fl oz) dry white wine

160g (5¾oz) cored and deseeded red pepper, cut into thin strips

160g (5¾oz) cored and deseeded yellow pepper, cut into thin strips

200g (7oz) Tenderstem broccoli, halved lengthways

100g (3½oz) half-fat crème fraîche

¼ tsp freshly grated nutmeg

200g (7oz) Reblochon cheese

pepper

COOK the sweet potatoes in a large saucepan of simmering water for 6–8 minutes until cooked through but not soft. Drain, then tip into a large baking dish (about 30 x 20cm/12 x 8in and 7cm/2¾in deep) and set aside.

PREHEAT the oven to 220°C (425°F), Gas Mark 7.

HEAT the olive oil in a large frying pan over a medium-high heat. Add the onions and fry for 5 minutes, stirring occasionally, until starting to brown. Add the lardons or bacon and cook for another 5 minutes, stirring occasionally.

POUR in the wine, stirring to deglaze the pan, then simmer for 5 minutes. Throw in the sliced peppers and broccoli, season generously with pepper and cook for another 3 minutes.

TIP the mixture into the baking dish, then toss together with the sweet potatoes, crème fraîche and nutmeg. Tear the cheese apart and dot over the top.

BAKE for 15 minutes, or until the cheese turns golden brown. Leave to cool for a few minutes, then serve.

RAINBOW TARTIFLETTE

SEE PAGE 143

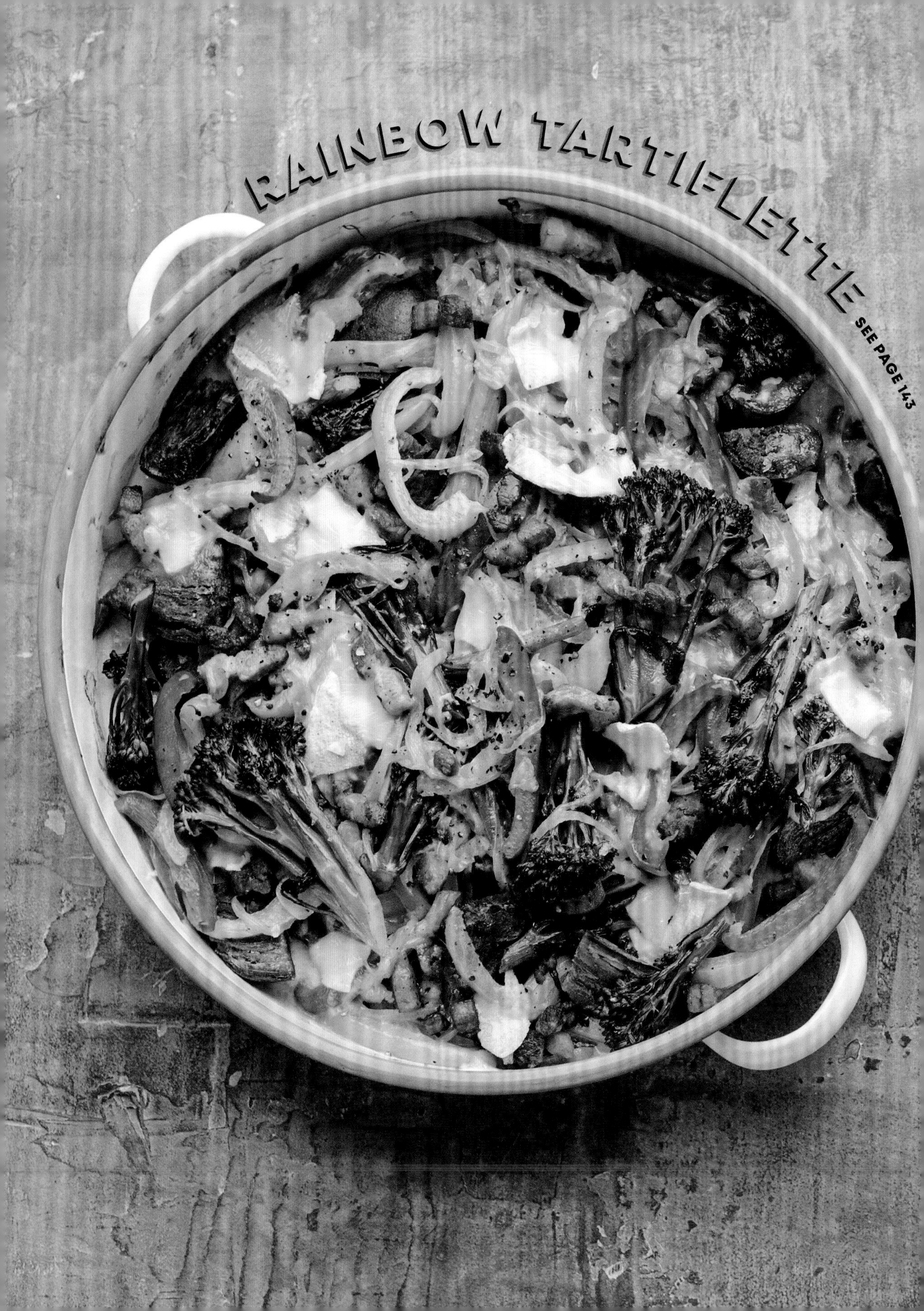

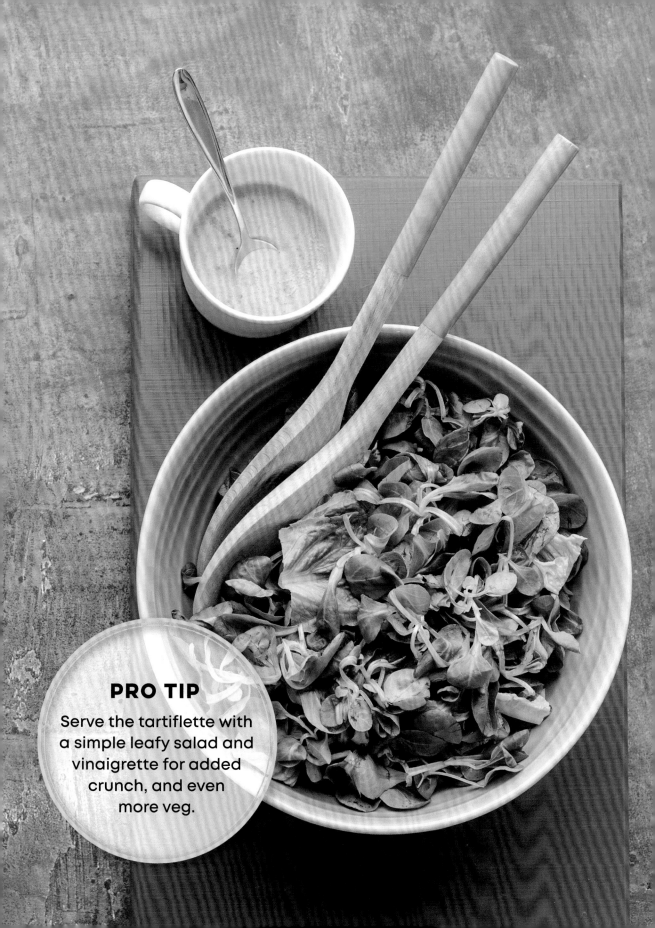

PRO TIP

Serve the tartiflette with a simple leafy salad and vinaigrette for added crunch, and even more veg.

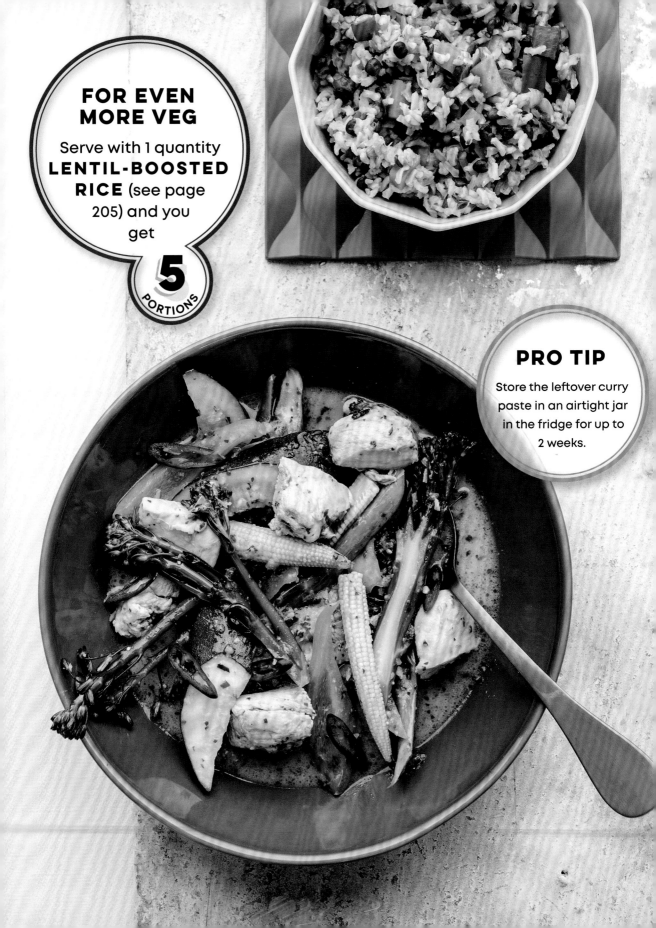

FOR EVEN MORE VEG

Serve with 1 quantity **LENTIL-BOOSTED RICE** (see page 205) and you get

5 PORTIONS

PRO TIP

Store the leftover curry paste in an airtight jar in the fridge for up to 2 weeks.

THAI GREEN CURRY

By now, you guys will know I am always up for a culinary short cut, so feel free to use shop-bought paste – you'll need 3 heaped tablespoons for this recipe – to make it even quicker. But, trust me, if you have the time to make your own paste from scratch it is totally worth it and will only take 10 minutes more.

Serves 4

Prep time 20 minutes

Cook time 25–30 minutes

1 tbsp extra virgin olive oil

450g (1lb) boneless, skinless chicken breasts, cut into chunks

300g (10½oz) trimmed courgettes, halved lengthways and cut into 2mm- (⅛in-) thick slices

400ml (14fl oz) can coconut milk

200g (7oz) cored, deseeded and sliced orange pepper

200g (7oz) baby sweetcorn, cut into 2.5cm (1in) pieces

200g (7oz) Tenderstem broccoli, halved lengthways and cut in half

1 tbsp fish sauce

juice of ½ lime

sliced red chillies, to garnish

Curry paste
(makes enough for 3 large curries)

2 lemon grass stalks, tough outer leaves removed and stalks trimmed

2 shallots, about 65g (2⅓oz) in total

10 large kaffir lime leaves, tough stalks removed

finely grated zest and juice of 1 lime

30g (1oz) garlic, crushed

15g (½oz) fresh root ginger, peeled

15g (½oz) fresh galangal, peeled (if you can't find it, use more ginger)

large handful of Thai basil leaves

1 tbsp ground coriander

1 tsp ground cumin

1 tbsp fish sauce

3 tbsp extra virgin olive oil

CUT the bottom 10cm (4in) from each lemon grass stalk, discarding the tops. Bash the stalks, then blitz with all the remaining curry paste ingredients in a food processor.

HEAT the olive oil in a large frying pan or wok over a medium-low heat. Tip in about a third of the curry paste (store the remainder, see Pro Tip opposite) and fry for 2 minutes, stirring frequently. Stir in the chicken and coat with the paste, then fry for 8–10 minutes, or until cooked through. Add the courgettes, stir well and cook for another 3 minutes.

POUR in the coconut milk and mix well, then bring to a simmer and cook for 3 minutes. Mix in the remaining veg, then cover and continue to cook for 5 minutes, or until the veg are cooked through but still crunchy.

STIR in the fish sauce and lime juice and garnish with sliced red chillies.

THAI YELLOW CURRY

There are very few things better in the world than hot prawn curry and cold, cold beer. With this recipe you can enjoy your curry *and* get 3 portions of fruit and veg along the way. Use 3 heaped tablespoons of shop-bought curry paste instead of homemade if you are pressed for time.

Serves 4
Prep time 15 minutes
Cook time 20–22 minutes

1 tbsp extra virgin olive oil

200g (7oz) butternut squash chunks

200g (7oz) cauliflower florets

400ml (14fl oz) can coconut milk

200g (7oz) raw peeled king prawns

200g (7oz) oyster mushrooms, cut into bite-sized pieces

200g (7oz) mangetout

juice of ½ lemon

dash of fish sauce

small handful of Thai basil leaves, torn

lime wedges, to serve

**Curry paste
(makes enough for 3 large curries)**

2 lemon grass stalks, tough outer leaves removed and stalks trimmed

2 shallots, about 65g (2⅓oz) in total

10 large kaffir lime leaves, tough stalks removed

30g (1oz) garlic, crushed

15g (½oz) fresh root ginger, peeled

15g (½oz) fresh galangal, peeled (if you can't find it, use more ginger)

5g (⅛oz) piece of fresh turmeric, peeled, or 1 tsp turmeric powder

1 tbsp tomato purée

1 tbsp ground coriander

1 tbsp ground cumin

½ tsp cinnamon

½ tsp freshly grated nutmeg

3 tbsp extra virgin olive oil

3 tbsp fish sauce

CUT the bottom 10cm (4in) from each lemon grass stalk, discarding the tops. Bash the stalks, then blitz with all the remaining curry paste ingredients in a food processor.

HEAT the olive oil in a large frying pan or wok over a medium heat. Add about a third of the curry paste (store the remainder, see Pro Tip on page 146) and fry for 2 minutes, stirring frequently. Stir the butternut squash and cauliflower into the paste, then fry for 10 minutes, stirring often.

POUR in the coconut milk and bring to a simmer, then cook for 5 minutes. Add the prawns, mushrooms and mangetout and cook for another 3–5 minutes until the prawns turn pink and are cooked through.

TAKE off the heat, then stir in the lemon juice and season with a dash of fish sauce, to taste. Stir through the Thai basil and serve with lime wedges.

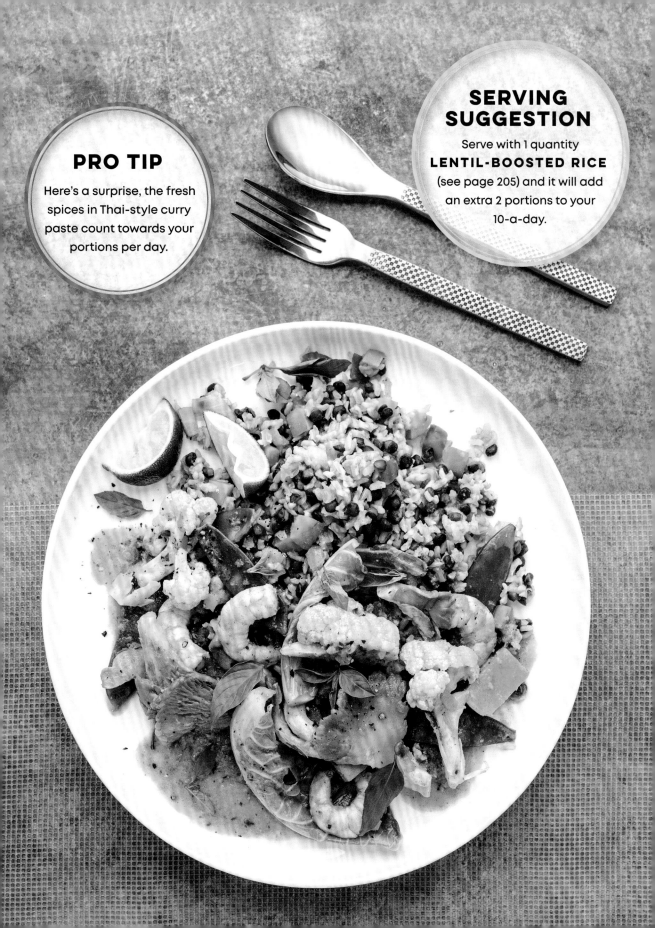

PRO TIP

Here's a surprise, the fresh spices in Thai-style curry paste count towards your portions per day.

SERVING SUGGESTION

Serve with 1 quantity **LENTIL-BOOSTED RICE** (see page 205) and it will add an extra 2 portions to your 10-a-day.

SPAGHETTI & MUSHROOM BALLS

Tangy, sweet and salty – I know this mix of flavours might sound a little off the wall, but boy does it work. Make a double dose of the mushroom mixture and you'll have dinner for tomorrow night sorted, too. Mmm, burgers…

Serves 4
Prep time 15 minutes
Cook time 15–20 minutes

1 x quantity Shiitake Burger mixture (see page 132), soaking water from the rehydrated mushrooms reserved

flour, for dusting

360g (12½oz) fresh spaghetti

320g (11¼oz) cavolo nero, sliced

2 tsp extra virgin olive oil

4 tbsp Greek yogurt

120g (4¼oz) pitted dates, sliced lengthways

3 garlic cloves, minced

1 large red chilli, finely sliced

2 tbsp capers

finely grated zest of 1 lemon

salt and pepper

PREHEAT the oven to 220°C (425°F), Gas Mark 7.

FORM the burger mixture into 24 golf-ball-sized spheres. Sprinkle some flour on to a large plate, then roll the balls in the flour and place about 1cm (½in) apart on a large baking sheet. Bake for 15–20 minutes until firm.

MEANWHILE, pour the reserved shiitake soaking water into a large saucepan and top up with boiling water to half-fill the pan. Bring to a simmer, then add the spaghetti and sliced cavolo nero and cook for 3 minutes, or to your liking.

DRAIN the pasta and veg, then return to the pan and stir in the remaining ingredients. Season with a little salt and a lot of pepper.

DIVIDE the pasta mixture among 4 large bowls, top each one with 6 mushroom balls and serve.

PRO TIP

Replace the fresh spaghetti with 200g (7oz) dried pasta, if you prefer. Just cook it for 4–5 minutes before adding the sliced cavolo nero to avoid overcooking the veg.

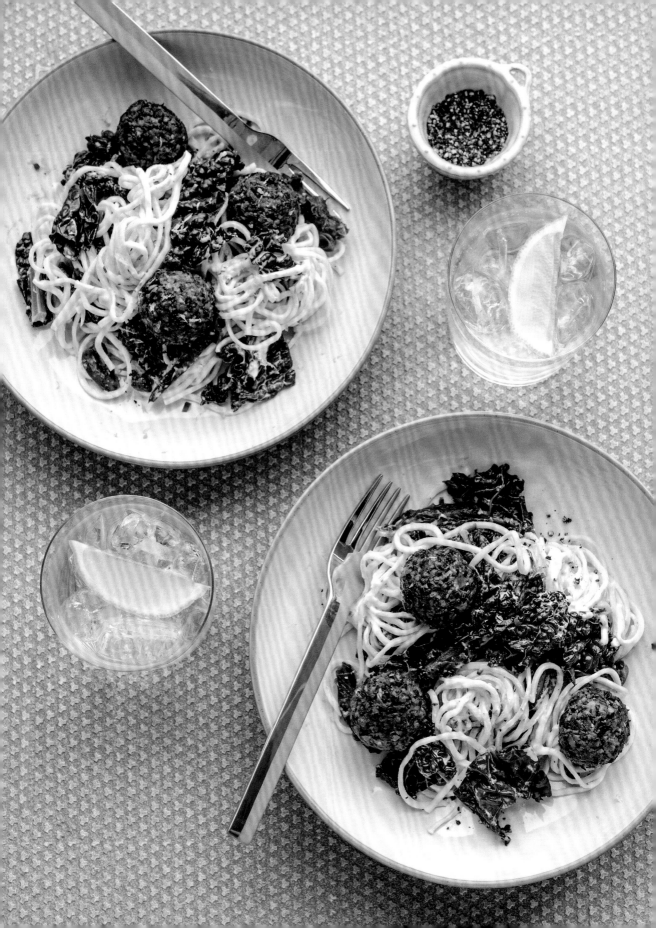

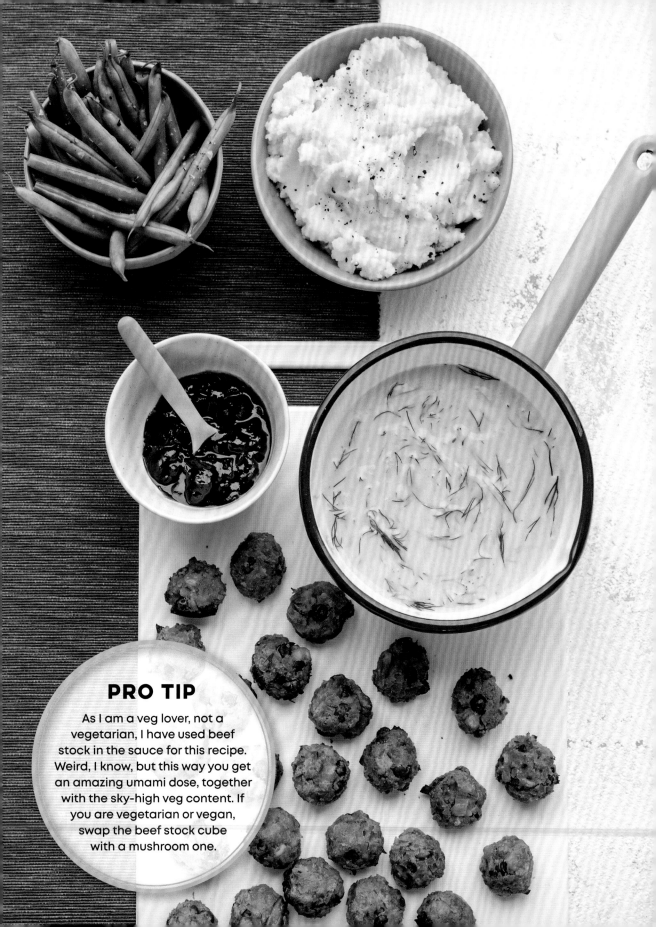

PRO TIP

As I am a veg lover, not a vegetarian, I have used beef stock in the sauce for this recipe. Weird, I know, but this way you get an amazing umami dose, together with the sky-high veg content. If you are vegetarian or vegan, swap the beef stock cube with a mushroom one.

SWEDISH NO-MEATBALLS

My mate Brontë runs one of the best cafés in central London, serving up a *smörgåsbord* of Scandi delights, including a modern veggie twist on Swedish meatballs. It's so good that the recipe is a closely guarded secret. So here's my attempt to recreate these with, you guessed it, even more of the good stuff. I was dubious as to whether these would work. But goodness me, do they! Lovely with parsnip mash, green beans and cranberry sauce.

Serves 4
Prep time 15 minutes
Cook time 55 minutes

Sauce

4 tbsp plain flour, plus extra for dusting
1 tbsp butter
500ml (18fl oz) milk
1 beef stock cube, crumbled
50ml (2fl oz) white wine
1 tsp chopped dill
½ tsp dried garlic granules
¼ tsp turmeric (for colour)

Meatballs

2 tbsp olive oil, plus extra for brushing
400g (14oz) finely chopped onions
300g (10½oz) frozen mixed vegetables
400g (14oz) can chickpeas, rinsed and drained
1 stock cube, crumbled (I usually use chicken)
½ tsp smoked paprika
½ tsp dried garlic granules
3 tbsp gram flour
1 tbsp finely chopped dill, to garnish

MIX the flour for the sauce with a little water to make a thin paste, then place in a saucepan with all the remaining sauce ingredients and combine well. Cook over a medium-high heat until thickened, whisking continuously to prevent any lumps forming. Reduce the heat to its lowest setting and cook for 5 minutes until thick and creamy. Take off the heat, cover and set aside.

HEAT the olive oil in a large frying pan over a medium heat, add the onions and mixed frozen veg and fry for 15 minutes until they are soft and starting to turn golden (this takes a little longer than normal as the veg are frozen).

USING a fork, mash the chickpeas together in a large mixing bowl until you have a rough paste. Set aside.

PREHEAT the oven to 200°C (400°F), Gas Mark 6. Line a large baking tray with nonstick baking paper.

FOLD the cooked veg and the remaining meatball ingredients into the chickpeas to form a dough. Shape spoonfuls of the mixture into little balls about 2.5cm (1in) in diameter, squeezing them gently with flour-dusted hands to compact them, then transfer to a plate dusted with flour (the flour makes this less of a sticky job) and roll them in it.

ARRANGE the balls in the prepared tray and brush with a little oil. Bake for 30 minutes until they start to turn golden brown and crisp, turning halfway through cooking.

WHEN the no-meatballs are nearly ready to serve, reheat the sauce over a low heat for 5 minutes.

REMOVE the balls from the oven and tip into the sauce. Serve immediately with a scattering of dill.

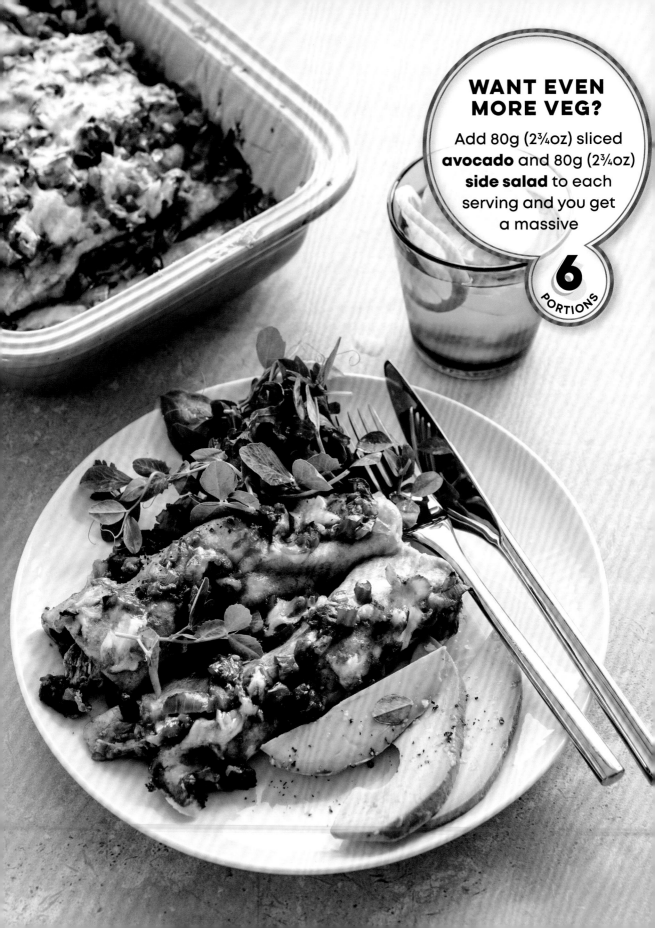

WANT EVEN MORE VEG?

Add 80g (2¾oz) sliced **avocado** and 80g (2¾oz) **side salad** to each serving and you get a massive

6
PORTIONS

CHEESY CHICKEN ENCHILADAS

Melty cheese, smoky paprika and creamy avocado, what more could you ask of a meal? Oh, 4 cleverly disguised portions of veg, that's what. A perfect restorative treat for a cold, dark winter's night that you need not feel the tiniest bit guilty about. Andalé!

Serves 4

Prep time 20 minutes

Cook time 50 minutes

400g (14oz) finely diced onions

300g (10½oz) cored, deseeded and finely diced red peppers

400g (14oz) can chopped tomatoes

250ml (9fl oz) water

1 chicken stock cube, crumbled

1 tbsp smoked paprika

1 tsp oregano

2 garlic cloves, minced

1 tsp cornflour, mixed with a little water to form a paste

300g (10½oz) ready-cooked roast chicken pieces (I get mine from the rotisserie counter)

400g (14oz) can black beans, rinsed and drained

8 soft corn tortillas

100g (3½oz) mature Cheddar cheese, coarsely grated

PLACE the onions, red peppers, tomatoes, measured water, stock cube, paprika and oregano in a saucepan. Bring to the boil, then reduce the heat and simmer for 25 minutes.

PREHEAT the oven to 220°C (425°F), Gas Mark 7.

STIR the garlic and cornflour paste into the sauce until completely combined, then cook for another minute or two until thickened. Transfer half of the mixture to a bowl and set aside. Stir the chicken and beans into the remaining sauce in the pan.

SPOON a few tablespoons of the chicken mixture into each tortilla, then roll them up and place seam-side down in a large baking dish (about 30 x 20cm/12 x 8in and 7cm/2¾in deep). Top with the reserved sauce and scatter over the cheese.

BAKE for 20 minutes until the chicken and beans are heated through and the cheese is melted.

CHICKEN POT PIE

Buttery pastry, creamy chicken and tasty veg are a perfect trifecta that make this pie such a great comfort food. With just a couple of tweaks you can up the veg even further to add extra sweetness and depth, giving each serving about 3 portions of veg. Serve it with one of the mash recipes on pages 200–204 and a side of sautéed green beans, if you like.

Serves 4

Prep time 15 minutes, plus standing

Cook time 50–60 minutes

1 tsp dried garlic granules

1 tsp onion powder

4 tbsp plain flour

4 tbsp cold water

1 tbsp olive oil

400g (14oz) boneless, skinless chicken thighs, cubed

350g (12oz) trimmed, cleaned and very finely sliced leeks

300g (10½oz) button mushrooms, very finely sliced

300g (10½oz) frozen mixed vegetables

300ml (10fl oz) milk, plus extra for brushing

50ml (2fl oz) sherry

1 tbsp chopped parsley

1 tsp chopped dill

2 chicken stock cubes, crumbled

1 sheet of ready-rolled puff pastry

PREHEAT the oven to 220°C (425°F), Gas Mark 7.

MIX together the garlic granules, onion powder, flour and measured water in a small bowl, then leave to stand for 20 minutes.

MEANWHILE, heat the olive oil in a large, shallow frying pan over a medium-high heat, add the chicken and fry for about 10 minutes, or until golden and cooked through. Remove from the pan and set aside.

TIP the remaining ingredients (except the pastry!) into the pan with the soaked garlic mixture and stir well. Bring to the boil, then reduce the heat and cook for 5–10 minutes until the sauce has thickened. Add the cooked chicken.

POUR the mixture into a 1.5-litre (2¾-pint) pie dish. Cut out a disc of pastry just a little larger than the top of the dish, then place on top of the filling. Press the pastry against the sides of the dish with a fork to crimp the edges, then brush the pastry lid with a little milk. Bake for 30–35 minutes, or until the pastry turns golden.

5-a-day in a single meal if served with a side of veg and mash.

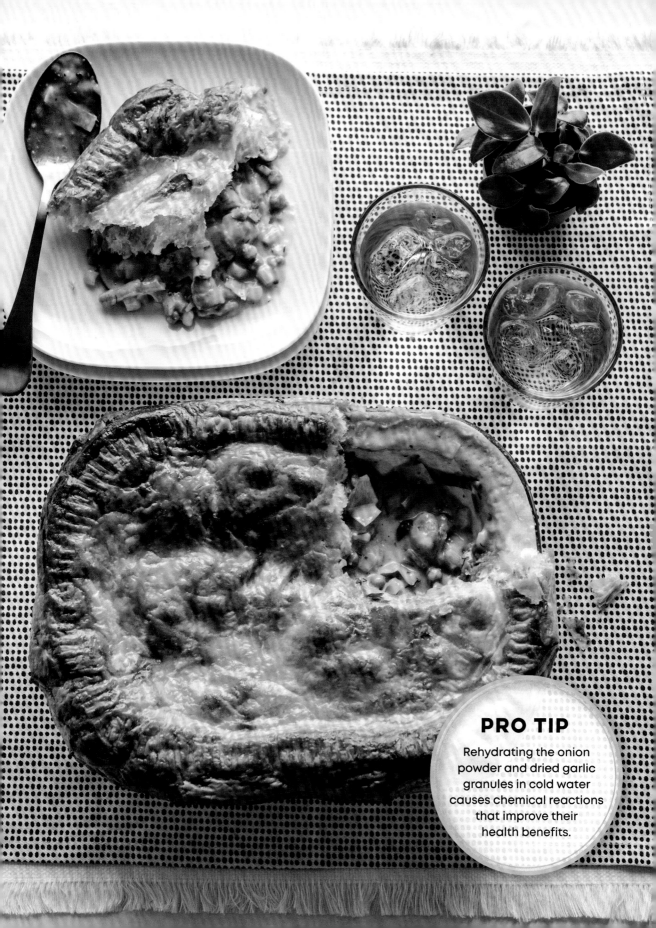

PRO TIP

Rehydrating the onion powder and dried garlic granules in cold water causes chemical reactions that improve their health benefits.

HADDOCK WITH RATATOUILLE

If you are looking for a light, fresh weeknight dinner, they really don't come any quicker than this. What else is there to say?

Serves 4

Prep time 10 minutes

Cook time 30–35 minutes

400g (14oz) frozen haddock fillets

½ lemon, sliced

3 large fresh bay leaves, torn along the edges in several places

Ratatouille

2 tbsp extra virgin olive oil

200g (7oz) diced onions

350g (12oz) diced aubergine

2 tbsp soy sauce

300g (10½oz) trimmed courgettes, cut into thin slices

160g (5¾oz) cored and deseeded red pepper, cut into thin strips

2 large fresh bay leaves, torn along the edges in several places

finely grated zest and juice of ½ lemon

400g (14oz) tomato passata

400g (14oz) can chickpeas, rinsed and drained

4 garlic cloves, crushed

2 tbsp herbes de Provence

pepper

To serve

couscous, pasta or brown rice

lemon wedges

a few flat leaf parsley sprigs, to garnish

START with the ratatouille. Heat the olive oil in a large flameproof casserole dish over a medium heat. Add the onions and fry for 5 minutes until they start to sweat. Add the diced aubergine and soy sauce and stir well. Cover with a lid and cook for 5 minutes.

STIR in the courgettes, red pepper, bay leaves, lemon juice and a dash of pepper. Re-cover and cook for another 10 minutes until all the veg have softened, stirring occasionally.

MIX in the passata, chickpeas, garlic and dried herbs, then re-cover and simmer gently for 10–15 minutes while you cook the fish.

BRING a large saucepan of water to the boil. Add the frozen fish, lemon slices and bay leaves, cover the pan and return to the boil, then reduce to a simmer and cook for about 10–15 minutes, or until the flesh flakes away easily. Remove the fish from the pan using a slotted spoon.

STIR the lemon zest into the ratatouille. Serve hot with the fish and couscous, pasta or rice and lemon wedges and garnish with a few sprigs of parsley.

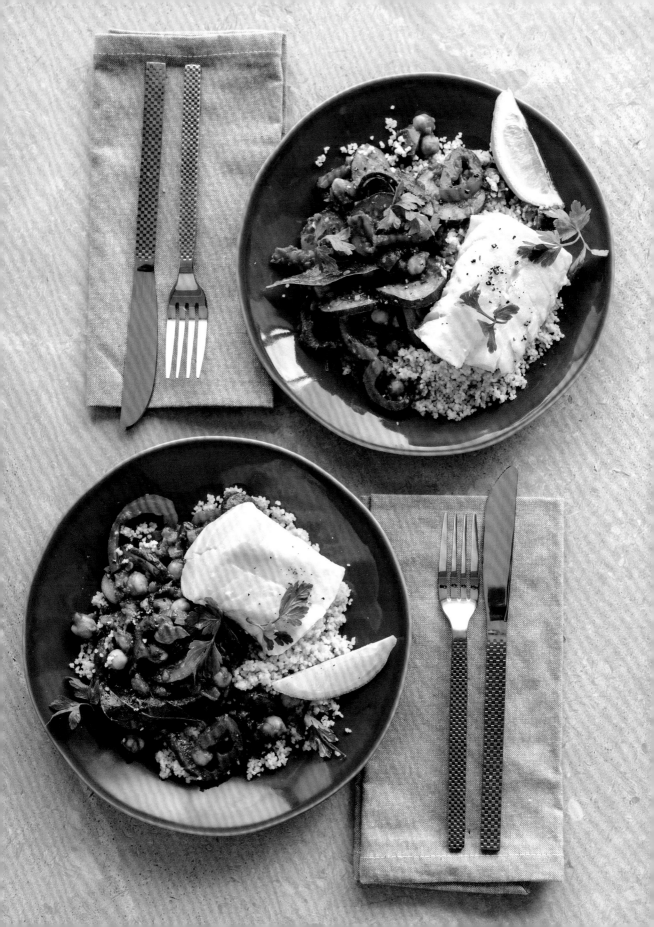

SPAGHETTI BOLOGNESE

I grew up on my mum's very British take on this Italian classic. It would probably be considered a heinous culinary crime to the foodies of Bologna, but boy does it taste good. I've added a simple salad to this 1980s recipe to give you a whopping 6 portions of veg in just one sitting! In fact, there is so much veg here, the total amount of meat is slashed by 50 per cent compared to some traditional recipes, but I promise you'll not miss it one bit.

Serves 4

Prep time 15 minutes

Cook time 40 minutes

400g (14oz) wholewheat spaghetti

Parmesan cheese shavings, to serve

Sauce

1 tbsp olive oil

200g (7oz) diced carrots

200g (7oz) cored, deseeded and diced red pepper

200g (7oz) chestnut mushrooms, diced

200g (7oz) diced red onions

200g (7oz) minced beef (5% fat)

50ml (2fl oz) sherry

1 tsp brown sugar

1 tsp mixed spice

1 tsp mixed herbs

1 beef stock cube, crumbled

2 x 400g (14oz) cans chopped tomatoes

Tomato salad

300g (10½oz) tomatoes, sliced

2 garlic cloves, minced

2 tsp olive oil

handful of basil leaves

salt and pepper

HEAT the olive oil in a large frying pan over a medium heat, add the carrots, red pepper, mushrooms, red onions and beef, breaking up the mince with a wooden spoon, and fry for 10 minutes until the veg have softened and the beef is browned.

TIP in all the remaining sauce ingredients, stir to combine and continue to simmer gently, uncovered, for 30 minutes.

ABOUT 10 minutes before the sauce cooking time is up, cook the spaghetti in a saucepan of boiling water according to the packet instructions until al dente.

MEANWHILE, toss together all the ingredients for the tomato salad.

DRAIN the pasta, then return it to the pan. Spoon over the sauce and tumble the tomato salad over the top. Bring to the table still in the pan to keep it warm and toss before serving. Serve with plenty of Parmesan cheese shavings.

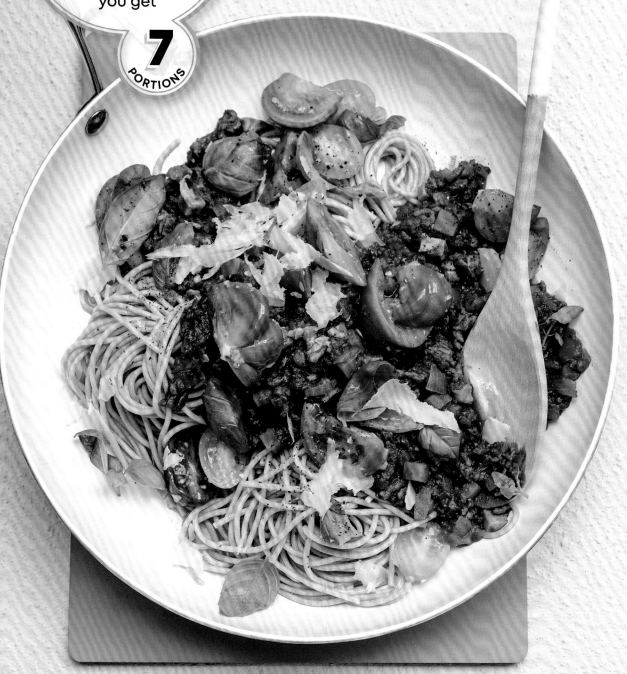

WANT EVEN MORE VEG?

Swap the beef for 100g (3½oz) **dried green lentils** plus 200ml (7fl oz) **water** and you get

7

PORTIONS

CHILLI CON CARNE

Dates, red wine and shiitake mushrooms in a chilli con carne? Yep. Foodie purists look away now. This fruit-and-veg-heavy version of an age-old Tex-Mex favourite might sound a little left field, but it totally works. In fact, it has so much tasty veg crammed into it that it contains just half the amount of beef in most regular recipes, but you would never know.

 PORTIONS PER SERVING **7**

Serves 4
Prep time 10 minutes
Cook time 40 minutes

1 tbsp extra virgin olive oil

400g (14oz) finely diced onions

320g (11¼oz) cored, deseeded and finely diced red peppers

250g (9oz) fresh shiitake mushrooms, finely sliced

100g (3½oz) tomato purée

400g (14oz) can chopped tomatoes

400g (14oz) can red kidney beans, rinsed and drained

50ml (2fl oz) red wine

50g (1¾oz) chopped dates

1 tbsp natural cocoa powder

1 tbsp smoked paprika

2 beef stock cubes, crumbled

1 tsp mixed spice

1 tsp dried garlic granules

250g (9oz) minced beef (5% fat)

To serve

cooked brown rice

1 large avocado, stoned, peeled and cubed

100g (3½oz) cherry tomatoes, halved

lemon wedges

100g (3½oz) Cheddar cheese, grated

HEAT the olive oil in a large saucepan over a medium heat. Add the onions, red peppers and shiitake and fry, stirring occasionally, until all the veg have softened and started to brown (the shiitake will kick out loads of water, so this will take about 30 minutes).

TIP in all the remaining ingredients and stir well, breaking up the mince with a wooden spoon. Bring to a simmer and cook for 10 minutes, stirring from time to time, until the mince is cooked through.

SERVE with brown rice, and the avocado, tomatoes, lemon wedges and heaps of grated cheese.

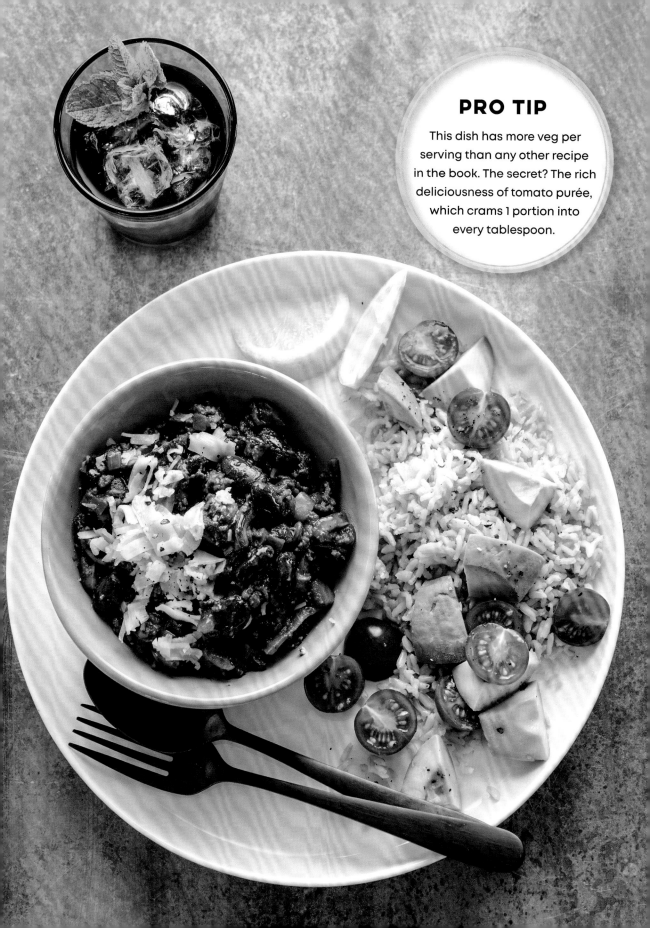

DESSERTS

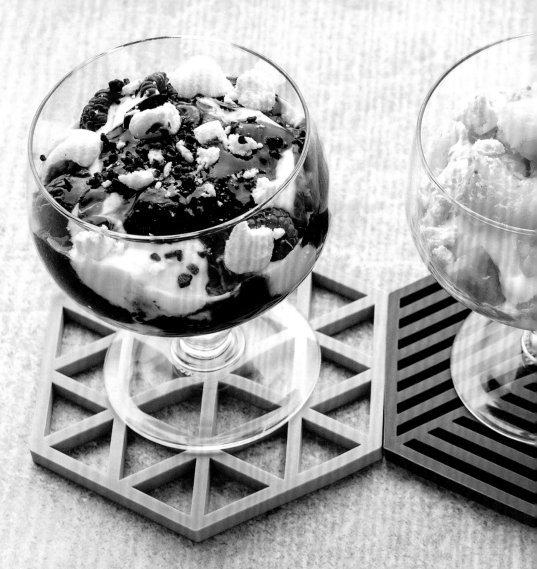

RED BERRY ETON MESS

This is a simple dessert that you can throw together in 10 minutes or less, to sneak in 2 extra fruit portions at the end of any meal and for only a modest amount of added sugar.

Serves 4
Prep time 10 minutes

320g (11¼oz) fresh or frozen raspberries

1 x quantity Strawberry & Cherry Compote (see page 58)

8 mini meringues

400g (14oz) Greek yogurt (5% fat)

freeze-dried raspberry sprinkles, to decorate

DIVIDE half the raspberries among 4 tumblers, followed by a third of the compote. Crumble 1 mini meringue into each glass.

SPOON half the yogurt among the tumblers, then top with another third of the compote. Add the remaining raspberries, then the rest of the yogurt. Top with the remaining compote, then crush another mini meringue over each glass.

DECORATE with freeze-dried raspberry sprinkles and serve.

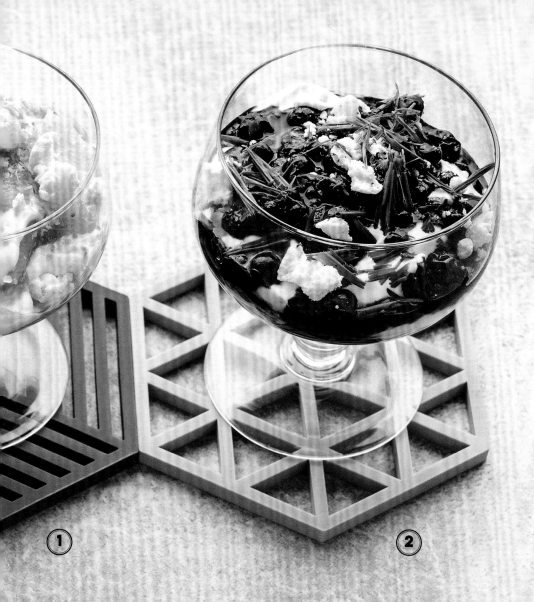

VARIATIONS

① TROPICAL MESS

Make the mess as opposite, replacing the raspberries with 320g (11¼oz) sliced **papaya** and the compote with 1 x quantity **Mango & Pineapple Compote** (see page 59). Omit the freeze-dried raspberries and sprinkle with a little **desiccated coconut**.

② BLACK FOREST MESS

Make the mess as opposite, replacing the raspberries with 320g (11¼oz) chopped **sour cherries** and the compote with 1 x quantity **Dark Berry Compote** (see page 59). Omit the freeze-dried raspberries and scatter over a few shavings of **dark chocolate**.

STRAWBERRY & ELDERFLOWER PIE

Yep. This might look as indulgent as anything from a window of a fancy French patisserie, but the sneaky use of ready-made pastry makes it as quick and convenient as it gets. And it still contains an astonishing 4 portions of fruit in each serving. You can replace the arrowroot with cornflour, but it will give a cloudy rather than crystal-clear set.

Serves 4

Prep time 15 minutes, plus cooling

Cook time 15–20 minutes

butter, for greasing

320g (11¼oz) sheet of ready-rolled shortcrust pastry

2 tbsp arrowroot

3 tbsp granulated stevia (baking blend), or to taste

350ml (12fl oz) apple and elderflower juice

1kg (2lb 4oz) hulled and quartered fresh strawberries

2 x 12g (½oz) sachets powdered gelatine

a few drops of natural red food colouring (optional)

Greek yogurt, to serve

PREHEAT the oven to 200°C (400°F), Gas Mark 6.

GREASE a deep 25cm (10in) pie dish with a little butter, then line it with the pastry. You'll want it to drape a little over the sides of the dish as it will shrink during cooking. Bake for 15–20 minutes, or until golden.

WHILE the pastry case is baking, blend the arrowroot, stevia, juice and 100g (3½oz) of the strawberries together in a blender, then pour into a saucepan and heat over a low heat. Sprinkle the gelatine powder over the surface of the mixture as it starts to steam, stirring to combine (always add the gelatine to the liquid, not the other way around). Simmer gently for a couple of minutes, stirring continuously, until the mixture begins to thicken, then leave to cool completely.

REMOVE the baked case from the oven and leave to cool completely, then break off any excess pastry that overlaps the dish.

TIP the gelatine mixture into a large mixing bowl and stir through 800g (1lb 12oz) of the strawberries and the food colouring, if using, until totally combined.

POUR the strawberry mixture into the cooled case and decorate with the remaining strawberries. Cover and chill for at least 1 hour until set.

VARIATIONS

① BLACK GRAPE & ELDERFLOWER PIE

Make the pie as opposite, replacing the strawberries with 1kg (2lb 4oz) halved **black grapes**.

② APRICOT & ELDERFLOWER PIE

Make the pie as opposite, replacing the strawberries with 1kg (2lb 4oz) stoned and quartered **apricots**.

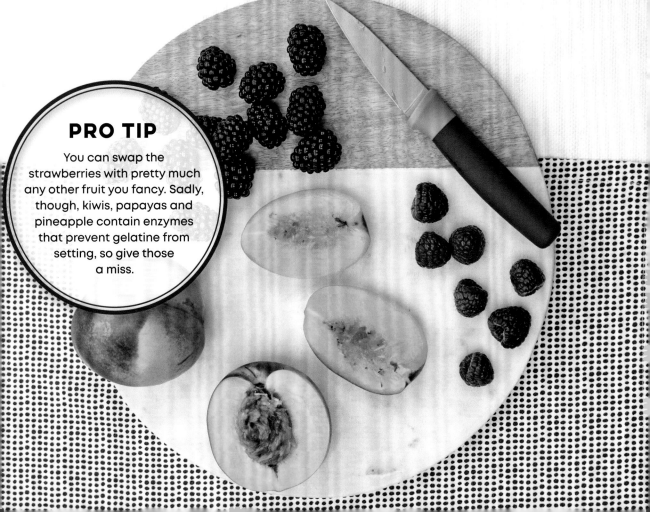

PRO TIP

You can swap the strawberries with pretty much any other fruit you fancy. Sadly, though, kiwis, papayas and pineapple contain enzymes that prevent gelatine from setting, so give those a miss.

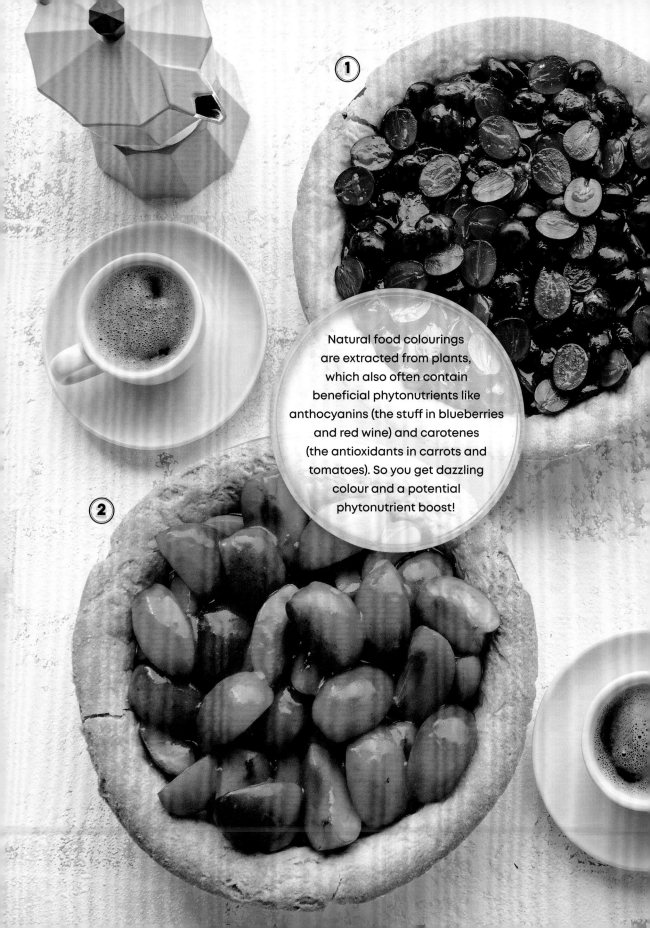

①

②

Natural food colourings are extracted from plants, which also often contain beneficial phytonutrients like anthocyanins (the stuff in blueberries and red wine) and carotenes (the antioxidants in carrots and tomatoes). So you get dazzling colour and a potential phytonutrient boost!

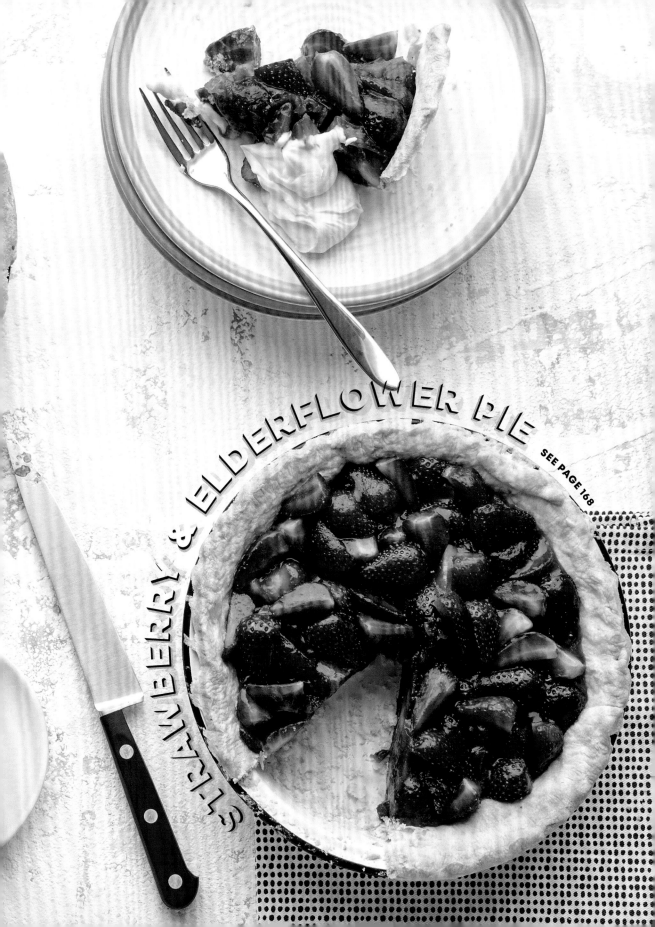

STRAWBERRY & ELDERFLOWER PIE SEE PAGE 168

ENGLISH GARDEN JELLY COCKTAIL

OK, I'm not ashamed to admit it. I have a nostalgia for the jelly shots of early noughties' university dorm rooms. Or at least my somewhat hazy memories of them. And, yes, chucking some fruit into this kitsch, student-days treat will (perhaps miraculously) count towards your daily intake. And why on earth not?

Serves 4

Prep time 15 minutes, plus setting

Cook time 5 minutes

7 gelatine leaves

600ml (20fl oz) apple juice

100ml (3½fl oz) vodka or gin

1 small bunch of large mint leaves (roughly the height of the glassware)

240g (8½oz) hulled and thinly sliced fresh strawberries

80g (2¾oz) cucumber, thinly sliced

SOAK the gelatine in cold water for 5 minutes.

MEANWHILE, pour the fruit juice and booze into a medium saucepan and heat to just below simmering point, then take off the heat.

SHAKE the excess liquid from the gelatine sheets, then stir into the liquid. Leave to cool for several minutes until warm rather than hot to the touch.

ARRANGE a few mint leaves around the edge of each glass, then divide a third of the warm liquid among the glasses.

DIVIDE a third of the strawberries carefully among the glasses, followed by half the cucumber. Add another layer of strawberries, then the rest of the cucumber and a final layer of strawberries.

POUR the remaining liquid into the glasses, then carefully transfer to the fridge and chill for 2–3 hours, or until set.

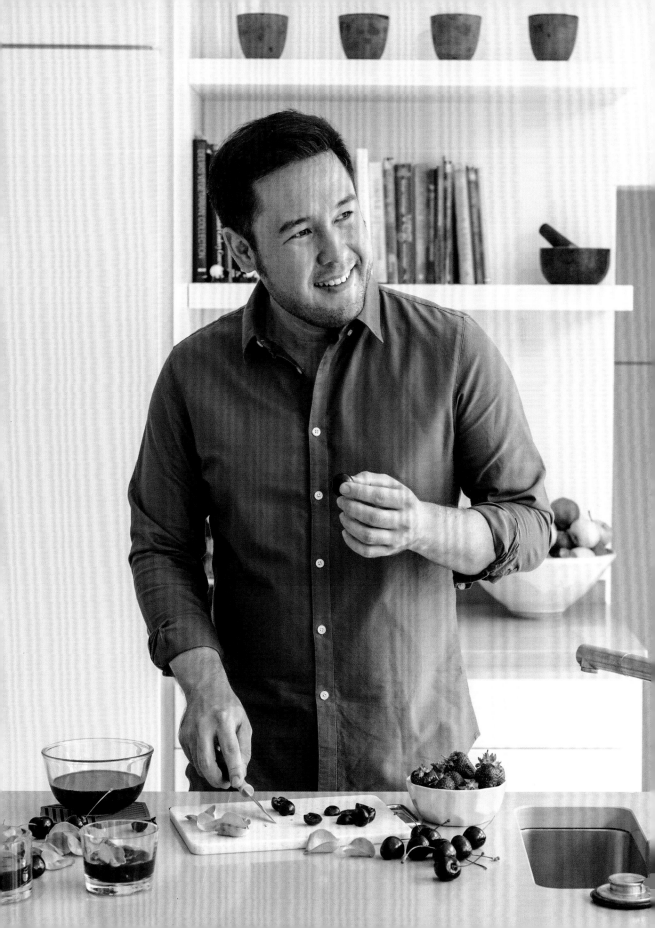

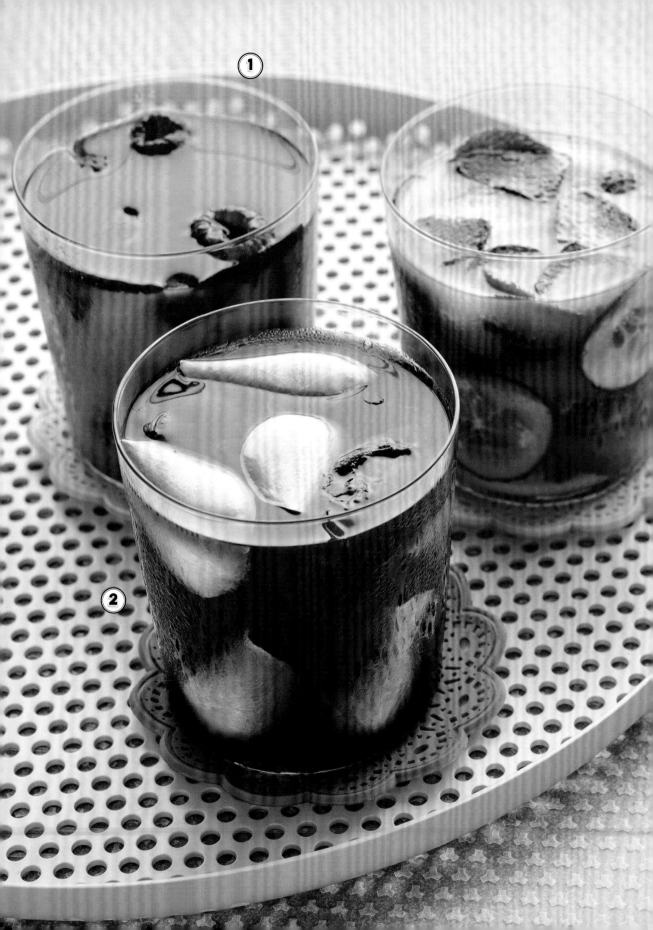

VARIATIONS

1 TEQUILA SUNRISE

Make the jelly cocktail as on page 172, replacing the apple juice and alcohol with 600ml (20fl oz) **orange juice** and 100ml (3½fl oz) **tequila**. Omit the mint, strawberries and cucumber. Toss 320g (11¼oz) **fresh raspberries** in 2 tsp **grenadine**, then divide half the raspberries among the glasses. Pour in all the warm liquid, then drop the remaining raspberries into the glasses. Chill as on page 172. Top with a thin layer of extra grenadine before serving.

2 SAKURA SURPRISE

Make the jelly cocktail as on page 172, replacing the apple juice and alcohol with 600ml (20fl oz) **purple grape juice** and 100ml (3½fl oz) **lychee liqueur**. Omit the mint, strawberries and cucumber. If liked, divide a small handful of **edible rose petals** around the bases of each glass. Quarter 320g (11¼oz) pitted **fresh cherries**, then divide half of them among the glasses. Pour in half of the warm liquid, then repeat with a few more rose petals, the remaining cherries and liquid. Chill as on page 172.

MANGO CUSTARD

This mango custard is delicious on its own (and provides 1 of your daily portions), or it can be used in place of regular custard in almost any recipe.

PORTION 1 PER SERVING

Serves 4
Prep time 2 minutes
Cook time 8 minutes

35g (1¼oz) custard powder
200ml (7fl oz) full-fat or semi-skimmed milk
320g (11¼oz) canned mango purée

MIX the custard powder with a small amount of the milk in a heatproof bowl to form a thick paste.

POUR the remaining milk into a medium saucepan, add the mango purée and heat until just below simmering point, stirring occasionally, then take off the heat.

STIR a quarter of the warm mixture into the custard paste to thin it, then pour it back into the pan and cook over a gentle heat, stirring constantly, until the mixture is simmering. Immediately remove the pan from the heat and serve hot.

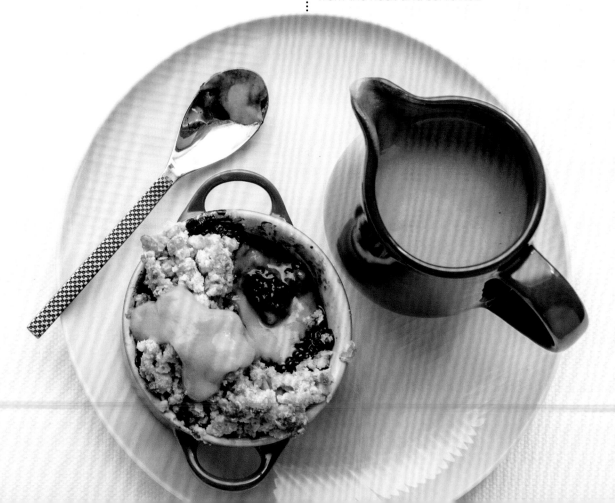

APPLE & BLACKBERRY CRUMBLE

It's amazing how a thin layer of crisp, crumbly topping can make what is essentially a giant dish of chopped fruit seem altogether more decadent. This no-added-sugar crumble with mango custard is super simple to make, delicious and crams in a full 3 portions of fruit and veg per serving.

Serves 4
Prep time 15 minutes
Cook time 30–35 minutes

1 x quantity Mango Custard (see opposite), to serve

Fruit layer
250g (9oz) cored apples, cut into 1.5cm (⅝in) chunks
250g (9oz) fresh or frozen blackberries
60g (2¼oz) raisins
2 tbsp dark rum
½ tsp ground allspice
15g (½oz) granulated stevia (baking blend)
2 tbsp cornflour

Topping
60g (2¼oz) rolled oats
60g (2¼oz) ground almonds
50g (1¾oz) granulated stevia (baking blend)
60g (2¼oz) cold unsalted butter, diced

PREHEAT the oven to 190°C (375°F), Gas Mark 5.

COMBINE all the fruit layer ingredients in a bowl, then transfer to 2 x 400ml (14fl oz) baking dishes.

PLACE the oats, almonds and stevia in a bowl, add the butter pieces and rub in with your fingertips until the mixture resembles coarse breadcrumbs. Sprinkle on top of the fruit, then press it in lightly.

BAKE for 30–35 minutes, or until the top is golden and crisp. Serve the crumble hot or cold, with hot Mango Custard.

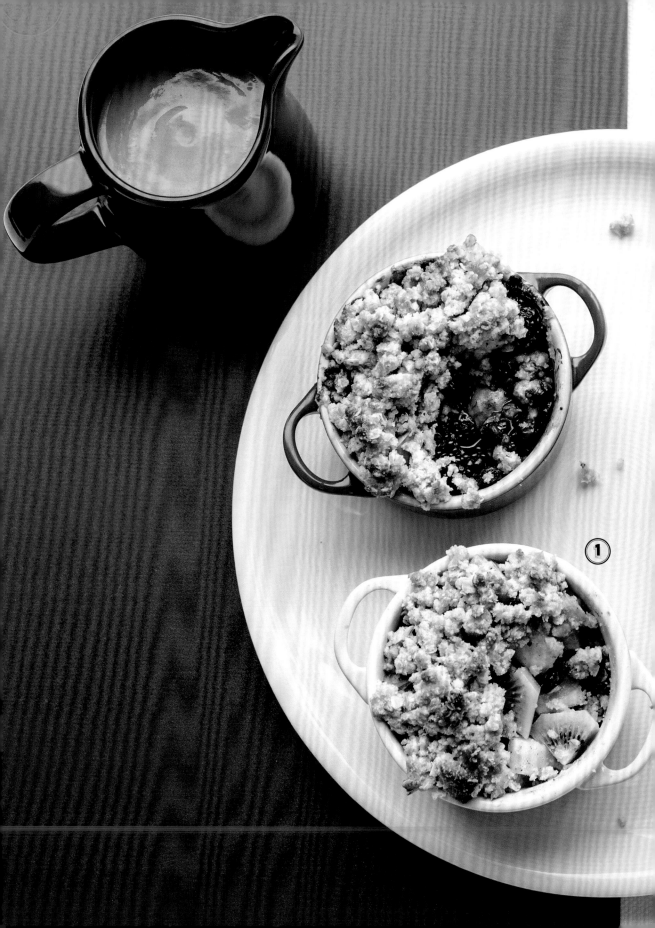

PRO TIP

It may sound a little weird using carrot in a sweet recipe that's not a cake, but just trust me on this one. The kids'll never know there's carrot in there!

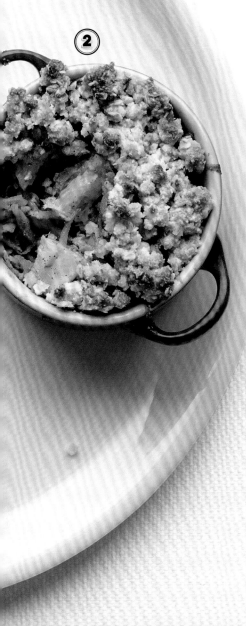

① TROPICAL CRUMBLE

Make the crumble as on page 177, replacing the apple and blackberries with 250g (9oz) peeled **kiwifruit** and 250g (9oz) skinned and cored **fresh pineapple**, both cut into 1.5cm (⅝in) chunks.

VARIATIONS

② CARROT CAKE CRUMBLE

Make the crumble as on page 177, replacing the apple and blackberries with 250g (9oz) finely grated **carrots** and 250g (9oz) **orange segments**, cut into 1.5cm (⅝in) cubes, and the rum with 2 tsp **vanilla bean paste**. Add 50g (1¾oz) **granulated stevia (baking blend)** to the fruit layer.

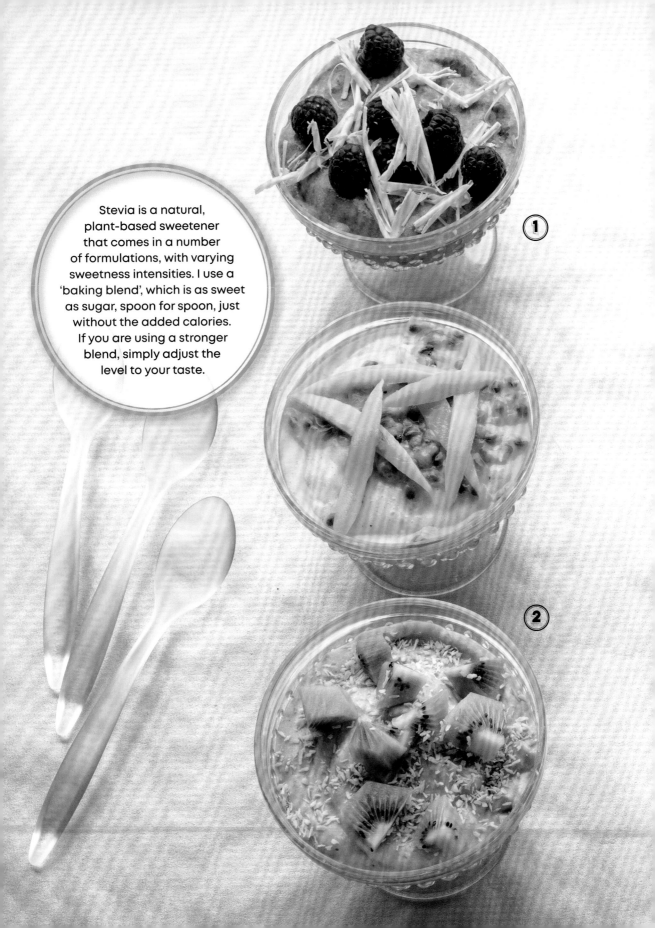

Stevia is a natural, plant-based sweetener that comes in a number of formulations, with varying sweetness intensities. I use a 'baking blend', which is as sweet as sugar, spoon for spoon, just without the added calories. If you are using a stronger blend, simply adjust the level to your taste.

1

2

MANGO & PASSION FRUIT MOUSSE

A deliciously light, airy mousse that packs in 2 of your daily portions, not to mention a dose of healthy protein and no added sugar. The basic recipe is super flexible, too, so you can replace the mango with 600g (1lb 5oz) of pretty much any fruit, except kiwis, papayas and pineapples, which can prevent gelatine from setting.

PORTIONS PER SERVING **2**

Serves 4

Prep time 10 minutes, plus cooling and setting

100ml (3½fl oz) hot water

12g (½oz) sachet powdered gelatine

600g (1lb 5oz) mango flesh

2 tbsp granulated stevia (baking blend)

2 tsp vanilla bean paste

200g (7oz) Greek yogurt

2 egg whites

2 passion fruit, halved

POUR the measured water into a small heatproof bowl and sprinkle over the gelatine. Stir vigorously until thoroughly combined, then leave to cool.

BLITZ 500g (1lb 2oz) of the mango with the stevia, vanilla, yogurt and cooled gelatine liquid in a blender or food processor until you have a smooth purée. Whisk the egg whites in a clean bowl until they form stiff peaks, then gently fold into the mango purée.

POUR into 4 glasses and chill for at least 2 hours, or until set.

DECORATE the set mousses with the remaining mango and the passion fruit pulp and serve.

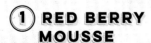
VARIATIONS

(1) RED BERRY MOUSSE

Make the mousse as above, replacing the mango with 500g (1lb 2oz) **strawberries**, adding all the strawberries to the blender or food processor, and replacing the passion fruit with 100g (3½oz) **raspberries** and 20g (¾oz) **white chocolate curls**.

(2) KIWI-CADO MOUSSE

Make the mousse as above, replacing the mango with 3 stoned and peeled **avocados** and the juice of ½ **lemon**, adding all the avocados to the blender or food processor, and replacing the passion fruit with 100g (3½oz) peeled and sliced **kiwifruit** and a sprinkling of **toasted desiccated coconut**.

STICKY TOFFEE PUDDINGS

My brother makes the best sticky toffee pudding in the world. His secret for extra gooey, deep, dark toffee goodness is adding loads more dates than most recipes suggest. Sorry for giving that one away, Pauly. But the funny thing about his recipe is that the extra sweetness from the dates means he has also reduced the sugar dramatically. So I thought, could you dispense with the sugar entirely? And guess what? You can! Here's my 60 per cent fruit and veg twist on his recipe that gives you 3 of your daily portions, sneakily disguised in the form of dessert.

Serves 4

Prep time 12 minutes

Cook time 8 minutes

1 tbsp melted butter, plus extra for greasing

about 125g (4½oz) mashed banana

100g (3½oz) finely grated carrot

100g (3½oz) chopped dates

1 large egg

1 tsp cinnamon

1 tsp ground ginger

1 tsp vanilla bean paste

125g (4½oz) self-raising wholemeal flour

1 tsp bicarbonate of soda

2 tsp black treacle, plus a little extra for drizzling

large pinch of salt

To serve

100g (3½oz) Greek yogurt

400g (14oz) fresh fruit of your choice

GREASE 4 large ramekins generously with butter.

STIR together all the ingredients in a large mixing bowl. Spoon the mixture into the prepared ramekins.

COOK each one separately in the microwave for 2 minutes on high.

SERVE with an extra drizzling of treacle, the Greek yogurt and fresh fruit.

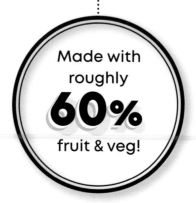

Made with roughly

60%

fruit & veg!

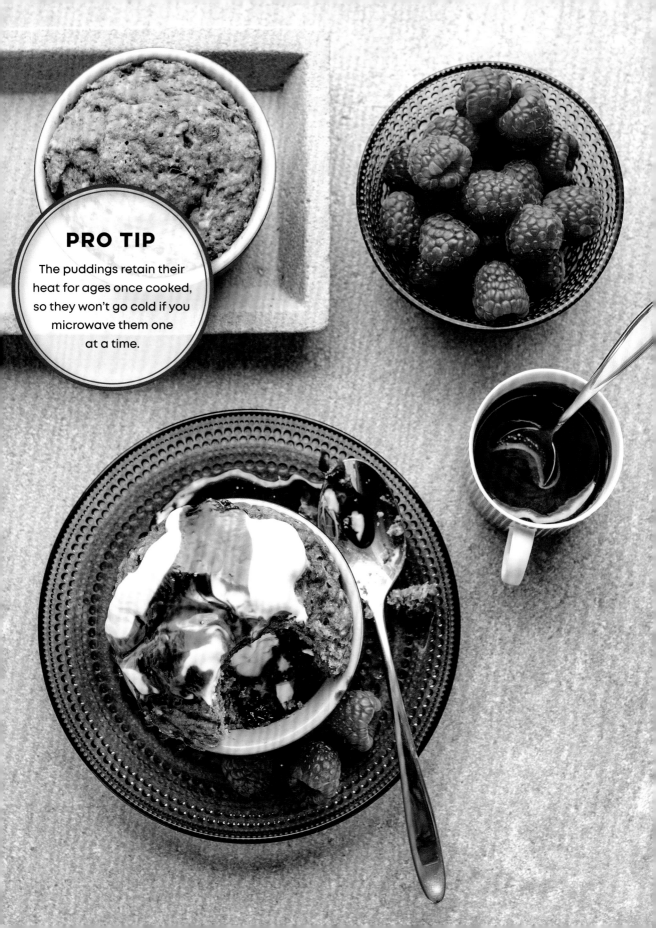

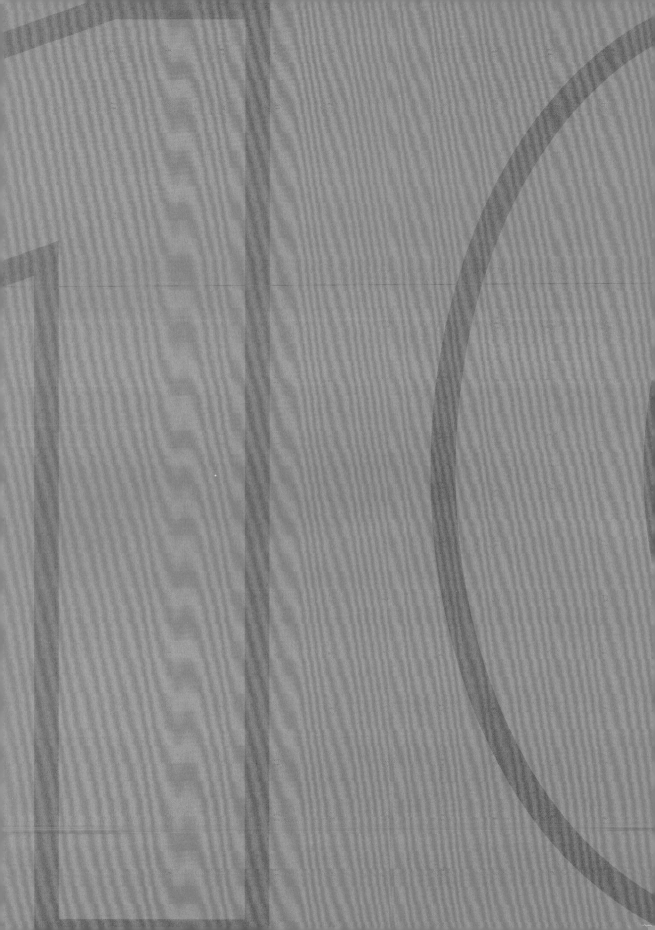

SNACKS, SIDES & SAUCES

PEANUT BUTTER, ORANGE & DATE COOKIES

Yes, I know it might sound too good to be true, but these cookies are indeed 75 per cent pure fruit and veg! In fact, just 2 of these tasty treats contain 1 of your daily fruit and veg portions. They are really quick to mix up, too, so you could be eating them in just 30 minutes from scratch, straight from the oven. Much like regular cookies, they are pretty calorie dense thanks to all that creamy peanut butter and sugary dried fruit, but are simultaneously packed with loads more nutrition. And the protein-rich nature of chickpeas means they will keep you fuller for longer too!

Makes 12
Prep time 10 minutes
Cook time 15–20 minutes

olive oil, for greasing
100g (3½oz) ripe peeled banana
60g (2¼oz) peanut butter (any type)
1 egg
2 tsp vanilla bean paste
200g (7oz) gram flour
150g (5½oz) chopped dates
finely grated zest of 1 orange
1 tsp bicarbonate of soda

PREHEAT the oven to 180°C (350°F), Gas Mark 4. Line a baking sheet with nonstick baking paper, then grease with olive oil.

PLACE the banana, peanut butter, egg and vanilla in a bowl and mash together until smooth. Tip in the remaining ingredients and stir to form a thick, sticky dough. It might look like there isn't quite enough liquid in the mix at first but, trust me, you'll get there.

GREASE your hands with a little olive oil, then scoop out tablespoonfuls of the mixture and roll into small balls. Arrange the balls on the prepared baking sheet, about 5cm (2in) apart. Dip a fork in oil, then use the back of it to gently flatten the balls.

BAKE for 15–20 minutes, or until the tops are golden brown. Transfer to a wire rack and leave to cool. The cookies will keep for up to 1 week in an airtight container.

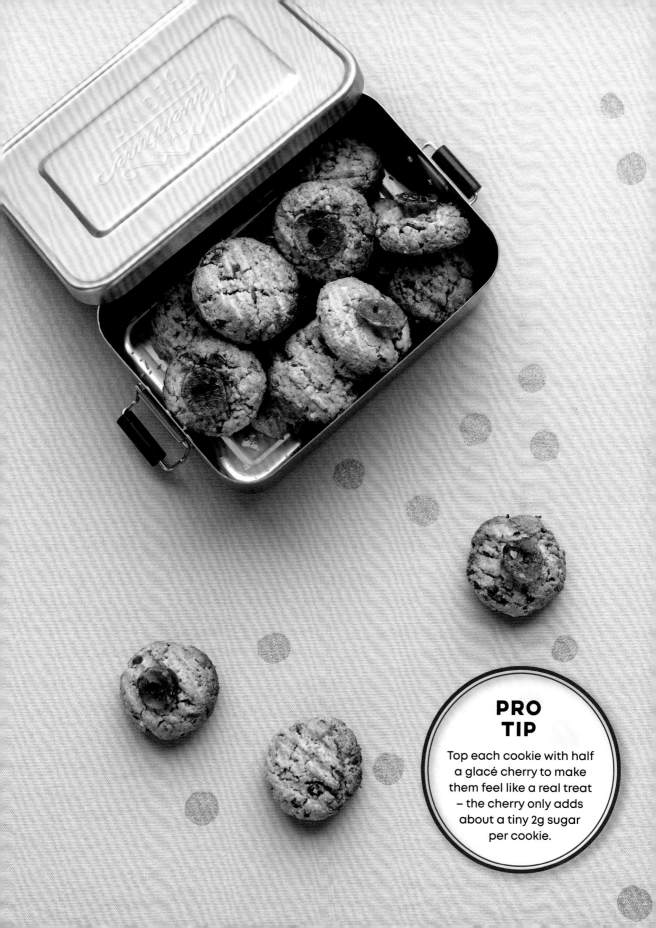

PRO TIP

Top each cookie with half a glacé cherry to make them feel like a real treat – the cherry only adds about a tiny 2g sugar per cookie.

CHEDDAR VEG SCONES

These plant-packed, rustic scones contain as much veg as they do flour, and only a tiny amount of fat compared to the regular kind. Yet the sky-high veg content keeps them deliciously moist and adds a slight, satisfying sweetness. Amazing as a side to soup with a little butter or just as they are.

Makes 10
Prep time 10 minutes
Cook time 35 minutes

1 tbsp olive oil

250g (9oz) frozen mixed veg

½ tsp dried garlic granules

½ tsp onion powder

25g (1oz) mature Cheddar cheese, grated, plus a little extra for sprinkling

100g (3½oz) self-raising flour, plus extra for dusting

150g (5½oz) wholemeal flour

1 tbsp baking powder

large pinch of salt

¼ tsp turmeric (for colour)

175ml (6fl oz) milk, plus extra for brushing

PREHEAT the oven to 220°C (425°F), Gas Mark 7 and line a baking sheet with nonstick baking paper.

HEAT the olive oil in a frying pan over a medium heat, add the frozen veg and fry for 10 minutes until completely cooked through.

TIP into a food processor with the remaining ingredients and pulse until the veg are finely chopped and a dough forms.

TURN the dough out on to a floured chopping board and shape into a flat rectangle, about a finger's width in height, then cut into 10 equal-sized squares.

TRANSFER the squares to the prepared sheet, brush with a little milk and sprinkle with a little grated cheese. Bake for 25 minutes, or until golden.

SERVE warm or cool. The scones will keep in an airtight container for up to 1 week.

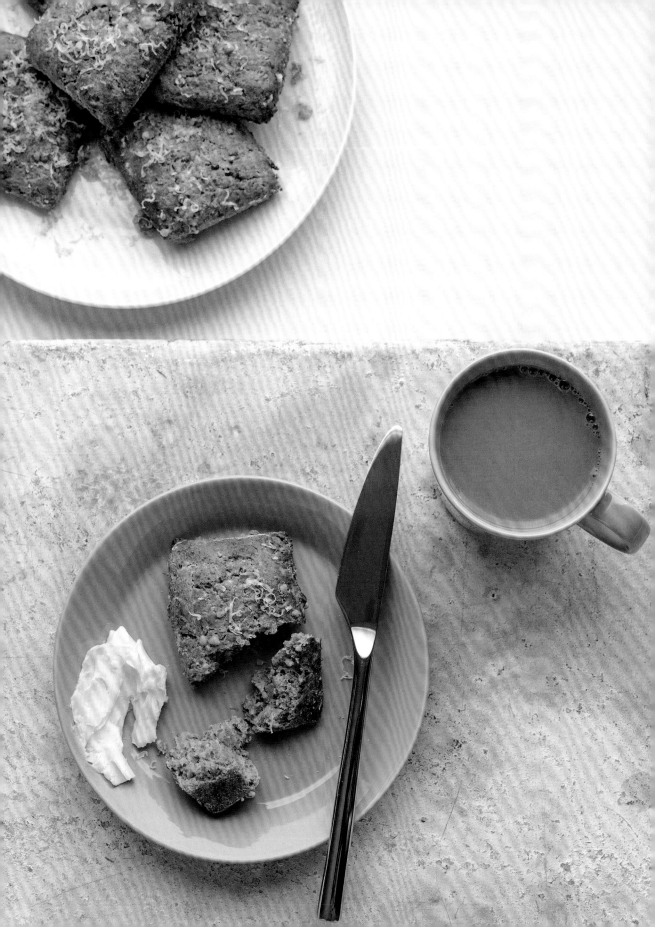

PUMPKIN & ONION SEED FLATBREAD

I always loved the idea of making my own bread but, not being a natural baker, the idea also filled me with fear. Fortunately, this simple flatbread recipe couldn't be any easier and contains almost the same amount of delicious, golden pumpkin as it does wholegrain flour, making it super filling and flavourful. Not to mention versatile!

Serves 4

Prep time 20 minutes, plus rising

Cook time 10–15 minutes

350g (12oz) very strong wholemeal bread flour, plus extra for dusting

7g (¼oz) sachet fast-action dried yeast

1 tsp sea salt

325g (11½oz) canned pumpkin purée

2 tsp clear honey

1 tbsp extra virgin olive oil, plus 1 tsp for frying and 1 tsp for brushing

½ tbsp onion seeds, for sprinkling

COMBINE all the dry ingredients except the onion seeds in a large mixing bowl.

PLACE the pumpkin purée in a microwavable bowl and heat in the microwave for 60–90 seconds until warm. Pour into the dry ingredients with the honey and olive oil, then mix the ingredients together with your fingers to form a fairly sticky dough. Knead the dough for a good 10 minutes.

COVER with clingfilm and leave to rise in a warm place for 1–2 hours until doubled in size.

SPRINKLE the onion seeds over the risen dough. Knock back the dough, incorporating the onion seeds as you knead. Divide the dough into 8 equal-sized balls. Form each ball into the shape of a pitta, about 5mm (¼in) thick, and dust with a little flour on both sides.

GREASE a large, shallow frying pan with the remaining olive oil and heat over a medium heat, then add up to 4 flatbreads and fry for 2–3 minutes on each side. Repeat with the remaining flatbreads.

SERVE warm, brushed with olive oil.

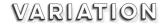

PESHWARI NAAN

Make the pumpkin dough as above, omitting the onion seeds, then knock it back and divide into 4 equal-sized balls. Form each ball into the shape of a thick crêpe, about 3mm (⅛in) thick, then rub ¼ tsp **cinnamon** and 1 tsp **ground almonds** over the tops, to about 1cm (½in) from the edges. Divide 30g (1oz) sliced pitted **dates** and 5g (⅛oz) **dried coconut flakes** among the flatbreads, sprinkling them over one side of each and leaving a 1cm (½in) gap from the edges. Fold the other half of dough over the filling, then pinch the edges together to seal (wet the edge with a little water if your dough isn't sticky enough). Flatten the stuffed flatbreads and work into a more rounded shape, then dust both sides with a little extra flour. Fry as above, adding 2 flatbreads to the pan at a time and cooking for 3 minutes on each side.

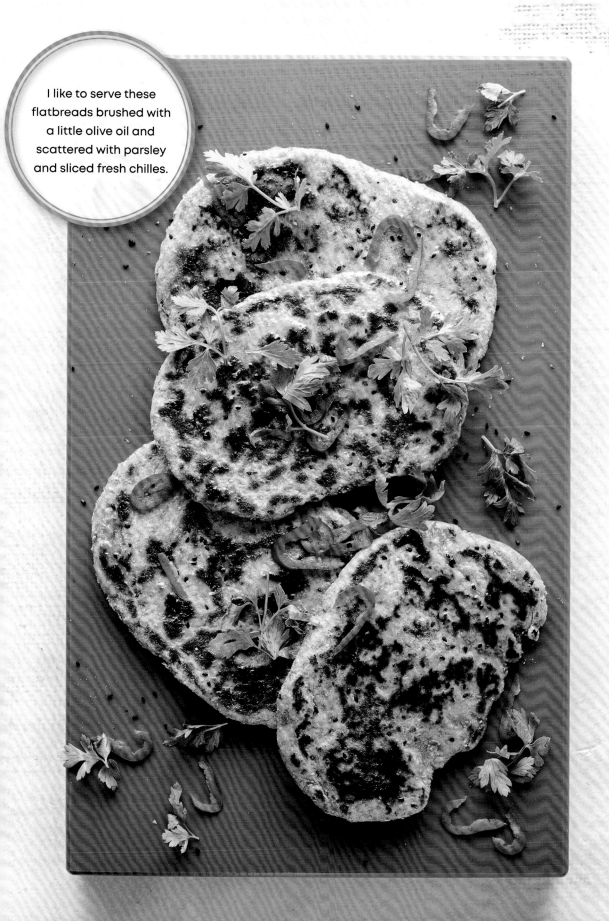

I like to serve these flatbreads brushed with a little olive oil and scattered with parsley and sliced fresh chilles.

PUMPKIN FARINATA

A chickpea flatbread originating in Genoa, with regional variations across the Med and Latin America. I like to add pumpkin to the batter to replace some of the water – it gives a gorgeous golden hue and sweet, comforting warmth, resulting in a protein-rich bread that is pretty much 100 per cent pure veg. Almost too good to be true, really. If a plant-based topping is added to this veggie-packed disc to create a tasty 'pizza' (Italian food purists, look away now), the fruit and veg content can be sent even higher, giving up to 4 portions per serving (see pages 102–103 for topping ideas).

Serves 4

Prep time 15 minutes, plus standing and cooling

Cook time 20 minutes

200ml (7fl oz) water

160g (5¾oz) canned pumpkin purée

1 tbsp extra virgin olive oil

½ tsp sea salt

160g (5¾oz) gram flour

Infused oil

3 rosemary sprigs, leaves finely chopped, plus extra to garnish

1 garlic clove, minced

½ tbsp extra virgin olive oil

PLACE the measured water, pumpkin purée, half the olive oil and the salt in a large bowl and whisk together until combined. Add the gram flour a little at a time, whisking constantly until smooth. Leave to stand for 30 minutes.

PREHEAT the oven to 220°C (425°F), Gas Mark 7. Combine all the infused oil ingredients in a small bowl, then set aside.

POUR the remaining oil into a 27cm (10¾in) diameter Pyrex dish and heat in the oven for 5 minutes. Remove the dish from the oven and carefully swirl the oil to ensure it evenly covers the dish, then give the batter a quick stir and pour into the hot oil.

PLACE in the top of the oven and bake for about 20 minutes until golden and resembling a giant Scotch pancake.

LEAVE the farinata to cool for 5 minutes, then brush with the infused oil. Slice into 16 pieces. Serve warm, garnished with extra rosemary.

MIGHTY MOLE

Here are my twists on the classic guacamole, without a hint of coriander in sight. #happywong

Serves 4

Prep time 10 minutes

2 large, ripe avocados, stoned and peeled

½ white onion, finely chopped

4 green bird's-eye chillies, finely chopped

2 heaped tbsp chopped dill, plus extra to garnish

2 heaped tbsp chopped parsley

1 tsp coarsely ground black pepper

2 tsp cider vinegar or lemon juice

To serve

1 tsp red chilli flakes

large pinch of sea salt flakes

SMASH the avocados roughly with a fork in a large bowl, then mix in all the remaining ingredients.

SPRINKLE over the chilli flakes, salt and extra dill and serve.

VARIATIONS

MILDER MOLE

Halve 1 **tomato** and scoop out and discard the seeds, then cut the remaining flesh into small cubes no bigger than 1cm (½in). Smash the avocados as above, then mix with the tomato, the finely grated zest and juice of 1 **lime** and 2 tbsp chopped **chives**. Season to taste with **salt** and **pepper** and garnish with a few extra chopped chives.

GUAC-MOLATA

Finely grate the zest of 2 **lemons**, reserving a little to garnish. Smash the avocados as above, then mix with most of the lemon zest and the juice of 1 of the lemons, 2 large minced **garlic cloves** and a large handful of **parsley**, finely chopped. Season with **salt** and **pepper** to taste, then garnish with an extra sprig of parsley and the reserved zest.

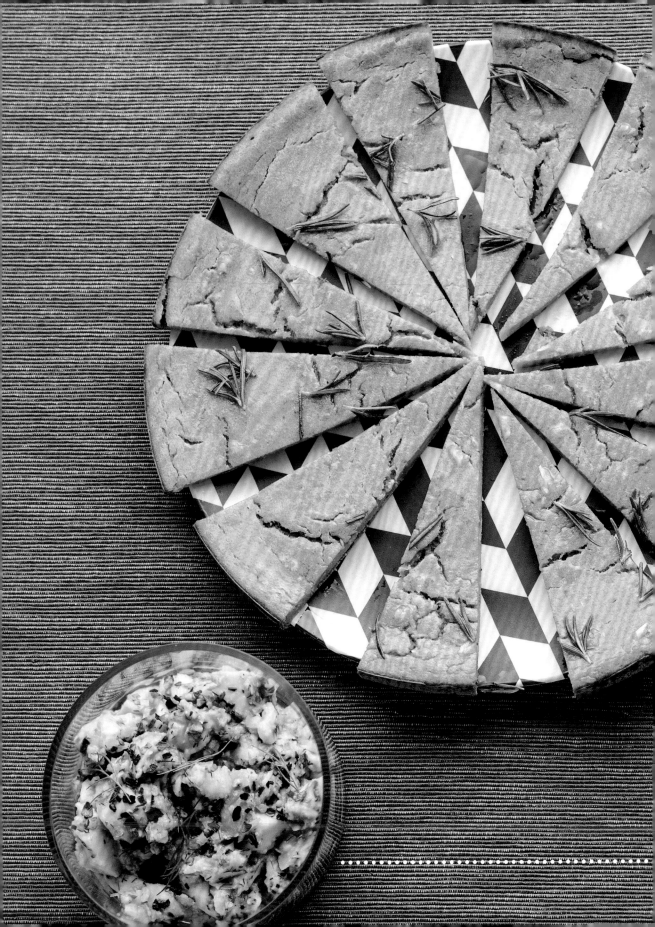

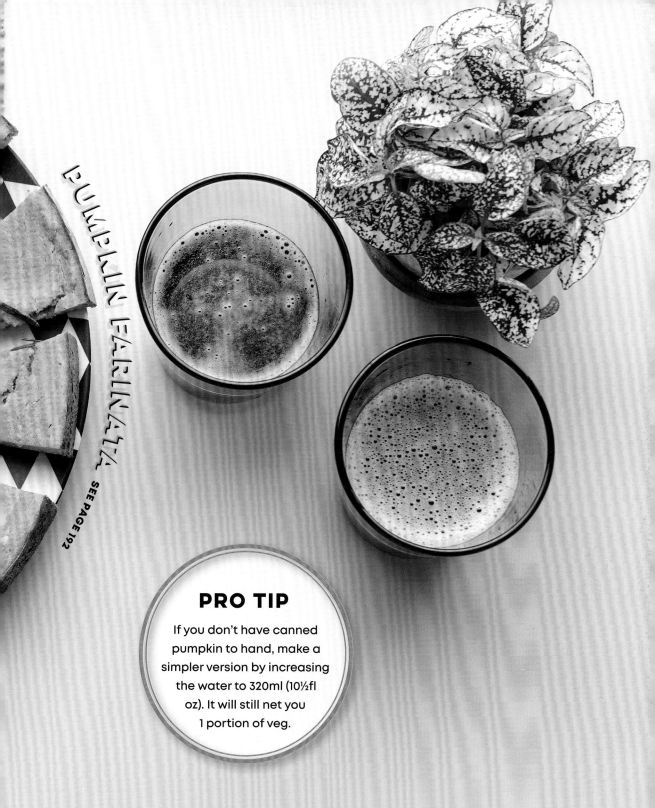

PUMPKIN FARINATA SEE PAGE 192

PRO TIP

If you don't have canned pumpkin to hand, make a simpler version by increasing the water to 320ml (10½fl oz). It will still net you 1 portion of veg.

MIGHTY MOLE SEE PAGE 193

BOOSTED BEETROOT HUMMUS

Take some shop-bought hummus, add more veg and you can halve its calories while dramatically boosting its flavour and colour. Reduced-fat hummus has a higher content of chickpeas than the standard stuff, making it a particularly rich source of veggies. Yum!

PORTION PER SERVING 1

Serves 4
Prep time 5 minutes, plus chilling

200g (7oz) tub reduced-fat hummus
200g (7oz) cooked beetroot
2 tsp caraway seeds
1 tsp black pepper

BLITZ the hummus and beetroot together in a food processor. Tip into a serving bowl, then stir in the caraway seeds and pepper.

CHILL in the fridge for at least 30 minutes, to allow the spices to infuse.

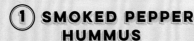

VARIATIONS

1 SMOKED PEPPER HUMMUS

Make the hummus as above, replacing the beetroot with 100g (3½oz) cored, deseeded and roughly chopped **red pepper** and the caraway and black pepper with 60g (2¼oz) **tomato purée** and 2 tsp **smoked paprika**.

2 MUSHY (CHICK)PEAS

Make the hummus as above, replacing the beetroot with a rinsed and drained 300g (10½oz) can **marrowfat peas** or **mushy peas**, and the caraway and black pepper with the finely grated zest of ½ **lemon**, 2 tsp **lemon juice**, 1 tbsp chopped **mint** leaves and 2 tsp **dried tarragon**. Season to taste with a little **salt** and **pepper**.

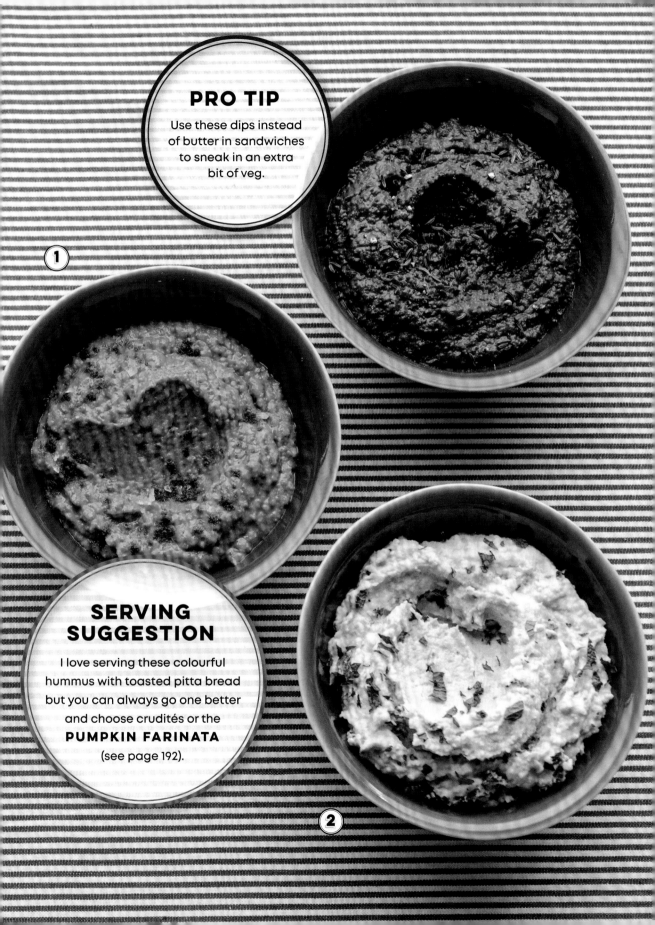

PRO TIP

Use these dips instead of butter in sandwiches to sneak in an extra bit of veg.

①

SERVING SUGGESTION

I love serving these colourful hummus with toasted pitta bread but you can always go one better and choose crudités or the **PUMPKIN FARINATA** (see page 192).

②

LOADED SWEET POTATO & PARSNIP FRIES

Yes, I am being serious. This unctuous dish of deliciousness offers up almost 4 portions of veg per serving, but it isn't excessive in fat or calories. Pushed for time? Swap the homemade fries for shop-bought sweet potato oven wedges (look out for the lower-fat ones) and get stuck in. These are particularly good served with super-hot chilli sauce and super-cold beer.

Serves 4

Prep time 15 minutes

Cook time 25 minutes

1 x quantity Sweet Potato & Parsnip Fries (see page 133)

1 x quantity Tomacado Salsa (see page 209)

120g (4¼oz) rinsed and drained canned black beans

2 spring onions, thinly sliced diagonally

4 fresh jalapeño chillies, thinly sliced into rings

large handful of grated Cheddar cheese

salt and pepper

COOK the sweet potato fries and make the salsa while they cook.

SCATTER the black beans over the fries, followed by the salsa, spring onions and jalapeños, then top generously with grated cheese and season well.

PLACE under a preheated hot grill until the cheese melts and begins to brown. Enjoy hot (or cold)!

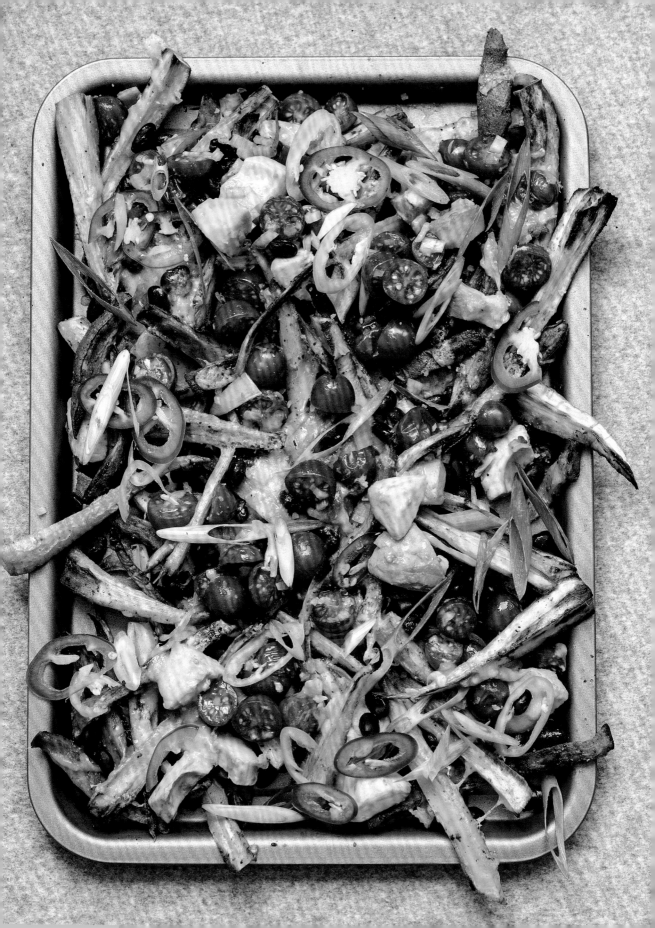

VEG-LOADED MASH

Swapping out up to half the spuds in a standard mash recipe is probably the easiest way to up the veg content in any dish. Making it in the microwave also means lightning fast results, loads less washing up and, as you are not boiling the potatoes, no loss of nutrients to the cooking water. This recipe works brilliantly, every time, with a whole range of more carby vegetables.

'HALF & HALF' MASH

Looks pretty much identical to regular mash, but with the subtly sweet smoothness of tasty parsnips, giving you a sneaky extra 1.5 portions per serving.

Serves 4

Prep time 10 minutes

Cook time 15 minutes

500g (1lb 2oz) unpeeled potatoes, such as Desiree, Vivaldi or Marabel, cut into chunks

500g (1lb 2oz) starchy veg, such as parsnips, sweet potatoes or pumpkin, cut into chunks, or canned cannellini beans, rinsed and drained

125ml (4fl oz) milk

large knob of butter

2 spring onions, very finely sliced

salt and pepper

POP the potatoes and starchy veg (but not the cannellini beans) into a large, microwavable bowl, cover loosely and cook on high for 5 minutes. Remove the bowl from the microwave using oven gloves and give the contents a good stir. Re-cover and microwave for another 10 minutes, or until the potatoes and other veg are totally soft when pricked with a fork.

ADD the milk and cannellini beans, if using, and mash everything together. Careful, the bowl will be very hot! Season well with salt and pepper, then top with the butter and spring onions.

COLCANNON

This isn't some new-fangled diet recipe, far from it, but an Irish favourite. Replacing 300g (10½oz) of the spuds in a normal mash recipe with buttery cabbage and tasty spring onions both slashes the calories and sneaks in an extra serving of veg per person.

Serves 4

Prep time 10 minutes

Cook time 15 minutes

700g (1lb 9oz) unpeeled potatoes, such as Desiree, Vivaldi or Marabel, cut into large chunks

100ml (3½fl oz) milk

large knob of butter

300g (10½oz) very finely sliced green cabbage or kale

10 spring onions, very finely sliced

salt and pepper

POP the potatoes and milk into a large microwavable bowl, cover loosely and cook on high for 5 minutes.

MEANWHILE, heat the butter in a frying pan, add the cabbage or kale and spring onions and fry gently for 2–3 minutes, or until the cabbage or kale wilts and turns a darker green.

REMOVE the bowl from the microwave using oven gloves and give the contents a good stir. Re-cover and microwave for another 10 minutes, or until the potatoes are totally soft when pricked with a fork.

MASH the potatoes and milk together. Careful, the bowl will be very hot! Fold in the cooked spring onions and cabbage or kale, season well with salt and pepper and serve.

PRO TIP

Don't bother to peel the spuds – the skin significantly increases the amount of nutrients like iron, calcium and protective polyphenols, not to mention providing loads more healthy fibre, which can make you feel fuller for longer. And all for less work! If the texture bothers you, simply slice the potatoes more thinly.

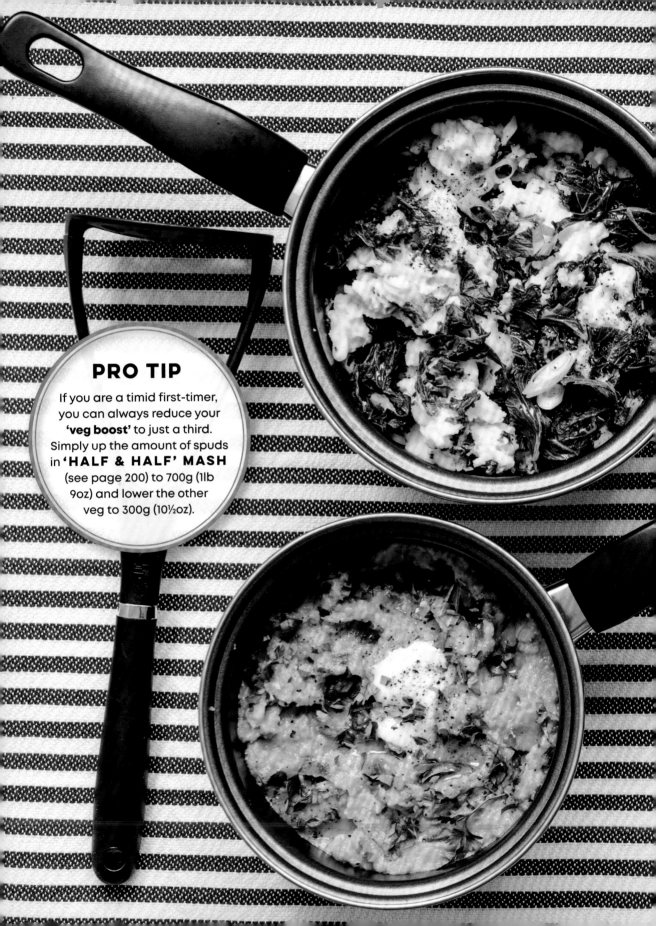

PRO TIP

If you are a timid first-timer, you can always reduce your **'veg boost'** to just a third. Simply up the amount of spuds in **'HALF & HALF' MASH** (see page 200) to 700g (1lb 9oz) and lower the other veg to 300g (10½oz).

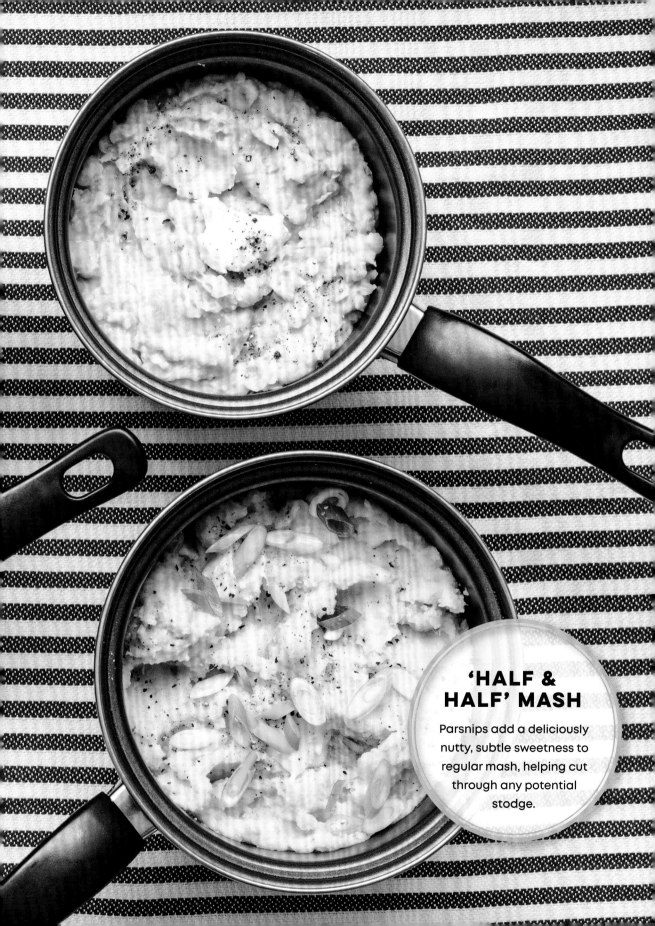

'HALF & HALF' MASH

Parsnips add a deliciously nutty, subtle sweetness to regular mash, helping cut through any potential stodge.

SPICED SWEET POTATO MASH

I know I risk messing with good old mash at my peril, but the smooth velvetiness of butter-mashed sweet potatoes makes a wonderful alternative to the regular kind. This simple substitution will give you roughly twice the fibre and one and a half times the amount of vitamin C, as well as over four times the vitamin A you need in a day. A pretty sweet deal in more ways than one!

Serves 4
Prep time 10 minutes
Cook time 15 minutes

1kg (2lb 4oz) unpeeled sweet potatoes, cut into 2.5cm (1in) cubes

125ml (4fl oz) milk

pinch of ground cardamom (a little goes a long way)

large knob of butter

1 tsp chopped parsley

salt and pepper

POP the sweet potatoes in a large microwavable bowl, cover loosely and cook on high for 5 minutes. Remove the bowl from the microwave using oven gloves and give the contents a good stir. Re-cover and microwave for another 10 minutes, or until the potatoes are totally soft when pricked with a fork.

ADD the milk and cardamom and mash everything together. Careful, the bowl will be very hot! Season well with salt and pepper, then serve topped with the butter and parsley.

WHITE BEAN & ONION MASH

OK, I know bean mash might seem a little 'out there', but the delicate creaminess of cannellini beans really does work as a spud substitute. An excellent source of satisfying protein, this is also probably the quickest type of mash to put together.

Serves 4
Prep time 5 minutes
Cook time 12 minutes

2 tbsp olive oil

300g (10½oz) finely diced onions

150ml (5oz) milk

2 garlic cloves, minced

3 x 400g (14oz) cans cannellini beans, rinsed and drained

salt and pepper

HEAT the olive oil in a large saucepan over a low heat, add the onions and fry gently for 10 minutes until softened and golden brown.

TIP in the milk, garlic and cannellini beans, stir together and cook for another minute or two, then take off the heat, mash and season well. The mixture will thicken up as it reaches serving temperature.

LENTIL-BOOSTED RICE

Whack all these ingredients in a pan and cook just as you would regular rice and you'll get loads of extra flavour plus 2 portions of veg snuck in.

Serves 4
Prep time 5 minutes
Cook time 25 minutes

200g (7oz) brown rice
200g (7oz) brown lentils, rinsed
500ml (18fl oz) water
150g (5½oz) cored, deseeded and diced red pepper
150g (5½oz) diced onion
150g (5½oz) diced carrots
¼ tsp salt

COMBINE all the ingredients in a large saucepan. Cover and bring to the boil, then immediately reduce the heat and simmer, still covered, for 20 minutes, or until the rice is cooked through and the veg are tender.

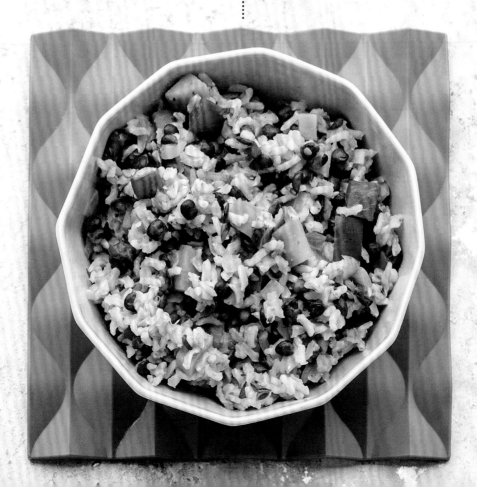

QUICK VEGGIE DHAL

Officially the easiest and fastest dhal recipe in the universe. Bung it all in one pan and go! So good and surprisingly versatile, you'll find yourself serving it with everything from curry to roast chicken, even sausage and mash.

Serves 4

Prep time 5 minutes

Cook time 20 minutes

320g (11¼oz) yellow mung dhal or other yellow lentils (check cooking times as these can vary), rinsed

1 tbsp extra virgin olive oil

400g (14oz) diced red onions

2 tsp cumin seeds

4 garlic cloves, minced

320g (11¼oz) tomatoes, chopped

2 tsp turmeric

2 chicken or vegetable stock cubes, crumbled

400ml (14fl oz) boiling water

200g (7oz) baby spinach leaves

pepper

POP the rinsed lentils into a large saucepan, pour over boiling water to cover 1cm (½in) above the lentils and bring to the boil. Boil rapidly for 1 minute. Skim off any scum with a spoon, then cover, reduce to a simmer and cook for 15 minutes, or until soft. Drain, then tip the lentils into a large bowl and set aside.

HEAT the olive oil in the lentil pan over a medium heat, add the diced onions and cumin seeds and fry for a few minutes until the onions begin to brown. Add the drained lentils with all the remaining ingredients except the spinach, bring to a simmer and cook for 1 minute. Stir well.

TAKE off the heat and stir in the spinach until the leaves start to wilt. Season with a little pepper and serve.

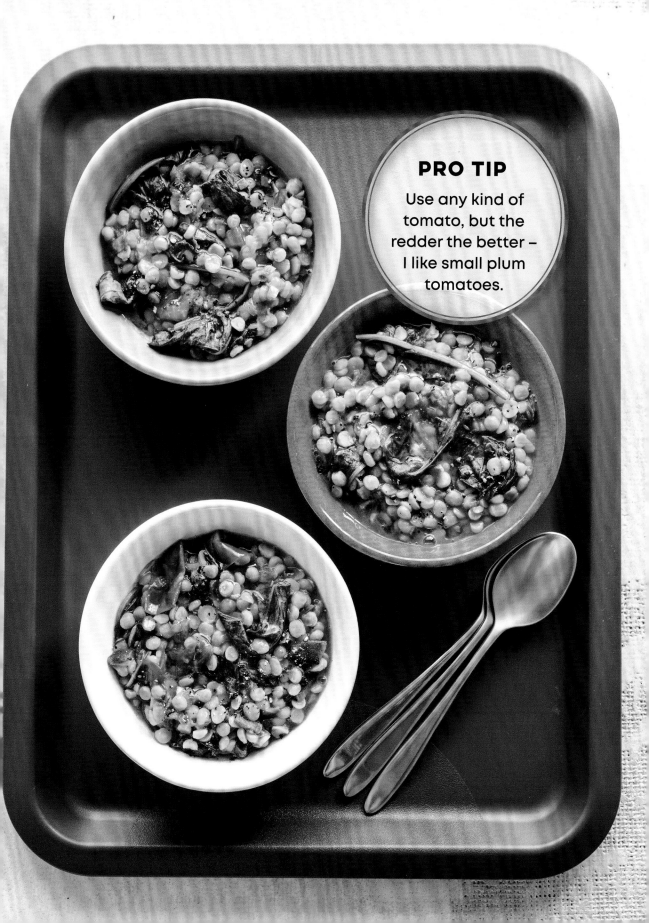

PRO TIP

Use any kind of tomato, but the redder the better – I like small plum tomatoes.

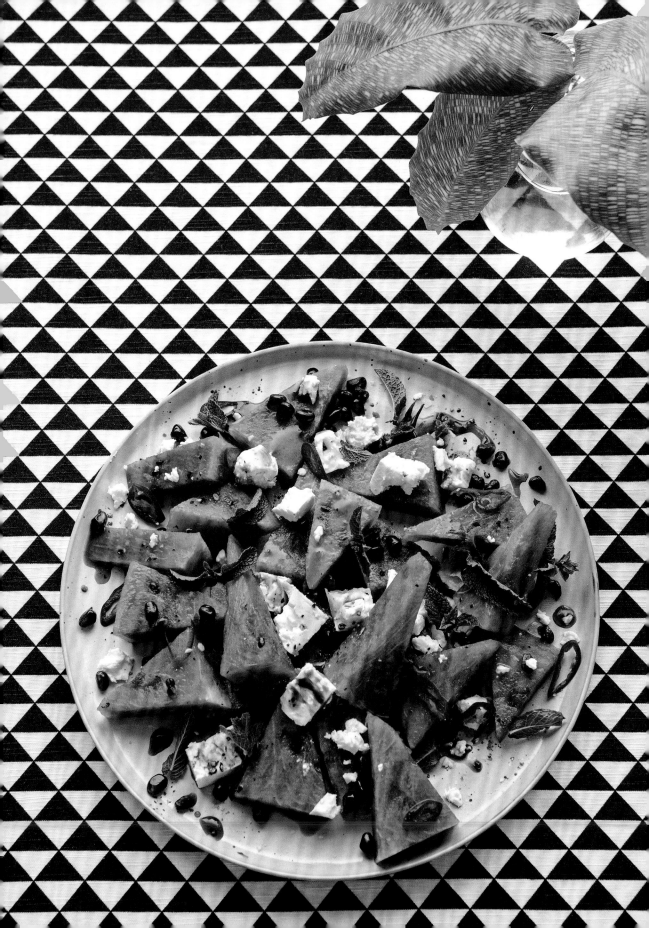

WATERMELON & FETA SALAD

The savoury fruit salad for your summer BBQ. Sort of a cross between a fruity salsa and fresh side salad, to me it's the taste of sunshine.

Serves 4

Prep time 10 minutes

600g (1lb 5oz) watermelon flesh, cut into wedges about 1.5cm (⅝in) thick

160g (5¾oz) feta cheese, cut into 2cm (¾in) chunks (or thereabouts)

250g (9oz) pomegranate seeds

2 red bird's-eye chillies, finely sliced

1 tbsp balsamic vinegar

1 tbsp clear honey

1 tbsp extra virgin olive oil

black pepper

PLACE the watermelon wedges in a large bowl, then add the feta, pomegranate seeds and chillies.

COMBINE the vinegar, honey and olive oil in a small bowl, then pour over the fruit and toss together.

SPRINKLE with a generous amount of black pepper and serve.

TOMACADO SALSA

One of my favourite flavour boosters, ever since I learned the recipe from my lovely landlady when running field research in Ecuador back in the early 2000s. So simple. So delicious.

Serves 4

Prep time 10 minutes, plus marinating

2 large avocados, stoned, peeled and cut into 2cm (¾in) chunks

350g (12oz) cherry tomatoes, halved

2 shallots, finely chopped

½ tbsp extra virgin olive oil

2 tbsp red wine vinegar or lime juice

salt and pepper

TOSS all the ingredients together in a non-reactive shallow bowl and leave to marinate for 15–20 minutes before serving.

KETCHUP

Making ketchup from scratch involves hours of simmering and a ton of sugar and salt. Alternatively, blitz a few store-cupboard staples together and have an almost 100 per cent fruit and veg condiment in minutes.

Serves 4

Prep time 5 minutes, plus soaking

50g (1¾oz) golden raisins

3 tbsp boiling water

2 tsp onion powder

2 tsp dried garlic granules

1 tsp mixed spice

200g (7oz) tomato purée

3 tbsp sherry vinegar

large pinch of salt, or to taste

PUT the golden raisins in a heatproof mug and pour in the measured water, which should cover them. Leave to soak for 10 minutes.

TIP the rehydrated fruit and soaking liquid into a food processor, add the remaining ingredients and blend to a smooth paste.

USE immediately or store the ketchup in an airtight container in the fridge for up to 1 week.

VARIATION

BBQ SAUCE

Make the ketchup as above, replacing the raisins with 50g (1¾oz) pitted **dates** and adding 1 tbsp **smoked paprika**, 1 tsp **liquid smoke** and 1 tsp **kecap manis** (sweet soy sauce) with all the other ingredients.

HARISSA CHILLI SAUCE

A fiery North African chilli sauce, based on a whole lot of veg. As delicious as it is versatile, making everything from sandwiches and salad to curries and soups extra tasty (and extra veg packed).

Serves 4
Prep time 10 minutes
Cook time 10 minutes

1 tbsp olive oil

150g (5½oz) cored, deseeded and chopped red pepper

150g (5½oz) chopped onion

4 red chillies, chopped

5 garlic cloves, minced

2 tsp ras el hanout (Moroccan spice mix)

2 tbsp tomato purée

2 tbsp lemon juice

½ tsp salt

HEAT the olive oil in a frying pan, add the red pepper, onion and chillies and fry for 10 minutes, or until the veg are soft and golden.

TRANSFER to a food processor with all the remaining ingredients and process until you have a smooth paste. Alternatively, pound together using a pestle and mortar.

SERVE warm or cold. Store the cooled harissa in an airtight container or jar in the fridge for up to 1 week.

FRESH MANGO CHUTNEY

This stuff is so good, I often make a double batch as I know it will likely all go in one meal (I have some very greedy mates as dinner guests) or I get to stuff some in sandwiches or scatter it on salads the next day.

Serves 4
Prep time 5 minutes
Cook time 17 minutes

1 tsp nigella seeds

1 tsp cumin seeds

½ tsp ground cardamom

pinch of salt

20g (¾oz) diced red bird's-eye chilli

50g (1¾oz) diced shallot

150ml (5fl oz) cider vinegar

250g (9oz) fresh mango flesh, diced

2 tbsp clear honey

2 tsp extra virgin olive oil

PLACE all the ingredients except the mango, honey and olive oil in a small frying pan and bring to the boil over a medium-high heat. Cook for 5 minutes until most of the vinegar has evaporated.

ADD the mango and honey and cook for another 10 minutes, stirring frequently.

TRANSFER to a food processor, add the olive oil and blitz briefly so the chutney stays slightly chunky.

SERVE immediately or keep the cooled chutney in a jar in the fridge for up to 2 weeks.

SAMBAL

It's kind of hard to describe sambal for those who haven't grown up with it. It's sort of halfway between a flavour-packed ketchup and a super-versatile curry paste. It's *the* go-to ingredient in South East Asia, both as a condiment to serve at the table and an indispensable ingredient to add instant flavour and depth to any dish you can imagine! Toss it in a pan while you are sautéeing any veg or meat, stir it into soups, stews and pasta sauces, or just use it like you would ketchup. As it's essentially 100 per cent veg, it counts towards your daily portions, too.

PORTIONS (2) PER SERVING

Serves 4
Prep time 10 minutes
Cook time 18–22 minutes

1 tbsp extra virgin olive oil

200g (7oz) finely diced onions

150g (5½oz) cored, deseeded and finely diced red pepper

2 large red chillies, finely diced

5 garlic cloves, minced

1 tsp brown sugar

1 thumb-sized piece of fresh root ginger, peeled and minced

1 tsp turmeric

1 tsp smoked paprika

2 heaped tsp yellow bean sauce (find this in your local Asian supermarket or online)

HEAT the olive oil in a frying pan, add the onions, red pepper, chillies, garlic, sugar and ginger and fry over a medium heat until the veg are completely softened and starting to turn golden brown. This will take about 15–20 minutes.

TIP in the remaining ingredients and cook for another minute or two.

SERVE warm or cold, either straight up, or, if you want to be really authentic, give it a few bashes using a pestle and mortar to turn it into a smooth paste.

USE immediately or store the cooled sambal in an airtight container or jar in the fridge for up to 1 week.

PRO TIP

Sambal will last a good week in the fridge, so I very often double or even triple this recipe so I always have some to hand.

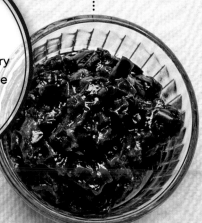

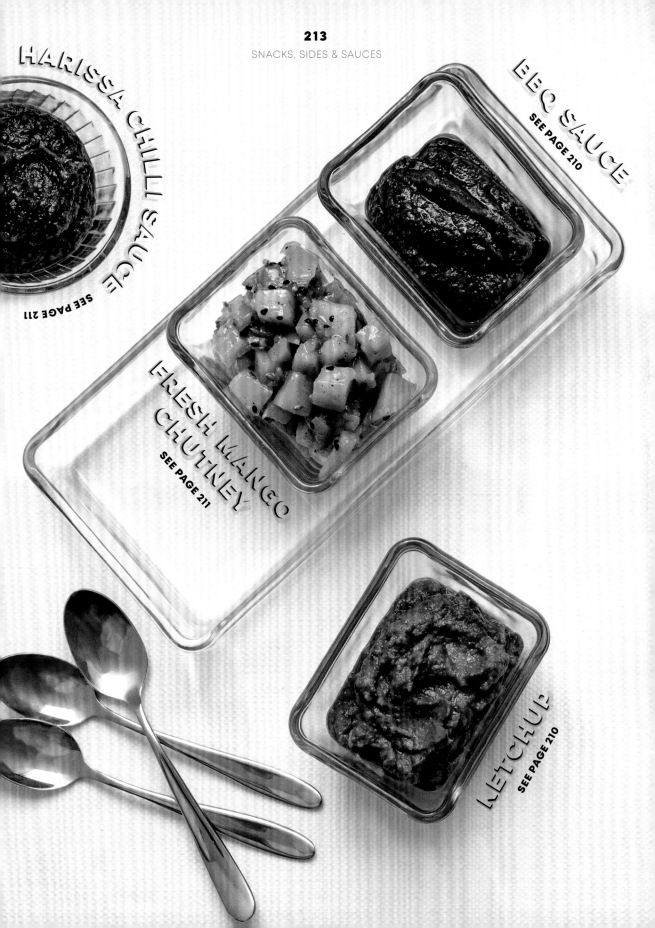

HARISSA CHILLI SAUCE
SEE PAGE 211

BBQ SAUCE
SEE PAGE 210

FRESH MANGO
CHUTNEY
SEE PAGE 211

KETCHUP
SEE PAGE 210

PUMPKIN DRESSING

I am forever looking for ways to sneak fruit and veg into everyday meals, and it turned out that one way is to blitz them into colourful, flavourful salad dressings (which also make great sauces, drizzles and dips). I first had this weird and wonderful concoction at, of all places, a motorway service station outside Osaka. This is my attempt to recreate (maybe even improve upon) this fresh, veggie-based dressing.

Serves 4

Prep time 5 minutes, plus infusing

200g (7oz) canned pumpkin purée
1 tbsp olive oil
½ tsp dried garlic granules
1 tsp clear honey
2 tbsp cider vinegar
2 tbsp water
½ tsp salt

MIX all the ingredients together in a large jug until smooth. Leave to stand for 10 minutes to allow the garlic to rehydrate and infuse.

USE immediately or store in a sealed jar in the fridge for up to 5 days.

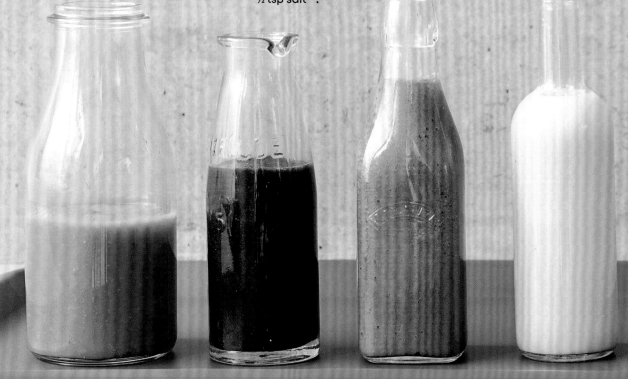

① ② ③

VARIATIONS

① BEETROOT DRESSING

Make the dressing as opposite, replacing the pumpkin with 200g (7oz) **cooked beetroot**, blitzed in a food processor.

② RASPBERRY DRESSING

Make the dressing as opposite, replacing the pumpkin with 200g (7oz) **fresh** or **frozen raspberries**, blitzed in a food processor.

③ MANGO DRESSING

Make the dressing as opposite, replacing the pumpkin with 200g (7oz) **fresh mango flesh**, blitzed in a food processor.

PICKLED CUCUMBER

Pickles don't normally count towards your daily fruit and veg portions due to their sky-high salt and sugar content. But this frankly ridiculously simple recipe avoids such high levels of salt and sugar and makes tasty, healthy veggie pickles that are ready to eat in just 30 minutes.

Serves 4
Prep time 5 minutes, plus pickling

200g (7oz) whole cucumber
300ml (10fl oz) white malt vinegar
1 tbsp caster sugar or granulated stevia (baking blend)
½ tsp chopped dill
½ tsp salt

SLICE the cucumber into long, thin ribbons using a vegetable peeler.

PACK the cucumber ribbons tightly into a medium Kilner jar, leaving as few gaps as possible.

ADD the remaining ingredients, then seal the jar and give it all a good shake. Your pickles will be ready to eat in 30 minutes, and can be stored for up to 2 weeks in the fridge.

VARIATIONS

PICKLED CAULIFLOWER

Make the pickled cauliflower using the method above, replacing the cucumber with 200g (7oz) **cauliflower florets** and the dill with ¼ tsp **turmeric**.

PICKLED CARROTS

Make the pickled carrots using the method above, replacing the cucumber with 200g (7oz) thinly sliced **carrots** and the dill with ½ tsp **caraway seeds**.

PICKLED JALAPEÑOS

Make the pickled jalapeños using the method above, replacing the cucumber with 200g (7oz) thinly sliced **fresh jalapeño chillies** and the dill with ½ tsp **coriander seeds**.

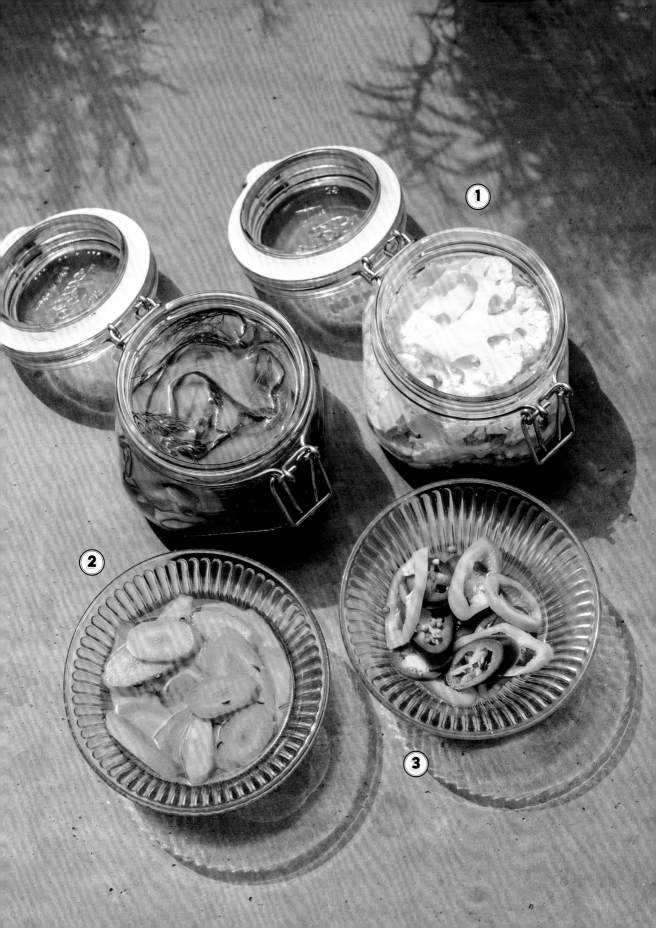

UK/US GLOSSARY

UK	US	UK	US
aubergine	eggplant	loaf tin	loaf pan
bacon rasher	bacon slice	mangetout	snow pea
baking paper	parchment paper	measuring jug	measuring cup
baking tray	baking sheet	minced beef	ground beef
BBQ	grill	mixed spice	apple pie spice
beetroot	beet	muslin	cheesecloth
bicarbonate of soda	baking soda		
black-eyed bean	black-eyed pea	orange pepper	orange bell pepper
black treacle	light molasses		
button mushroom	white mushroom	passata	puréed canned tomatoes
		pastry	dough
cake tin	cake pan	pickled cucumber	dill pickle
case (pastry)	shell	plain flour	all-purpose flour
casserole	Dutch oven	pollack	pollock
cavolo nero	Tuscan kale	pudding	dessert
chestnut mushroom	cremini mushroom	pulses	legumes
chopping board	cutting board		
chilli/chillies	chili/chiles	rapeseed oil	canola oil
chilli flakes	red pepper flakes	red pepper	red bell pepper
chips	French fries	rocket	arugula
clingfilm	plastic wrap		
cocoa powder	unsweetened cocoa powder	salad leaves	greens
		self-raising flour	self-rising flour
cornflour	cornstarch	semi-skimmed milk	reduced-fat milk
courgette	zucchini	shortcrust pastry	basic pie dough
crisps	potato chips	soya milk	soy milk
		spring onion	scallion
dark chocolate	semisweet chocolate	spud	potato
double cream	heavy cream	stick blender	immersion blender
		stock	broth
fast-action dried yeast	active dry yeast	stock cube	bouillon cube
		sultana	golden raisin
French bean	green bean	swede	rutabaga
fresh root ginger	fresh ginger	sweetcorn	corn
fridge	refrigerator		
frying pan	skillet	takeaway	takeout
full-fat milk	whole milk	tea towel	dish towel
		tomato purée	tomato paste
green pepper	green bell pepper		
grill	broiler	wholemeal flour	whole wheat flour
		wire rack	cooling rack
ice lolly	Popsicle		
icing sugar	confectioners' sugar	yellow pepper	yellow bell pepper
king prawn	jumbo shrimp		
kitchen foil	aluminum foil		
kitchen paper	paper towel		
knob of butter	piece of butter		

INDEX

ABOUT THE AUTHOR

James Wong is a Kew-trained botanist, science writer and broadcaster based in London. Graduating with a Master of Science degree in Ethnobotany in 2006, he pursued his key research interests of under-utilized crop species and traditional food systems through field work in rural Ecuador, Java and southern China.

He is the author of the best-selling books *Grow Your Own Drugs*, *Homegrown Revolution* and, for Mitchell Beazley, *RHS Grow for Flavour* (more than 60,000 copies sold) and *How to Eat Better* (more than 80,000 copies sold). He has presented BBC2's award-winning series *Grow Your Own Drugs* and co-presented, with Dr Michael Mosley, *The Secrets of Your Food* – a major BBC series on the science of food. He has a column in the *Observer* magazine.

With his obsession for food almost eclipsing his love of plants, James's small London garden serves as a testing station for all manner of crops from around the world.

THE NUTRITION CONSULTANTS

Rosie Saunt RD & Helen West RD, The Rooted Project: Nutrition and wellness is a booming industry with a critical problem at its core: anyone can call themselves a guru and dole out advice to the public. The Rooted Project is an award-winning enterprise founded by registered dietitians Rosie Saunt and Helen West. They love food, but hate nutri-nonsense and have made it their mission to empower people to choose what goes on their plates with the latest science-backed info.

ACKNOWLEDGEMENTS

You might only see one guy on the cover, but the truth is that creating a book is a great big team effort. And here's the part where I reveal the amazing people who helped make it happen, in no particular order.

Thanks to my wonderful team of foodies: Chris 'Ffitfood' Warlow, who helped me develop and test the recipes, accepting my last-minute changes and countless fussy demands, always with endless enthusiasm; and the lovely food stylists Sian Henley and Megan Davies, who calmly turned mountains of ingredients into sensational-looking dishes each shoot day, as if by magic, like fairy godmothers.

I am perpetually indebted to the super-talented photographer Jason Ingram and his assitant Jamie Murray for bringing the dishes to life. I can't believe it's the third book we've done together!

Speaking of long-time work buddies, a huge 'thank you' is in order to the wonderful art director Yasia Williams-Leedham, who not only has turned pages of raw text into a visual treat, but also has talked me down from more than one culinary ledge!

And let's not forget the science geeks, dietitians Rosie Saunt and Helen West of the Rooted Project, who helped me with the masses of research the book is based on and kept me on the straight and narrow. They are total foodie geniuses.

With my terrible grammar and spelling, this book just wouldn't be the same without Clare Churly, Jo Murray and Leanne Bryan, with their ridiculous gift for getting things right each and every time. Nor would the book look as good as it does without the creative attention of designer Geoff Fennell.

Finally, a very special thanks to my publisher Alison Starling, who gives me such a rare amount of creative freedom and support.

You guys are all wonderful!

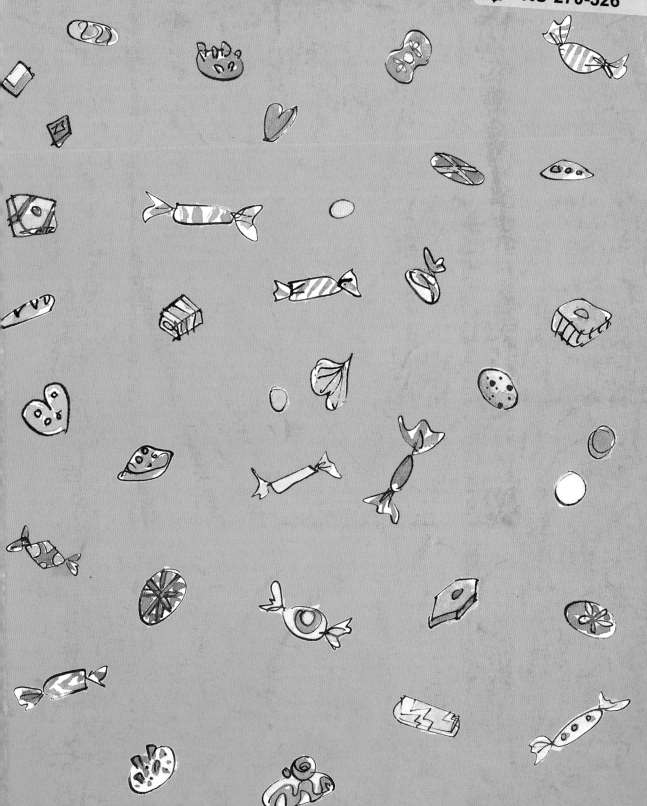

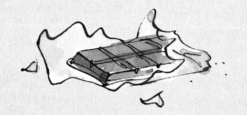

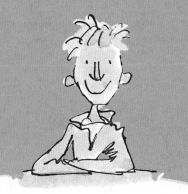

THIS BOOK BELONGS TO

. . . .

~ For Theo ~

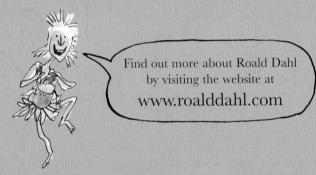

Find out more about Roald Dahl
by visiting the website at
www.roalddahl.com

PUFFIN BOOKS

Published by the Penguin Group

Penguin Books Ltd, 80 Strand, London WC2R 0RL, England

Penguin Group (USA) Inc., 375 Hudson Street, New York, New York 10014, USA

Penguin Group (Canada), 90 Eglinton Avenue East, Suite 700, Toronto, Ontario, Canada M4P 2Y3
(a division of Pearson Penguin Canada Inc.)

Penguin Ireland, 25 St Stephen's Green, Dublin 2, Ireland (a division of Penguin Books Ltd)

Penguin Group (Australia), 707 Collins Street, Melbourne, Victoria 3008, Australia
(a division of Pearson Australia Group Pty Ltd)

Penguin Books India Pvt Ltd, 11 Community Centre, Panchsheel Park, New Delhi – 110 017, India

Penguin Group (NZ), 67 Apollo Drive, Rosedale, Auckland 0632, New Zealand
(a division of Pearson New Zealand Ltd)

Penguin Books (South Africa) (Pty) Ltd, Block D, Rosebank Office Park, 181 Jan Smuts Avenue,
Parktown North, Gauteng 2193, South Africa

Penguin Books Ltd, Registered Offices: 80 Strand, London WC2R 0RL, England

puffinbooks.com

First published in the USA by Alfred A. Knopf, Inc., 1964
Published in Great Britain by George Allen & Unwin 1967
Published by Puffin Books 1973
Reissued with new illustrations 1995
Colour edition published by Viking 1997
Colour edition published by Puffin Books 2004
This edition published 2014
001

Filmset in Bembo and QuentinBlake
Made and printed in China

British Library Cataloguing in Publication Data
A CIP catalogue record for this book is available from the British Library

ISBN: 978–0–141–33437–0

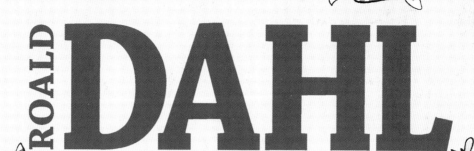

ROALD DAHL

ILLUSTRATED BY QUENTIN BLAKE

Charlie and the Chocolate Factory

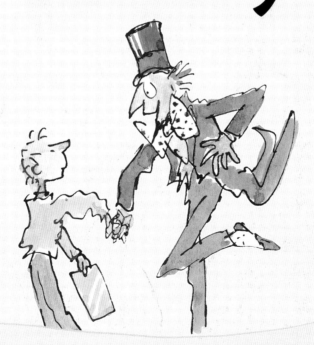

PUFFIN

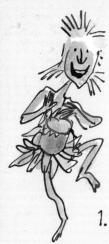

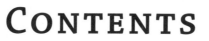

CONTENTS

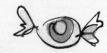

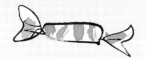

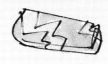

There are five children in this book:

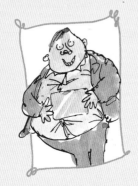

AUGUSTUS GLOOP
A greedy boy

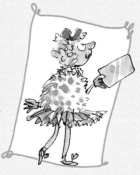

VERUCA SALT
A girl who is spoiled by her parents

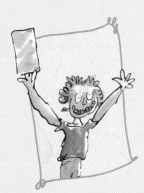

VIOLET BEAUREGARDE
A girl who chews gum all day long

MIKE TEAVEE
A boy who does nothing but watch television

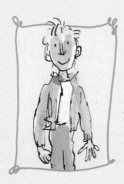

and

CHARLIE BUCKET
The hero

CHAPTER ONE
Here Comes Charlie

These two very old people are the father and mother of Mr Bucket. Their names are Grandpa Joe and Grandma Josephine.

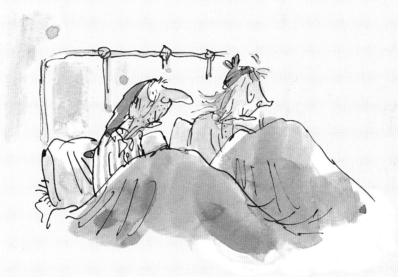

And *these* two very old people are the father and mother of Mrs Bucket. Their names are Grandpa George and Grandma Georgina.

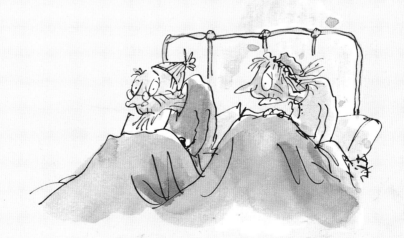

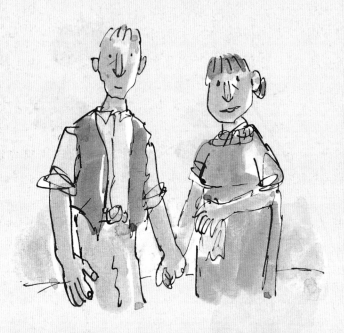

This is Mr Bucket. This is Mrs Bucket.

Mr and Mrs Bucket have a small boy whose name is Charlie Bucket.

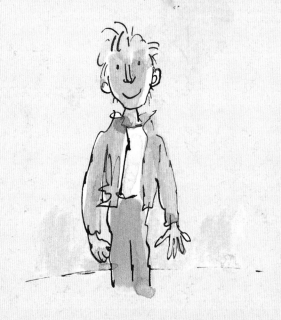

This is Charlie.

How d'you do? And how d'you do? And how d'you do again?

He is pleased to meet you.

Here Comes Charlie

The whole of this family – the six grown-ups (count them) and little Charlie Bucket – live together in a small wooden house on the edge of a great town.

The house wasn't nearly large enough for so many people, and life was extremely uncomfortable for them all. There were only two rooms in the place altogether, and there was only one bed. The bed was given to the four old grandparents because they were so old and tired. They were so tired, they never got out of it.

Grandpa Joe and Grandma Josephine on this side, Grandpa George and Grandma Georgina on this side.

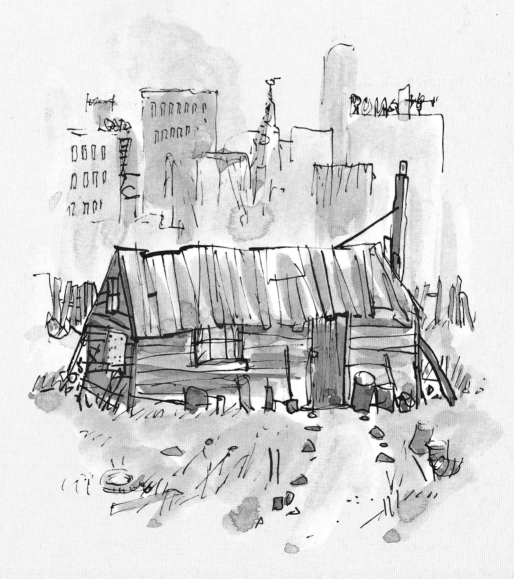

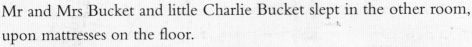

Mr and Mrs Bucket and little Charlie Bucket slept in the other room, upon mattresses on the floor.

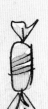

In the summertime, this wasn't too bad, but in the winter, freezing cold draughts blew across the floor all night long, and it was awful.

There wasn't any question of them being able to buy a better house – or even one more bed to sleep in. They were far too poor for that.

Mr Bucket was the only person in the family with a job. He worked in a toothpaste factory, where he sat all day long at a bench and screwed the little caps on to the tops of the tubes of toothpaste after the tubes had been filled. But a toothpaste cap-screwer is never paid very much money, and poor Mr Bucket, however hard he worked, and however fast he screwed on the caps, was never able to make enough to buy one half of the things that so large a family needed. There wasn't even enough money to buy proper food for them all. The only meals they could afford were bread and margarine for breakfast, boiled potatoes and cabbage for lunch, and cabbage soup for supper. Sundays were a bit better. They all looked forward to Sundays because then, although they had exactly the same, everyone was allowed a second helping.

The Buckets, of course, didn't starve, but every one of them – the two old grandfathers, the two old grandmothers, Charlie's father, Charlie's mother, and especially little Charlie himself – went about from morning till night with a horrible empty feeling in their tummies.

Charlie felt it worst of all. And although his father and mother often went without their own share of lunch or supper so that they could give it to him, it still wasn't nearly enough for a growing boy. He desperately wanted something more filling and satisfying than cabbage and cabbage soup. The one thing he longed for more than anything else was . . . CHOCOLATE.

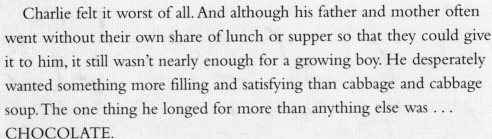

Walking to school in the mornings, Charlie could see great slabs of chocolate piled up high in the shop windows, and he would stop and stare and press his nose against the glass, his mouth watering like mad.

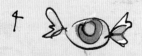

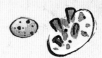
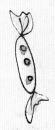

Many times a day, he would see other children taking bars of creamy chocolate out of their pockets and munching them greedily, and *that*, of course, was *pure* torture.

Only once a year, on his birthday, did Charlie Bucket ever get to taste a bit of chocolate. The whole family saved up their money for that special occasion, and when the great day arrived, Charlie was always presented with one small chocolate bar to eat all by himself. And each time he received it, on those marvellous birthday mornings, he would place it carefully in a small wooden box that he owned, and treasure it as though it were a bar of solid gold; and for the next few days, he would

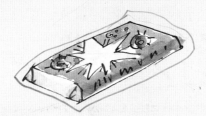

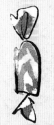

allow himself only to look at it, but never to touch it. Then at last, when he could stand it no longer, he would peel back a *tiny* bit of the paper wrapping at one corner to expose a *tiny* bit of chocolate, and then he would take a *tiny* nibble – just enough to allow the lovely sweet taste to spread out slowly over his tongue. The next day, he would take another tiny nibble, and so on, and so on. And in this way, Charlie would make his sixpenny bar of birthday chocolate last him for more than a month.

But I haven't yet told you about the one awful thing that tortured little Charlie, the lover of chocolate, more than *anything* else. This thing, for him, was far, far worse than seeing slabs of chocolate in the shop windows or watching other children munching bars of creamy chocolate right in front of him. It was the most terrible torturing thing you could imagine, and it was this:

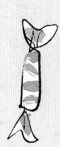

In the town itself, actually within *sight* of the house in which Charlie lived, there was an ENORMOUS CHOCOLATE FACTORY!

Just imagine that!

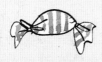

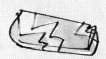

And it wasn't simply an ordinary enormous chocolate factory, either. It was the largest and most famous in the whole world! It was WONKA'S FACTORY, owned by a man called Mr Willy Wonka, the greatest inventor and maker of chocolates that there has ever been. And what a tremendous, marvellous place it was! It had huge iron gates leading into it, and a high wall surrounding it, and smoke belching from its chimneys, and strange whizzing sounds coming from deep inside it. And outside the walls, for half a mile around in every direction, the air was scented with the heavy rich smell of melting chocolate!

Twice a day, on his way to and from school, little Charlie Bucket had to walk right past the gates of the factory. And every time he went by, he would begin to walk very, very slowly, and he would hold his nose high in the air and take long deep sniffs of the gorgeous chocolatey smell all around him.

Oh, how he loved that smell!

And oh, how he wished he could go inside the factory and see what it was like!

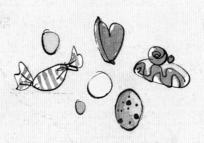

CHAPTER TWO

Mr Willy Wonka's Factory

In the evenings, after he had finished his supper of watery cabbage soup, Charlie always went into the room of his four grandparents to listen to their stories, and then afterwards to say good night.

Every one of these old people was over ninety. They were as shrivelled as prunes, and as bony as skeletons, and throughout the day, until Charlie made his appearance, they lay huddled in their one bed, two at either end, with nightcaps on to keep their heads warm, dozing the time away with nothing to do. But as soon as they heard the door opening, and heard Charlie's voice saying, 'Good evening, Grandpa Joe and Grandma Josephine, and Grandpa George and Grandma Georgina,' then all four of them would suddenly sit up, and their old wrinkled faces would light up with smiles of pleasure – and the talking would begin. For they loved this little boy. He was the only bright thing in their lives, and his evening visits were something that they looked forward to all day long. Often, Charlie's mother and father would come in as well, and stand by the door, listening to the stories that the old people told; and thus, for perhaps half an hour every night, this room would become a happy place, and the whole family would forget that it was hungry and poor.

One evening, when Charlie went in to see his grandparents, he said to them, 'Is it *really* true that Wonka's Chocolate Factory is the biggest in the world?'

'*True?*' cried all four of them at once. 'Of course it's true! Good heavens, didn't you know *that*? It's about *fifty* times as big as any other!'

'And is Mr Willy Wonka *really* the cleverest chocolate maker in the world?'

'My *dear* boy,' said Grandpa Joe, raising himself up a little higher on his pillow, 'Mr Willy Wonka is the most *amazing*, the most *fantastic*, the most *extraordinary* chocolate maker the world has ever seen! I thought *everybody* knew that!'

'I knew he was famous, Grandpa Joe, and I knew he was very clever . . .'

'*Clever!*' cried the old man. 'He's more than that! He's a *magician* with chocolate! He can make *anything* – anything he wants! Isn't that a fact, my dears?'

The other three old people nodded their heads slowly up and down, and said, '*Absolutely* true. *Just* as true as can be.'

And Grandpa Joe said, 'You mean to say I've never *told* you about Mr Willy Wonka and his factory?'

'Never,' answered little Charlie.

'Good heavens above! I don't know what's the matter with me!'

'Will you tell me now, Grandpa Joe, please?'

'I certainly will. Sit down beside me on the bed, my dear, and listen carefully.'

Grandpa Joe was the oldest of the four grandparents. He was ninety-six and a half, and that is just about as old as anybody can be. Like all extremely old people, he was delicate and weak, and throughout the day he spoke very little. But in the evenings, when Charlie, his beloved grandson, was in the room, he seemed in some marvellous way to grow quite young again. All his tiredness fell away from him, and he became as eager and excited as a young boy.

'Oh, what a man he is, this Mr Willy Wonka!' cried Grandpa Joe. 'Did you know, for example, that he has himself invented more than two hundred new kinds of chocolate bars, each with a different centre, each far sweeter and creamier and more delicious than anything the other chocolate factories can make!'

'Perfectly true!' cried Grandma Josephine. 'And he sends them to *all* the four corners of the earth! Isn't that so, Grandpa Joe?'

'It is, my dear, it is. And to all the kings and presidents of the world as well. But it isn't only chocolate bars that he makes. Oh, dear me, no! He has some really *fantastic* inventions up his sleeve, Mr Willy Wonka has! Did you know that he's invented a way of making chocolate ice cream so that it stays cold for hours and hours without being in the refrigerator? You can even leave it lying in the sun all morning on a hot day and it won't go runny!'

'But that's *impossible*!' said little Charlie, staring at his grandfather.

'Of course it's impossible!' cried Grandpa Joe. 'It's completely *absurd*! But Mr Willy Wonka has done it!'

'Quite right!' the others agreed, nodding their heads. 'Mr Wonka has done it.'

'And then again,' Grandpa Joe went on speaking very slowly now so that Charlie wouldn't miss a word, 'Mr Willy Wonka can make marshmallows that taste of violets, and rich caramels that change colour every ten seconds as you suck them, and little feathery sweets that melt away deliciously the moment you put them between your lips. He can make chewing-gum that never loses its taste, and sugar balloons that you can blow up to enormous sizes before you pop them with a pin and gobble them up. And, by a most secret method, he can make lovely blue birds' eggs with black spots on them, and when you put one of these in your mouth, it gradually gets smaller and smaller until suddenly there is nothing left except a tiny little pink sugary baby bird sitting on the tip of your tongue.'

Grandpa Joe paused and ran the point of his tongue slowly over his lips. 'It makes my mouth water just *thinking* about it,' he said.

'Mine, too,' said little Charlie. 'But *please* go on.'

While they were talking, Mr and Mrs Bucket, Charlie's mother and father, had come quietly into the room, and now both were standing just inside the door, listening.

'Tell Charlie about that crazy Indian prince,' said Grandma Josephine. 'He'd like to hear that.'

'You mean Prince Pondicherry?' said Grandpa Joe, and he began chuckling with laughter.

'*Completely* dotty!' said Grandpa George.

'But *very* rich,' said Grandma Georgina.

'What did he do?' asked Charlie eagerly.

'Listen,' said Grandpa Joe, 'and I'll tell you.'

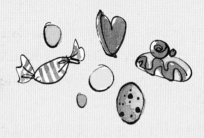

CHAPTER THREE

Mr Wonka and the Indian Prince

'Prince Pondicherry wrote a letter to Mr Willy Wonka,' said Grandpa Joe, 'and asked him to come all the way out to India and build him a colossal palace entirely out of chocolate.'

'Did Mr Wonka do it, Grandpa?'

'He did, indeed. And what a palace it was! It had one hundred rooms, and *everything* was made of either dark or light chocolate! The bricks were chocolate, and the cement holding them together was chocolate, and the windows were chocolate, and all the walls and ceilings were made of chocolate, so were the carpets and the pictures and the furniture and the beds; and when you turned on the taps in the bathroom, hot chocolate came pouring out.

'When it was all finished, Mr Wonka said to Prince Pondicherry, "I warn you, though, it won't last very long, so you'd better start eating it right away."

' "Nonsense!" shouted the Prince. "I'm not going to eat my palace! I'm not even going to nibble the staircase or lick the walls! I'm going to *live* in it!"

'But Mr Wonka was right, of course, because soon after this, there came a very hot day with a boiling sun, and the whole palace began to melt, and then it sank slowly to the ground, and the crazy prince, who was dozing in the living room at the time, woke up to find himself swimming around in a huge brown sticky lake of chocolate.'

Little Charlie sat very still on the edge of the bed, staring at his grandfather.

Charlie's face was bright, and his eyes were stretched so wide you could see the whites all around. 'Is all this *really* true?' he asked. 'Or are you pulling my leg?'

'It's true!' cried all four of the old people at once. 'Of course it's true! Ask anyone you like!'

'And I'll tell you something else that's true,' said Grandpa Joe, and now he leaned closer to Charlie, and lowered his voice to a soft, secret whisper. '*Nobody . . . ever . . . comes . . . out!*'

'Out of where?' asked Charlie.

'*And . . . nobody . . . ever . . . goes . . . in!*'

'In *where*?' cried Charlie.

'Wonka's factory, of course!'

'Grandpa, what *do* you mean?'

'I mean *workers*, Charlie.'

'Workers?'

'All factories,' said Grandpa Joe, 'have workers streaming in and out of the gates in the mornings and evenings – except Wonka's! Have *you* ever seen a single person going into that place – or coming out?'

Little Charlie looked slowly around at each of the four old faces, one after the other, and they all looked back at him. They were friendly smiling faces, but they were also quite serious. There was no sign of joking or leg-pulling on any of them.

'Well? Have *you*?' asked Grandpa Joe.

'I . . . I really don't know, Grandpa,' Charlie stammered. 'Whenever I walk past the factory, the gates seem to be closed.'

'Exactly!' said Grandpa Joe.

'But there *must* be people working there . . .'

'Not *people*, Charlie. Not *ordinary* people, anyway.'

'Then who?' cried Charlie.

'Ah-ha . . . That's it, you see . . . That's another of Mr Willy Wonka's clevernesses.'

'Charlie, dear,' Mrs Bucket called out from where she was standing by the door, 'it's time for bed. That's enough for tonight.'

'But, Mother, I *must* hear . . .'

'Tomorrow, my darling . . .'

'That's right,' said Grandpa Joe, 'I'll tell you the rest of it tomorrow evening.'

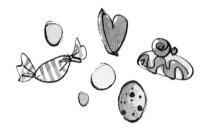

CHAPTER FOUR
The Secret Workers

The next evening, Grandpa Joe went on with his story.

'You see, Charlie,' he said, 'not so very long ago there used to be thousands of people working in Mr Willy Wonka's factory. Then one day, all of a sudden, Mr Wonka had to ask *every single one of them* to leave, to go home, never to come back.'

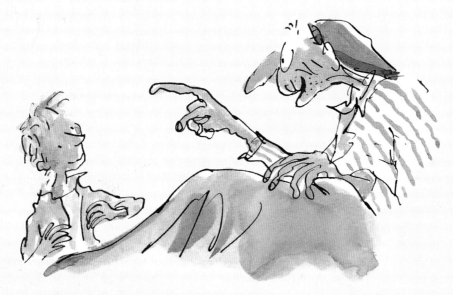

'But why?' asked Charlie.

'Because of spies.'

'Spies?'

'Yes. All the other chocolate makers, you see, had begun to grow jealous of the wonderful sweets that Mr Wonka was making, and they started sending in spies to steal his secret recipes. The spies took jobs in the Wonka factory, pretending that they were ordinary workers, and while they were there, each one of them found out exactly how a certain special thing was made.'

'And did they go back to their own factories and tell?' asked Charlie.

'They must have,' answered Grandpa Joe, 'because soon after that, Fickelgruber's factory started making an ice cream that would never melt, even in the hottest sun. Then Mr Prodnose's factory came out with a chewing-gum that never lost its flavour however much you chewed it. And then Mr Slugworth's factory began making sugar balloons that you could blow up to huge sizes before you popped them with a pin and gobbled them up. And so on, and so on. And Mr Willy Wonka tore his beard and shouted, "This is terrible! I shall be ruined! There are spies everywhere! I shall have to close the factory!" '

'But he didn't do that!' Charlie said.

'Oh, yes he did. He told *all* the workers that he was sorry, but they would have to go home. Then, he shut the main gates and fastened them with a chain. And suddenly, Wonka's giant chocolate factory became silent and deserted. The chimneys stopped smoking, the machines stopped whirring, and from then on, not a single chocolate or sweet was made. Not a soul went in or out, and even Mr Willy Wonka himself disappeared completely.

'Months and months went by,' Grandpa Joe went on, 'but still the factory remained closed. And everybody said, "Poor Mr Wonka. He was so nice. And he made such marvellous things. But he's finished now. It's all over."

'Then something astonishing happened. One day, early in the morning, thin columns of white smoke were seen to be coming out of the tops of the tall chimneys of the factory! People in the town stopped and stared. "What's going on?" they cried. "Someone's lit the furnaces! Mr Wonka must be opening up again!" They ran to the gates, expecting

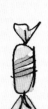

to see them wide open and Mr Wonka standing there to welcome his workers back.

'But no! The great iron gates were still locked and chained as securely as ever, and Mr Wonka was nowhere to be seen.

' "But the factory *is* working!" the people shouted. "Listen! You can hear the machines! They're all whirring again! And you can smell the smell of melting chocolate in the air!" '

Grandpa Joe leaned forward and laid a long bony finger on Charlie's knee, and he said softly, 'But most mysterious of all, Charlie, were the shadows in the windows of the factory. The people standing on the street outside could see small dark shadows moving about behind the frosted glass windows.'

'Shadows of whom?' said Charlie quickly.

'That's exactly what everybody else wanted to know.

' "The place is full of workers!" the people shouted. "But nobody's gone in! The gates are locked! It's crazy! Nobody ever comes out, either!"

'But there was no question at all,' said Grandpa Joe, 'that the factory was running. And it's gone on running ever since, for these last ten years. What's more, the chocolates and sweets it's been turning out have become more fantastic and delicious all the time. And of course now when Mr Wonka invents some new and wonderful sweet, neither Mr Fickelgruber nor Mr Prodnose nor Mr Slugworth nor anybody else is able to copy it. No spies can go into the factory to find out how it is made.'

'But Grandpa, *who*,' cried Charlie, '*who* is Mr Wonka using to do all the work in the factory?'

'Nobody knows, Charlie.'

'But that's *absurd*! Hasn't someone asked Mr Wonka?'

'Nobody sees him any more. He never comes out. The only things that come out of that place are chocolates and sweets. They come out through a special trap door in the wall, all packed and addressed, and they are picked up every day by Post Office trucks.'

'But Grandpa, what *sort* of people are they that work in there?'

'My dear boy,' said Grandpa Joe, 'that is one of the great mysteries of the chocolate-making world. We know only one thing about them. They are very small. The faint shadows that sometimes appear behind the windows, especially late at night when the lights are on, are those of *tiny* people, people no taller than my knee . . .'

'There aren't any such people,' Charlie said.

Just then, Mr Bucket, Charlie's father, came into the room. He was home from the toothpaste factory, and he was waving an evening newspaper rather excitedly. 'Have you heard the news?' he cried. He held up the paper so that they could see the huge headline. The headline said:

WONKA FACTORY TO BE OPENED AT LAST TO LUCKY FEW

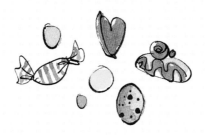

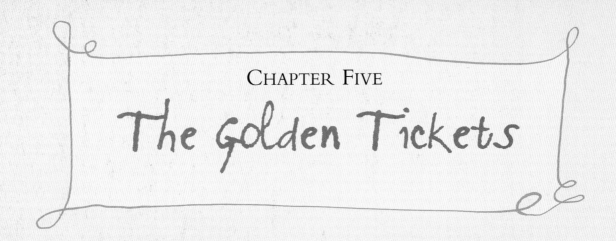

CHAPTER FIVE

The Golden Tickets

'You mean people are actually going to be allowed to go inside the factory?' cried Grandpa Joe. 'Read us what it says – quickly!'

'All right,' said Mr Bucket, smoothing out the newspaper. 'Listen.'

Evening Bulletin

Mr Willy Wonka, the confectionery genius whom nobody has seen for the last ten years, sent out the following notice today:

I, Willy Wonka, have decided to allow five children – just *five*, mind you, and no more – to visit my factory this year. These lucky five will be shown around personally by me, and they will be allowed to see all the secrets and the magic of my factory. Then, at the end of the tour, as a special present, all of them will be given enough chocolates and sweets to last them for the rest of their lives! So watch out for the Golden Tickets! Five Golden Tickets have been printed on golden paper, and these five Golden Tickets have been hidden underneath the ordinary wrapping paper of five ordinary bars of chocolate. These five chocolate bars may be anywhere – in any shop in any street in any town in any country in the world – upon any counter where Wonka's Sweets are sold. And the five lucky finders of these five Golden Tickets are the *only* ones who will be allowed to visit my factory and see what it's like *now* inside! Good luck to you all, and happy hunting! (Signed Willy Wonka.)

'The man's dotty!' muttered Grandma Josephine.

'He's brilliant!' cried Grandpa Joe. 'He's a magician! Just imagine what will happen now! The whole world will be searching for those Golden Tickets! Everyone will be buying Wonka's chocolate bars in the hope of finding one! He'll sell more than ever before! Oh, how exciting it would be to find one!'

'And all the chocolate and sweets that you could eat for the rest of your life – *free*!' said Grandpa George. 'Just imagine that!'

'They'd have to deliver them in a truck!' said Grandma Georgina.

'It makes me quite ill to think of it,' said Grandma Josephine.

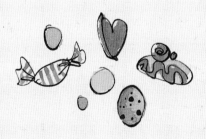

'Nonsense!' cried Grandpa Joe. 'Wouldn't it be *something*, Charlie, to open a bar of chocolate and see a Golden Ticket glistening inside!'

'It certainly would, Grandpa. But there isn't a hope,' Charlie said sadly. 'I only get one bar a year.'

'You never know, darling,' said Grandma Georgina. 'It's your birthday next week. You have as much chance as anybody else.'

'I'm afraid that simply isn't true,' said Grandpa George. 'The kids who are going to find the Golden Tickets are the ones who can afford to buy bars of chocolate every day. Our Charlie gets only one a year. There isn't a hope.'

CHAPTER SIX

The First Two Finders

The very next day, the first Golden Ticket was found. The finder was a boy called Augustus Gloop, and Mr Bucket's evening newspaper carried a large picture of him on the front page. The picture showed a nine-year-old boy who was so enormously fat he looked as though he had been blown up with a powerful pump. Great flabby folds of fat bulged out from every part of his body, and his face was like a monstrous ball of dough with two small greedy curranty eyes peering out upon the world. The town in which Augustus Gloop lived, the newspaper said, had gone wild with excitement over their hero. Flags were flying from all the windows, children had been given a holiday from school, and a parade was being organized in honour of the famous youth.

'I just *knew* Augustus would find a Golden Ticket,' his mother had told the newspapermen. 'He eats *so many* bars of chocolate a day that it was almost *impossible* for him *not* to find one. Eating is his hobby, you know. That's *all* he's interested in. But still, that's better than being a *hooligan* and shooting off *zip guns* and things like that in his spare time, isn't it? And what I always say is, he wouldn't go on eating like he does unless he *needed* nourishment, would he? It's all *vitamins*, anyway. What a *thrill* it will be for him to visit Mr Wonka's marvellous factory! We're just as *proud* as anything!'

'What a revolting woman,' said Grandma Josephine.

'And what a repulsive boy,' said Grandma Georgina.

'Only four Golden Tickets left,' said Grandpa George. 'I wonder who'll get *those*.'

And now the whole country, indeed, the whole world, seemed suddenly to be caught up in a mad chocolate-buying spree, everybody searching frantically for those precious remaining tickets. Fully grown women were seen going into sweet shops and buying ten Wonka bars at a time, then tearing off the wrappers on the spot and peering eagerly underneath for a glint of golden paper. Children were taking hammers and smashing their piggy banks and running out to the shops with handfuls of money. In one city, a famous gangster robbed a bank of a thousand pounds and spent the whole lot on Wonka bars that same afternoon. And when the police entered his house to arrest him, they found him sitting on the floor amidst mountains of chocolate, ripping off the wrappers with the blade of a long dagger. In far-off Russia, a woman called Charlotte Russe claimed to have found the second ticket, but it turned out to be a clever fake. The famous English scientist, Professor Foulbody, invented a machine which would tell you at once, without opening the wrapper of a bar of chocolate, whether or not there was a Golden Ticket hidden underneath it. The machine had a mechanical arm that shot out with tremendous force and grabbed hold of anything that had the slightest bit of gold inside it, and for a moment, it looked like the answer to everything. But unfortunately, while the Professor was showing off the machine to the public at the sweet counter of a large department store, the mechanical arm shot out and made a grab for the gold filling in the back tooth of a duchess who was standing near by. There was an ugly scene, and the machine was smashed by the crowd.

Suddenly, on the day before Charlie Bucket's birthday, the newspapers announced that the second Golden Ticket had been found. The lucky person was a small girl called Veruca Salt who lived with her rich parents in a great city far away. Once again Mr Bucket's evening newspaper carried a big picture of the finder. She was sitting between her beaming father and mother in the living room of their house, waving the Golden Ticket above her head, and grinning from ear to ear.

Veruca's father, Mr Salt, had eagerly explained to the newspapermen exactly how the ticket was found. 'You see, boys,' he had said, 'as soon as

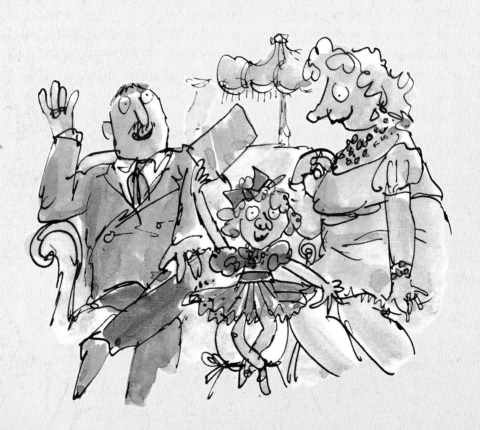

my little girl told me that she simply *had* to have one of those Golden Tickets, I went out into the town and started buying up all the Wonka bars I could lay my hands on. *Thousands* of them, I must have bought. *Hundreds* of thousands! Then I had them loaded on to trucks and sent directly to my own factory. I'm in the peanut business, you see, and I've got about a hundred women working for me over at my place, shelling peanuts for roasting and salting. That's what they do all day long, those women, they sit there shelling peanuts. So I says to them, "Okay, girls," I says, "from now on, you can stop shelling peanuts and start shelling the wrappers off these chocolate bars instead!" And they did. I had every worker in the place yanking the paper off those bars of chocolate full speed ahead from morning till night.

'But three days went by, and we had no luck. Oh, it was terrible! My little Veruca got more and more upset each day, and every time I went home she would scream at me, "*Where's my Golden Ticket! I want my Golden Ticket!*" And she would lie for hours on the floor, kicking and yelling in the most disturbing way. Well, I just hated to see my little girl feeling unhappy like that, so I vowed I would keep up the search until I'd got her what she wanted. Then suddenly . . . on the evening of the fourth day, one of my women workers yelled, "I've got it! A Golden Ticket!" And I said, "Give it to me, quick!" and she did, and I rushed it home and gave it to my darling Veruca, and now she's all smiles, and we have a happy home once again.'

'That's even worse than the fat boy,' said Grandma Josephine.

'She needs a really good spanking,' said Grandma Georgina.

'I don't think the girl's father played it quite fair, Grandpa, do you?' Charlie murmured.

'He spoils her,' Grandpa Joe said. 'And no good can ever come from spoiling a child like that, Charlie, you mark my words.'

'Come to bed, my darling,' said Charlie's

mother. 'Tomorrow's your birthday, don't forget that, so I expect you'll be up early to open your present.'

'A Wonka chocolate bar!' cried Charlie. 'It is a Wonka bar, isn't it?'

'Yes, my love,' his mother said. 'Of course it is.'

'Oh, wouldn't it be wonderful if I found the third Golden Ticket inside it?' Charlie said.

'Bring it in here when you get it,' Grandpa Joe said. 'Then we can all watch you taking off the wrapper.'

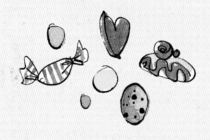

CHAPTER SEVEN
Charlie's Birthday

'Happy birthday!' cried the four old grandparents, as Charlie came into their room early the next morning.

Charlie smiled nervously and sat down on the edge of the bed. He was holding his present, his only present, very carefully in his two hands. WONKA'S WHIPPLE-SCRUMPTIOUS FUDGEMALLOW DELIGHT, it said on the wrapper.

The four old people, two at either end of the bed, propped themselves up on their pillows and stared with anxious eyes at the bar of chocolate in Charlie's hands.

Mr and Mrs Bucket came in and stood at the foot of the bed, watching Charlie.

The room became silent. Everybody was waiting now for Charlie to start opening his present. Charlie looked down at the bar of chocolate. He ran his fingers slowly back and forth along the length of it, stroking it lovingly, and the shiny paper wrapper made little sharp crackly noises in the quiet room.

Then Mrs Bucket said gently, 'You mustn't be too disappointed, my darling, if you don't find what you're looking for underneath that wrapper. You really can't expect to be as lucky as all that.'

'She's quite right,' Mr Bucket said.

Charlie didn't say anything.

'After all,' Grandma Josephine said, 'in the whole wide world there are only three tickets left to be found.'

'The thing to remember,' Grandma Georgina said, 'is that whatever happens, you'll still have the bar of chocolate.'

'Wonka's Whipple-Scrumptious Fudgemallow Delight!' cried Grandpa George. 'It's the best of them all! You'll just *love* it!'

'Yes,' Charlie whispered. 'I know.'

'Just forget all about those Golden Tickets and enjoy the chocolate,' Grandpa Joe said. 'Why don't you do that?'

They all knew it was ridiculous to expect this one poor little bar of chocolate to have a magic ticket inside it, and they were trying as gently and as kindly as they could to prepare Charlie for the disappointment. But there was one other thing that the grown-ups also knew, and it was this: that however *small* the chance might be of striking lucky, *the chance was there*.

The chance *had* to be there.

This particular bar of chocolate had as much chance as any other of having a Golden Ticket.

And that was why all the grandparents and parents in the room were actually just as tense and excited as Charlie was, although they were pretending to be very calm.

'You'd better go ahead and open it up, or you'll be late for school,' Grandpa Joe said.

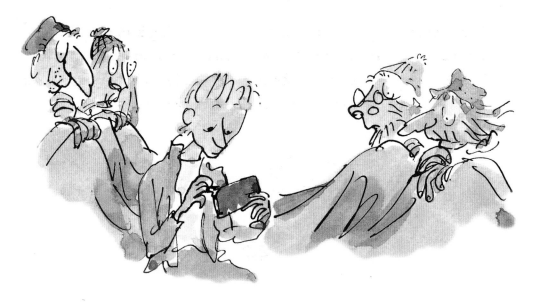

Charlie's Birthday

'You might as well get it over with,' Grandpa George said.

'Open it, my dear,' Grandma Georgina said. 'Please open it. You're making me jumpy.'

Very slowly, Charlie's fingers began to tear open one small corner of the wrapping paper.

The old people in the bed all leaned forward, craning their scraggy necks.

Then suddenly, as though he couldn't bear the suspense any longer, Charlie tore the wrapper right down the middle . . . and on to his lap, there fell . . . a light-brown creamy-coloured bar of chocolate.

There was no sign of a Golden Ticket anywhere.

'Well – that's *that*!' said Grandpa Joe brightly. 'It's just what we expected.'

Charlie looked up. Four kind old faces were watching him intently from the bed. He smiled at them, a small sad smile, and then he shrugged his shoulders and picked up the chocolate bar and held it out to his mother, and said, 'Here, Mother, have a bit. We'll share it. I want everybody to taste it.'

'Certainly not!' his mother said.

And the others all cried, 'No, no! We wouldn't dream of it! It's *all* yours!'

'*Please*,' begged Charlie, turning round and offering it to Grandpa Joe.

But neither he nor anyone else would take even a tiny bit.

'It's time to go to school, my darling,' Mrs Bucket said, putting an arm around Charlie's skinny shoulders. 'Come on, or you'll be late.'

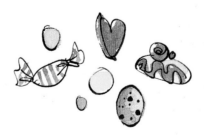

CHAPTER EIGHT
Two More Golden Tickets Found

That evening, Mr Bucket's newspaper announced the finding of not only the third Golden Ticket, but the fourth as well. **TWO GOLDEN TICKETS FOUND TODAY**, screamed the headlines. **ONLY ONE MORE LEFT**.

'All right,' said Grandpa Joe, when the whole family was gathered in the old people's room after supper, 'let's hear who found them.'

'The third ticket,' read Mr Bucket, holding the newspaper up close to his face because his eyes were bad and he couldn't afford glasses, 'the third ticket was found by a Miss Violet Beauregarde. There was great excitement in the Beauregarde household when our reporter arrived to interview the lucky young lady – cameras were clicking and flashbulbs were flashing and people were pushing and jostling and trying to get a bit closer to the famous girl. And the famous girl was standing on a chair in the living room waving the Golden Ticket madly at arm's length as though she were flagging a taxi. She was talking very fast and very loudly to everyone, but it was not easy to hear all that she said because she was chewing so ferociously upon a piece of gum at the same time.

' "I'm a gum chewer, normally," she shouted, "but when I heard about these ticket things of Mr Wonka's, I gave up gum and started on chocolate bars in the hope of striking lucky. *Now*, of course, I'm back on gum. I just *adore* gum. I can't do without it. I munch it all day long except for a few minutes at mealtimes when I take it out and stick it behind my ear for safekeeping. To tell you the truth, I simply wouldn't feel *comfortable* if I didn't have that little wedge of gum to chew on every moment of the day, I really wouldn't. My mother says it's not ladylike and it looks ugly to see a girl's jaws going up and down like mine do all the time, but I don't agree. And who's she to criticize, anyway, because if you ask me, I'd say that *her* jaws are going up and down almost as much as mine are just from *yelling* at me every minute of the day."

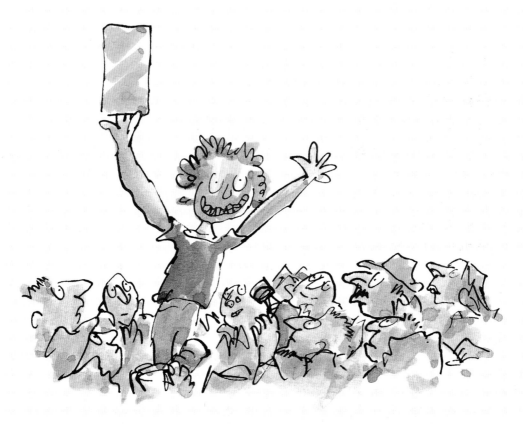

' "Now, Violet," Mrs Beauregarde said from a far corner of the room where she was standing on the piano to avoid being trampled by the mob.

' "All right, Mother, keep your hair on!" Miss Beauregarde shouted. "And now," she went on, turning to the reporters again, "it may interest you to know that this piece of gum I'm chewing right at this moment is one I've been working on for over *three months solid*. That's a record, that is. It's beaten the record held by my best friend, Miss Cornelia Prinzmetel. And was she furious! It's my most treasured possession now, this piece of gum is. At night-time, I just stick it on the end of the bedpost, and it's as good as ever in the mornings – a bit hard at first, maybe, but it soon softens up again after I've given it a few good chews. Before I started chewing for the world record, I used to change my piece of gum once a day. I used to do it in our lift on the way home from school. Why the lift? Because I liked sticking the gooey piece that I'd just finished with on to one of the control buttons. Then the next person who came along and pressed the button got my old gum on the end of his or her finger. Ha-ha! And what a racket they kicked up, some of them. You get the best results with women who have expensive gloves on. Oh yes, I'm thrilled to be going to Mr Wonka's factory. And I understand that afterwards he's going to give me enough gum to last me for the rest of my whole life. Whoopee! Hooray!" '

'*Beastly* girl,' said Grandma Josephine.

'Despicable!' said Grandma Georgina. 'She'll come to a sticky end one day, chewing all that gum, you see if she doesn't.'

'And who got the fourth Golden Ticket?' Charlie asked.

'Now, let me see,' said Mr Bucket, peering at the newspaper again. 'Ah yes, here we are. The fourth Golden Ticket,' he read, 'was found by a boy called Mike Teavee.'

'Another bad lot, I'll be bound,' muttered Grandma Josephine.

'Don't interrupt, Grandma,' said Mrs Bucket.

'The Teavee household,' said Mr Bucket, going on with his reading, 'was crammed, like all the others, with excited visitors when our reporter arrived, but young Mike Teavee, the lucky winner, seemed extremely annoyed by the whole business. "Can't you fools see I'm watching television?" he said angrily. "I wish you wouldn't interrupt!"

'The nine-year-old boy was seated before an enormous television set, with his eyes glued to

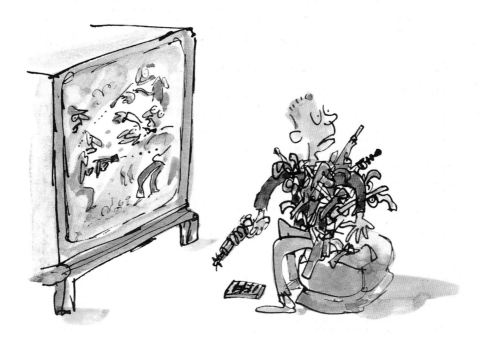

the screen, and he was watching a film in which one bunch of gangsters was shooting up another bunch of gangsters with machine guns. Mike Teavee himself had no less than eighteen toy pistols of various sizes hanging from belts around his body, and every now and again he would leap up into the air and fire off half a dozen rounds from one or another of these weapons.

' "Quiet!" he shouted, when someone tried to ask him a question. "Didn't I *tell* you not to interrupt! This show's an absolute whiz-banger! It's terrific! I watch it every day. I watch all of them every day, even the rotten ones, where there's no shooting. I like the gangsters best. They're terrific, those gangsters! Especially when they start pumping each other full of lead, or flashing the old stilettos, or giving each other the one-two-three with their knuckledusters! Gosh, what wouldn't I give to be doing that myself! It's the *life*, I tell you! It's terrific!" '

'That's quite enough!' snapped Grandma Josephine. 'I can't *bear* to listen to it!'

31

'Nor me,' said Grandma Georgina. 'Do *all* children behave like this nowadays – like these brats we've been hearing about?'

'Of course not,' said Mr Bucket, smiling at the old lady in the bed. 'Some do, of course. In fact, quite a lot of them do. But not *all*.'

'And now there's only *one ticket left*!' said Grandpa George.

'Quite so,' sniffed Grandma Georgina. 'And just as sure as I'll be having cabbage soup for supper tomorrow, that ticket'll go to some nasty little beast who doesn't deserve it!'

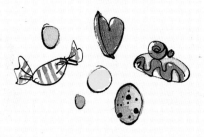

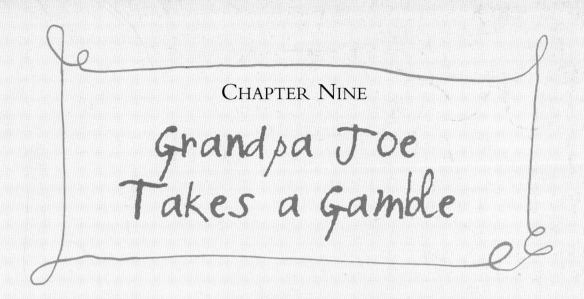

CHAPTER NINE

Grandpa Joe Takes a Gamble

The next day, when Charlie came home from school and went in to see his grandparents, he found that only Grandpa Joe was awake. The other three were all snoring loudly.

'Ssshh!' whispered Grandpa Joe, and he beckoned Charlie to come closer. Charlie tiptoed over and stood beside the bed. The old man gave Charlie a sly grin, and then he started rummaging under his pillow with one hand; and when the hand came out again, there was an ancient leather purse clutched in the fingers. Under cover of the bedclothes, the old man opened the purse and tipped it upside down. Out fell a single silver sixpence. 'It's my secret hoard,' he whispered. 'The others don't know I've got it. And now, you and I are going to have one more fling at finding that last ticket. How about it, eh? But you'll have to help me.'

'Are you *sure* you want to spend your money on that, Grandpa?' Charlie whispered.

'Of course I'm sure!' spluttered the old man excitedly. 'Don't stand there arguing! I'm as keen as you are to find that ticket! Here – take the money and run down the street to the nearest shop and buy the first Wonka bar you see and bring it straight back to me, and we'll open it together.'

Charlie took the little silver coin, and slipped quickly out of the room. In five minutes, he was back.

'Have you got it?' whispered Grandpa Joe, his eyes shining with excitement.

Charlie nodded and held out the bar of chocolate. WONKA'S NUTTY CRUNCH SURPRISE, it said on the wrapper.

'Good!' the old man whispered, sitting up in the bed and rubbing his hands. 'Now – come over here and sit close to me and we'll open it together. Are you ready?'

'Yes,' Charlie said. 'I'm ready.'

'All right. You tear off the first bit.'

'No,' Charlie said, 'you paid for it. You do it all.'

The old man's fingers were trembling most terribly as they fumbled with the wrapper. 'We don't have a hope, really,' he whispered, giggling a bit. 'You do know we don't have a hope, don't you?'

'Yes,' Charlie said. 'I know that.'

They looked at each other, and both started giggling nervously.

'Mind you,' said Grandpa Joe, 'there is just that *tiny* chance that it *might* be the one, don't you agree?'

'Yes,' Charlie said. 'Of course. Why don't you open it, Grandpa?'

'All in good time, my boy, all in good time. Which end do you think I ought to open first?'

'That corner. The one furthest from you. Just tear off a *tiny* bit, but not quite enough for us to see anything.'

'Like that?' said the old man.

'Yes. Now a little bit more.'

'You finish it,' said Grandpa Joe. 'I'm too nervous.'

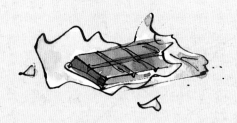

'No, Grandpa. You must do it yourself.'

'Very well, then. Here goes.' He tore off the wrapper.

They both stared at what lay underneath. It was a bar of chocolate – nothing more.

All at once, they both saw the funny side of the whole thing, and they burst into peals of laughter.

'What on earth's going on!' cried Grandma Josephine, waking up suddenly.

'Nothing,' said Grandpa Joe. 'You go on back to sleep.'

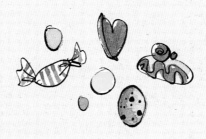

CHAPTER TEN

The Family Begins to Starve

During the next two weeks, the weather turned very cold. First came the snow. It began very suddenly one morning just as Charlie Bucket was getting dressed for school. Standing by the window, he saw the huge flakes drifting slowly down out of an icy sky that was the colour of steel.

By evening, it lay four feet deep around the tiny house, and Mr Bucket had to dig a path from the front door to the road.

After the snow, there came a freezing gale that blew for days and days without stopping. And oh, how bitter cold it was! Everything that Charlie touched seemed to be made of ice, and each time he stepped outside the door, the wind was like a knife on his cheek.

Inside the house, little jets of freezing air came rushing in through the sides of the windows and under the doors, and there was no place to go to escape them. The four old ones lay silent and huddled in their bed, trying to keep the cold out of their bones. The excitement over the Golden Tickets had long since been forgotten. Nobody in the family gave a thought now to anything except the two vital problems of trying to keep warm and trying to get enough to eat.

There is something about very cold weather that gives one an enormous appetite. Most of us find ourselves beginning to crave rich steaming stews and hot apple pies and all kinds of delicious warming dishes; and because we are all a great deal luckier than we realize, we usually get what we want – or near enough. But Charlie Bucket never got what he wanted because the family couldn't afford it, and as the cold weather went on and on, he became ravenously and desperately hungry. Both bars of chocolate, the birthday one and the one Grandpa Joe had bought, had long since been nibbled away, and all he got now were those thin, cabbagy meals three times a day.

Then all at once, the meals became even thinner.

The reason for this was that the toothpaste factory, the place where Mr Bucket worked, suddenly went bust and had to close down. Quickly, Mr Bucket tried to get another job. But he had no luck. In the end, the only way in which he managed to earn a few pennies was by shovelling snow in the streets. But it wasn't enough to buy even a quarter of the food that seven people needed. The situation became desperate. Breakfast was a single slice of bread for each person now, and lunch was maybe half a boiled potato.

Slowly but surely, everybody in the house began to starve.

And every day, little Charlie Bucket, trudging through the snow on his way to school, would have to pass Mr Willy Wonka's giant chocolate factory. And every day, as he came near to it, he would lift his small pointed nose high in the air and sniff the wonderful sweet smell of melting chocolate. Sometimes, he would stand motionless outside the gates for several minutes on end, taking deep swallowing breaths as though he were trying to *eat* the smell itself.

'That child,' said Grandpa Joe, poking his head up from under the blanket one icy morning, 'that child has *got* to have more food. It doesn't matter about us. We're too old to bother with. But a *growing boy*! He can't go on like this! He's beginning to look like a skeleton!'

'What can one *do*?' murmured Grandma Josephine miserably. 'He refuses to take any of ours. I hear his mother tried to slip her own piece of bread on to his plate at breakfast this morning, but he wouldn't touch it. He made her take it back.'

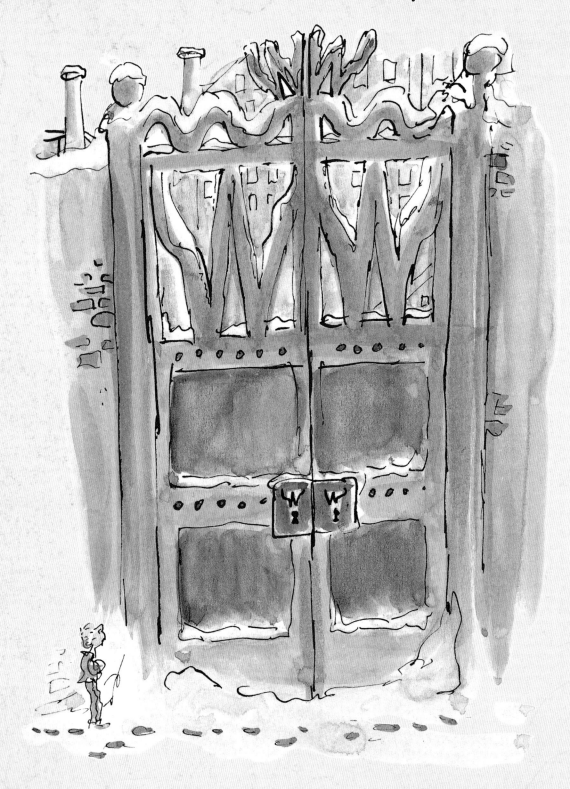

The Family Begins to Starve

'He's a fine little fellow,' said Grandpa George. 'He deserves better than this.'

The cruel weather went on and on.

And every day, Charlie Bucket grew thinner and thinner. His face became frighteningly white and pinched. The skin was drawn so tightly over the cheeks that you could see the shapes of the bones underneath. It seemed doubtful whether he could go on much longer like this without becoming dangerously ill.

And now, very calmly, with that curious wisdom that seems to come so often to small children in times of hardship, he began to make little changes here and there in some of the things that he did, so as to save his strength. In the mornings, he left the house ten minutes earlier so that he could walk slowly to school, without ever having to run. He sat quietly in the classroom during break, resting himself, while the others rushed outdoors and threw snowballs and wrestled in the snow. Everything he did now, he did slowly and carefully, to prevent exhaustion.

Then one afternoon, walking back home with the icy wind in his face (and incidentally feeling hungrier than he had ever felt before), his eye was caught suddenly by something silvery lying in the gutter, in the snow. Charlie stepped off the kerb and bent down to examine it. Part of it was buried under the snow, but he saw at once what it was.

It was a fifty-pence piece!

Quickly he looked around him.

Had somebody just dropped it?

No – that was impossible because of the way part of it was buried.

Several people went hurrying past him on the pavement, their chins sunk deep in the collars of their coats, their feet crunching in the snow. None of them was searching for any money; none of them was taking the slightest notice of the small boy crouching in the gutter.

Then was it *his*, this fifty pence?

Could he *have* it?

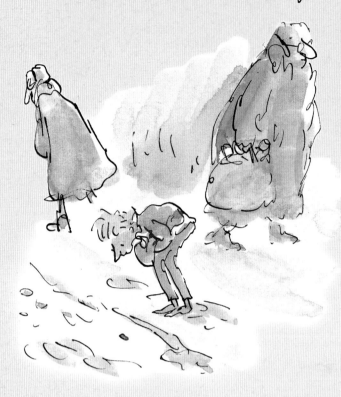

Carefully, Charlie pulled it out from under the snow. It was damp and dirty, but otherwise perfect.

A WHOLE fifty pence!

He held it tightly between his shivering fingers, gazing down at it. It meant one thing to him at that moment, only *one* thing. It meant FOOD.

Automatically, Charlie turned and began moving towards the nearest shop. It was only ten paces away . . . it was a newspaper and stationery shop, the kind that sells almost everything, including sweets and cigars . . . and what he would *do*, he whispered quickly to himself . . . he would buy one luscious bar of chocolate and eat it *all* up, every bit of it, right then and there . . . and the rest of the money he would take straight back home and give to his mother.

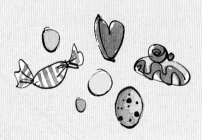

CHAPTER ELEVEN
The Miracle

Charlie entered the shop and laid the damp fifty pence on the counter.

'One Wonka's Whipple-Scrumptious Fudgemallow Delight,' he said, remembering how much he had loved the one he had on his birthday.

The man behind the counter looked fat and well-fed. He had big lips and fat cheeks and a very fat neck. The fat around his neck bulged out all around the top of his collar like a rubber ring. He turned and reached behind him for the chocolate bar, then he turned back again and handed it to Charlie. Charlie grabbed it and quickly tore off the wrapper and took an enormous bite. Then he took another . . . and another . . . and oh, the joy of being able to cram large pieces of something sweet and solid into one's mouth! The sheer blissful joy of being able to fill one's mouth with rich solid food!

'You look like you wanted that one, sonny,' the shopkeeper said pleasantly.

Charlie nodded, his mouth bulging with chocolate.

The shopkeeper put Charlie's change on the counter. 'Take it easy,' he said. 'It'll give you a tummy ache if you swallow it like that without chewing.'

Charlie went on wolfing the chocolate. He couldn't stop. And in less than half a minute, the whole thing had disappeared down his throat. He was quite out of breath, but he felt marvellously, extraordinarily happy. He reached out a hand to take the change. Then he paused. His eyes were just above the level of the counter. They were staring at the

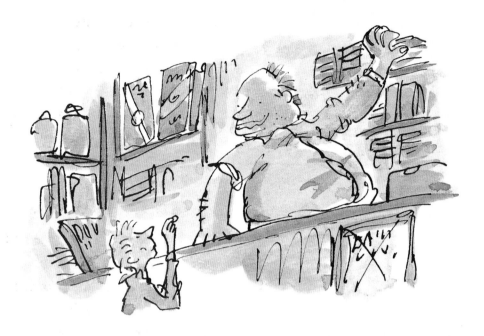

silver coins lying there. The coins were all five-penny pieces. There were nine of them altogether. Surely it wouldn't matter if he spent just one more . . .

'I think,' he said quietly, 'I think . . . I'll have just one more of those chocolate bars. The same kind as before, please.'

'Why not?' the fat shopkeeper said, reaching behind him again and taking another Whipple-Scrumptious Fudgemallow Delight from the shelf. He laid it on the counter.

Charlie picked it up and tore off the wrapper . . . and *suddenly* . . . from underneath the wrapper . . . there came a brilliant flash of gold.

Charlie's heart stood still.

'It's a Golden Ticket!' screamed the shopkeeper, leaping about a foot in the air. 'You've got a Golden Ticket! You've found the last Golden Ticket! Hey, would you believe it! Come and look at this, everybody! The kid's found Wonka's last Golden Ticket! There it is! It's right here in his hands!'

The Miracle

It seemed as though the shopkeeper might be going to have a fit. 'In my shop, too!' he yelled. 'He found it right here in my own little shop! Somebody call the newspapers quick and let them know! Watch out now, sonny! Don't tear it as you unwrap it! That thing's precious!'

In a few seconds, there was a crowd of about twenty people clustering around Charlie, and many more were pushing their way in from the street. Everybody wanted to get a look at the Golden Ticket and at the lucky finder.

'Where is it?' somebody shouted. 'Hold it up so all of us can see it!'

'There it is, there!' someone else shouted. 'He's holding it in his hands! See the gold shining!'

'How did *he* manage to find it, I'd like to know?' a large boy shouted angrily. '*Twenty* bars a day I've been buying for weeks and weeks!'

'Think of all the free stuff he'll be getting too!' another boy said enviously. 'A lifetime supply!'

'He'll need it, the skinny little shrimp!' a girl said, laughing.

Charlie hadn't moved. He hadn't even unwrapped the Golden Ticket from around the chocolate. He was standing very still, holding it tightly with both hands while the crowd pushed and shouted all around him. He felt quite dizzy. There was a peculiar floating sensation coming over him, as though he were floating up in the air like a balloon. His feet didn't seem to be touching the ground at all. He could hear his heart thumping away loudly somewhere in his throat.

At that point, he became aware of a hand resting lightly on his shoulder, and when he looked up, he saw a tall man standing over him. 'Listen,' the man whispered. 'I'll buy it from you. I'll give you fifty pounds. How about it, eh? And I'll give you a new bicycle as well. Okay?'

'Are you *crazy*?' shouted a woman who was standing equally close. 'Why, I'd give him *two hundred* pounds for that ticket! You want to sell that ticket for two hundred pounds, young man?'

'That's *quite* enough of that!' the fat shopkeeper shouted, pushing his way through the crowd and taking Charlie firmly by the arm. 'Leave the kid alone, will you! Make way there! Let him out!' And to Charlie, as he led him to the door, he whispered, 'Don't you let *anybody* have it! Take it straight home, quickly, before you lose it! Run all the way and don't stop till you get there, you understand?'

Charlie nodded.

'You know something,' the fat shopkeeper said, pausing a moment and smiling at Charlie, 'I have a feeling you needed a break like this. I'm awfully glad you got it. Good luck to you, sonny.'

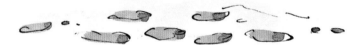

'Thank you,' Charlie said, and off he went, running through the snow as fast as his legs would go. And as he flew past Mr Willy Wonka's factory, he turned and waved at it and sang out, 'I'll be seeing you! I'll be seeing you soon!' And five minutes later he arrived at his own home.

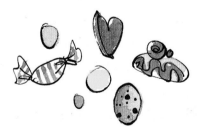

CHAPTER TWELVE

What It Said on the Golden Ticket

Charlie burst through the front door, shouting, '*Mother! Mother! Mother!*'

Mrs Bucket was in the old grandparents' room, serving them their evening soup.

'*Mother!*' yelled Charlie, rushing in on them like a hurricane. 'Look! I've got it! Look, Mother, look! The last Golden Ticket! It's mine! I found some money in the street and I bought two bars of chocolate and the second one had the Golden Ticket and there were *crowds* of people all around me wanting to see it and the shopkeeper rescued me and I ran all the way home and here I am! IT'S THE FIFTH GOLDEN TICKET, MOTHER, AND I'VE FOUND IT!'

Mrs Bucket simply stood and stared, while the four old grandparents, who were sitting up in bed balancing bowls of soup on their laps, all dropped their spoons with a clatter and froze against their pillows.

For about ten seconds there was absolute silence in the room. Nobody dared to speak or move. It was a magic moment.

Then, very softly, Grandpa Joe said, 'You're pulling our legs, Charlie, aren't you? You're having a little joke?'

'I am *not!*' cried Charlie, rushing up to the bed and holding out the large and beautiful Golden Ticket for him to see.

Grandpa Joe leaned forward and took a close look, his nose almost

45

touching the ticket. The others watched him, waiting for the verdict.

Then very slowly, with a slow and marvellous grin spreading all over his face, Grandpa Joe lifted his head and looked straight at Charlie. The colour was rushing to his cheeks, and his eyes were wide open, shining with joy, and in the centre of each eye, right in the very centre, in the black pupil, a little spark of wild excitement was slowly dancing. Then the old man took a deep breath, and suddenly, with no warning whatsoever, an explosion seemed to take place inside him. He threw up his arms and yelled '*Yippeeeeeeee!*' And at the same time, his long bony body rose up out of the bed and his bowl of soup went flying into the face of Grandma Josephine, and in one fantastic leap, this old fellow of ninety-six and a half, who hadn't been out

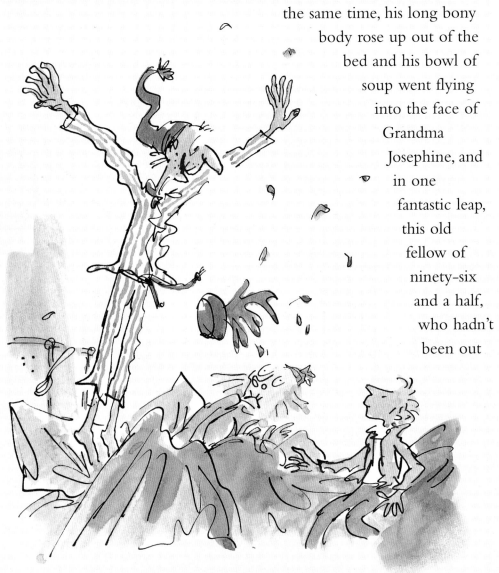

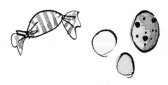

of bed these last twenty years, jumped on to the floor and started doing a dance of victory in his pyjamas.

'Yippeeeeeeeeee!' he shouted. 'Three cheers for Charlie! Hip, hip, hooray!'

At this point, the door opened, and Mr Bucket walked into the room. He was cold and tired, and he looked it. All day long, he had been shovelling snow in the streets.

'*Cripes!*' he cried. 'What's going on in here?'

It didn't take them long to tell him what had happened.

'I don't believe it!' he said. 'It's not possible.'

'Show him the ticket, Charlie!' shouted Grandpa Joe, who was still dancing around the floor like a dervish in his striped pyjamas. 'Show your father the fifth and last Golden Ticket in the world!'

'Let me see it, Charlie,' Mr Bucket said, collapsing into a chair and holding out his hand. Charlie came forward with the precious document.

It was a very beautiful thing, this Golden Ticket, having been made, so it seemed, from a sheet of pure gold hammered out almost to the thinness of paper. On one side of it, printed by some clever method in jet-black letters, was the invitation itself – from Mr Wonka.

'Read it aloud,' said Grandpa Joe, climbing back into bed again at last. 'Let's all hear exactly what it says.'

Mr Bucket held the lovely Golden Ticket up close to his eyes. His hands were trembling slightly, and he seemed to be overcome by the whole business. He took several deep breaths. Then he cleared his throat, and said, 'All right, I'll read it. Here we go:

'*Greetings to you*, the lucky finder of this Golden Ticket, from Mr Willy Wonka! I shake you warmly by the hand! Tremendous things are in store for you! Many wonderful surprises await you! For now, I do invite you to come to my factory and be my guest for one whole day – you and all others who are lucky enough to find my Golden Tickets. I, Willy Wonka, will conduct you around the factory myself, showing you everything that there is to see, and afterwards, when it is time to leave, you will be escorted home by a procession of large trucks. These trucks, I can promise you, will be loaded with enough delicious eatables to last you and your entire household for many years. If, at any time thereafter, you should run out of supplies, you have only to come back to the factory and show this Golden Ticket, and I shall be happy to refill your cupboard with whatever you want. In this way, you will be able to keep yourself supplied with tasty morsels for the rest of your life. But this is by no means the most exciting thing that will happen on the day of your visit. I am preparing other surprises that are even more marvellous and more fantastic for you and for all my beloved Golden Ticket holders – mystic and marvellous surprises that will entrance, delight, intrigue, astonish, and perplex you beyond measure. In your wildest dreams you could not imagine that such things could happen to you! Just wait and see! And now, here are your instructions: the day I have chosen for the visit is the first day in the month of February. On this day, and on no other, you must come to the factory gates at ten o'clock sharp in the morning. Don't be late! And you are allowed to bring with you either one or two members of your own family to look after you and to ensure that you don't get into mischief. One more thing – be certain to have this ticket with you, otherwise you will not be admitted.

(Signed) **Willy Wonka.**

What It Said on the Golden Ticket

'The first day of *February*!' cried Mrs Bucket. 'But that's *tomorrow*! Today is the last day of January. *I know it is!*'

'Cripes!' said Mr Bucket. 'I think you're right!'

'You're just in time!' shouted Grandpa Joe. 'There's not a moment to lose. You must start making preparations at once! Wash your face, comb your hair, scrub your hands, brush your teeth, blow your nose, cut your nails, polish your shoes, iron your shirt, and for heaven's sake, get all that mud off your pants! You must get ready, my boy! You must get ready for the biggest day of your life!'

'Now don't over-excite yourself, Grandpa,' Mrs Bucket said. 'And don't fluster poor Charlie. We must all try to keep very calm. Now the first thing to decide is this – who is going to go with Charlie to the factory?'

'I will!' shouted Grandpa Joe, leaping out of bed once again. 'I'll take him! I'll look after him! You leave it to me!'

Mrs Bucket smiled at the old man, then she turned to her husband and said, 'How about you, dear? Don't you think *you* ought to go?'

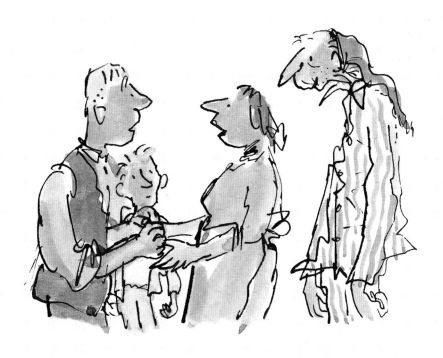

'Well . . .' Mr Bucket said, pausing to think about it, 'no . . . I'm not so sure that I should.'

'But you *must*.'

'There's no *must* about it, my dear,' Mr Bucket said gently. 'Mind you, I'd *love* to go. It'll be tremendously exciting. But on the other hand . . . I believe that the person who really *deserves* to go most of all is Grandpa Joe himself. He seems to know more about it than we do. Provided, of course, that he feels well enough . . .'

'Yippeeeeee!' shouted Grandpa Joe, seizing Charlie by the hands and dancing round the room.

'He certainly *seems* well enough,' Mrs Bucket said, laughing. 'Yes . . . perhaps you're right after all. Perhaps Grandpa Joe should be the one to go with him. I certainly can't go myself and leave the other three old people all alone in bed for a whole day.'

'Hallelujah!' yelled Grandpa Joe. 'Praise the Lord!'

At that point, there came a loud knock on the front door. Mr Bucket went to open it, and the next moment, swarms of newspapermen and photographers were pouring into the house. They had tracked down the finder of the fifth Golden Ticket, and now they all wanted to get the full story for the front pages of the morning papers. For several hours, there was complete pandemonium in the little house, and it must have been nearly midnight before Mr Bucket was able to get rid of them so that Charlie could go to bed.

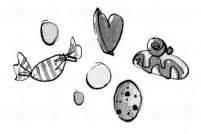

CHAPTER THIRTEEN

The Big Day Arrives

The sun was shining brightly on the morning of the big day, but the ground was still white with snow and the air was very cold.

Outside the gates of Wonka's factory, enormous crowds of people had gathered to watch the five lucky ticket holders going in. The excitement was tremendous. It was just before ten o'clock. The crowds were pushing and shouting, and policemen with arms linked were trying to hold them back from the gates.

Right beside the gates, in a small group that was carefully shielded from the crowds by the police, stood the five famous children, together with the grown-ups who had come with them.

The tall bony figure of Grandpa Joe could be seen standing quietly among them, and beside him, holding tightly on to his hand, was little Charlie Bucket himself.

All the children, except Charlie, had both their mothers and fathers with them, and it was a good thing that they had, otherwise the whole party might have got out of hand. They were so eager to get going that their parents were having to hold them back by force to prevent them from climbing over the gates. 'Be patient!' cried the fathers. 'Be still! It's not *time* yet! It's not ten o'clock!'

Behind him, Charlie Bucket could hear the shouts of the people in the crowd as they pushed and fought to get a glimpse of the famous children.

'There's Violet Beauregarde!' he heard someone shouting. 'That's her all right! I can remember her face from the newspapers!'

'And you know what?' somebody else shouted back. 'She's still chewing that dreadful old piece of gum she's had for three months! You look at her jaws! They're still working on it!'

'Who's the big fat boy?'

'That's Augustus Gloop!'

'So it is!'

'Enormous, isn't he!'

'Fantastic!'

'Who's the kid with a picture of The Lone Ranger stencilled on his windcheater?'

'That's Mike Teavee! He's the television fiend!'

'He must be crazy! Look at all those toy pistols he's got hanging all over him!'

'The one I want to see is Veruca Salt!' shouted another voice in the crowd. 'She's the girl whose father bought up half a million chocolate bars and then made the workers in his peanut factory unwrap every one of them until they found a Golden Ticket! He gives her anything

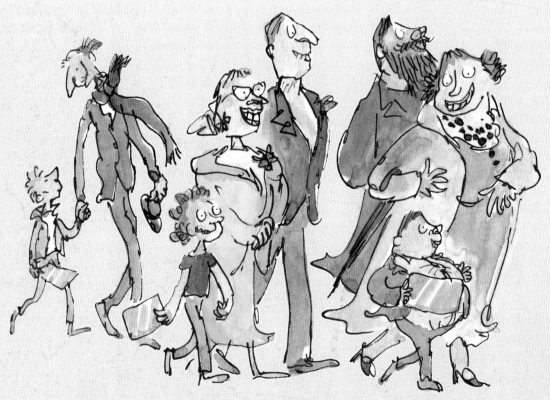

she wants! Absolutely anything! She only has to start screaming for it and she gets it!'

'Dreadful, isn't it?'

'Shocking, I call it!'

'Which do you think is her?'

'That one! Over there on the left! The little girl in the silver mink coat!'

'Which one is Charlie Bucket?'

'Charlie Bucket? He must be that skinny little shrimp standing beside the old fellow who looks like a skeleton. Very close to us. Just there! See him?'

'Why hasn't he got a coat on in this cold weather?'

'Don't ask me. Maybe he can't afford to buy one.'

'Goodness me! He must be freezing!'

Charlie, standing only a few paces away from the speaker, gave Grandpa Joe's hand a squeeze, and the old man looked down at Charlie and smiled.

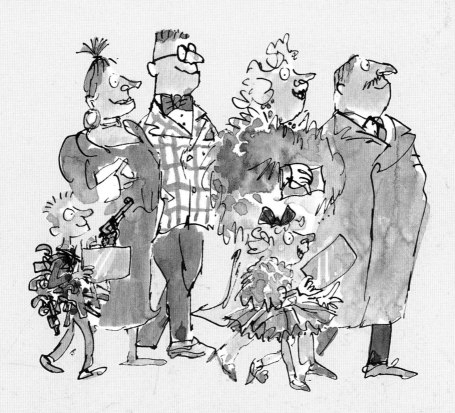

Somewhere in the distance, a church clock began striking ten.

Very slowly, with a loud creaking of rusty hinges, the great iron gates of the factory began to swing open.

The crowd became suddenly silent. The children stopped jumping about. All eyes were fixed upon the gates.

'*There he is!*' somebody shouted. '*That's him!*'

And so it was!

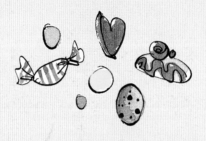

CHAPTER FOURTEEN

Mr Willy Wonka

Mr Wonka was standing all alone just inside the open gates of the factory.

And what an extraordinary little man he was!

He had a black top hat on his head.

He wore a tail coat made of a beautiful plum-coloured velvet.

His trousers were bottle green.

His gloves were pearly grey.

And in one hand he carried a fine gold-topped walking cane.

Covering his chin, there was a small, neat, pointed black beard – a goatee. And his eyes – his eyes were most marvellously bright. They seemed to be sparkling and twinkling at you all the time. The whole face, in fact, was alight with fun and laughter.

And oh, how clever he looked! How quick and sharp and full of life! He kept making quick jerky little movements with his head, cocking it this way and that, and taking everything in with those bright twinkling eyes. He was like a squirrel in the quickness of his movements, like a quick clever old squirrel from the park.

Suddenly, he did a funny little skipping dance in the snow, and he spread his arms wide, and he smiled at the five children who were clustered near the gates, and he called out, 'Welcome, my little friends! Welcome to the factory!'

His voice was high and flutey. 'Will you come forward one at a time, please,' he called out, 'and bring your parents. Then show me your Golden Ticket and give me your name. Who's first?'

The big fat boy stepped up. 'I'm Augustus Gloop,' he said.

'Augustus!' cried Mr Wonka, seizing his hand and pumping it up and down with terrific force. 'My *dear* boy, how *good* to see you! Delighted! Charmed! Overjoyed to have you with us! And *these* are your parents? How *nice*! Come in! Come in! That's right! Step through the gates!'

Mr Wonka was clearly just as excited as everybody else.

'My name,' said the next child to go forward, 'is Veruca Salt.'

'My *dear* Veruca! How *do* you do? What a pleasure this is! You *do* have an interesting name, don't you? I always thought that a verruca was a sort of wart that you got on the sole of your foot! But I must be wrong, mustn't I? How pretty you look in that lovely mink coat! I'm so glad you could come! Dear me, this is going to be *such* an exciting day! I *do* hope you enjoy it! I'm sure you *will*! I *know* you will! Your father? How *are* you, Mr Salt? And Mrs Salt? Overjoyed to see you! Yes, the ticket is *quite* in order! Please go in!'

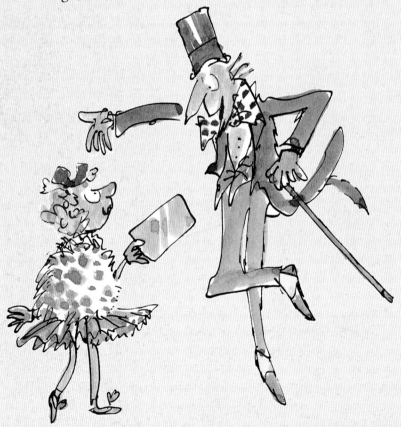

The next two children, Violet Beauregarde and Mike Teavee, came forward to have their tickets examined and then to have their arms practically pumped off their shoulders by the energetic Mr Wonka.

And last of all, a small nervous voice whispered, 'Charlie Bucket.'

'Charlie!' cried Mr Wonka. 'Well, well, well! So *there* you are! You're the one who found your ticket only yesterday, aren't you? Yes, yes. I read *all* about it in this morning's papers! *Just* in time, my dear boy! I'm so glad! So happy for you! And this? Your grandfather? Delighted to meet you, sir! Overjoyed! Enraptured! Enchanted! All right! Excellent! Is everybody in now? Five children? Yes! Good! Now will you please follow me! Our tour is about to begin! But *do* keep together! *Please* don't wander off by yourselves! I shouldn't like to lose any of you at *this* stage of the proceedings! Oh, dear me, no!'

Charlie glanced back over his shoulder and saw the great iron entrance gates slowly closing behind him. The crowds on the outside were still pushing and shouting. Charlie took a last look at them. Then, as the gates closed with a clang, all sight of the outside world disappeared.

'Here we are!' cried Mr Wonka, trotting along in front of the group. 'Through this big red door, please! *That's* right! It's nice and warm inside! I have to keep it warm inside the factory because of the workers! My workers are used to an *extremely* hot climate! They can't stand the cold! They'd perish if they went outdoors in this weather! They'd freeze to death!'

'But who *are* these workers?' asked Augustus Gloop.

'All in good time, my dear boy!' said Mr Wonka, smiling at Augustus. 'Be patient! You shall see everything as we go along! Are all of you inside? Good! Would you mind closing the door? Thank you!'

Charlie Bucket found himself standing in a long corridor that stretched away in front of him as far as he could see. The corridor was so wide that a car could easily have been driven along it. The walls were pale pink, the lighting was soft and pleasant.

'How lovely and warm!' whispered Charlie.

'I know. And what a marvellous smell!' answered Grandpa Joe, taking a long deep sniff. All the most wonderful smells in the world seemed to be mixed up in the air around them – the smell of roasting coffee and burnt sugar and melting chocolate and mint and violets and crushed hazelnuts and apple blossom and caramel and lemon peel . . .

And far away in the distance, from the heart of the great factory, came a muffled roar of energy as though some monstrous gigantic machine were spinning its wheels at breakneck speed.

'Now *this*, my dear children,' said Mr Wonka, raising his voice above the noise, 'this is the main corridor. Will you please hang your coats and hats on those pegs over there, and then follow me. *That's* the way! Good! Everyone ready? Come on, then! Here we go!' He trotted off rapidly down the corridor with the tails of his plum-coloured velvet coat flapping behind him, and the visitors all hurried after him.

It was quite a large party of people, when you came to think of it. There were nine grown-ups and five children, fourteen in all. So you can imagine that there was a good deal of pushing and shoving as they hustled and bustled down the passage, trying to keep up with the swift little figure in front of them. 'Come *on*!' cried Mr Wonka. 'Get a move on, please! We'll *never* get round today if you dawdle like this!'

Soon, he turned right off the main corridor into another slightly narrower passage.

Then he turned left.

Then left again.

Then right.

Then left.

Then right.

Then right.

Then left.

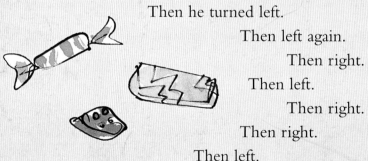

The place was like a gigantic rabbit warren, with passages leading this way and that in every direction.

'Don't you let go my hand, Charlie,' whispered Grandpa Joe.

'Notice how all these passages are sloping downwards!' called out Mr Wonka. 'We are now going underground! *All* the most important rooms in my factory are deep down below the surface!'

'Why is that?' somebody asked.

'There wouldn't be *nearly* enough space for them up on top!' answered Mr Wonka. 'These rooms we are going to see are *enormous*! They're larger than football fields! No building in the *world* would be big enough to house them! But down here, underneath the ground, I've got *all* the space I want. There's no limit – so long as I hollow it out.'

Mr Wonka turned right.

He turned left.

He turned right again.

The passages were sloping steeper and steeper downhill now.

Then suddenly, Mr Wonka stopped. In front of him, there was a shiny metal door. The party crowded round. On the door, in large letters, it said:

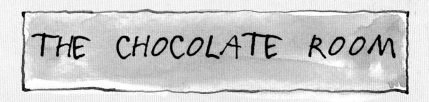

THE CHOCOLATE ROOM

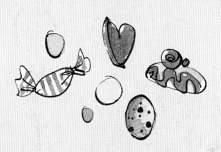

CHAPTER FIFTEEN
The Chocolate Room

'An important room, this!' cried Mr Wonka, taking a bunch of keys from his pocket and slipping one into the keyhole of the door. '*This* is the nerve centre of the whole factory, the heart of the whole business! And so *beautiful*! I *insist* upon my rooms being beautiful! I can't *abide* ugliness in factories! *In* we go, then! But *do* be careful, my dear children! Don't lose your heads! Don't get over-excited! Keep very calm!'

Mr Wonka opened the door. Five children and nine grown-ups pushed their ways in – and *oh*, what an amazing sight it was that now met their eyes!

They were looking down upon a lovely valley. There were green meadows on either side of the valley, and along the bottom of it there flowed a great brown river.

What is more, there was a tremendous waterfall halfway along the river – a steep cliff over which the water curled and rolled in a solid sheet, and then went crashing down into a boiling churning whirlpool of froth and spray.

Below the waterfall (and this was the most astonishing sight of all), a whole mass of enormous glass pipes were dangling down into the river from somewhere high up in the ceiling! They really were *enormous*, those pipes. There must have been a dozen of them at least, and they were sucking up the brownish muddy water from the river and carrying it away to goodness knows where. And because they were made of glass, you could see the liquid flowing and bubbling along inside them, and

The Chocolate Room

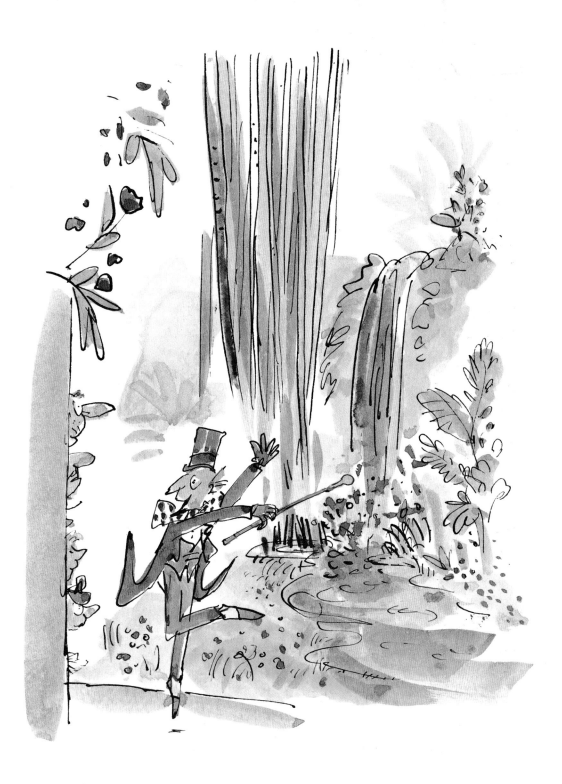

above the noise of the waterfall, you could hear the never-ending suck-suck-sucking sound of the pipes as they did their work.

Graceful trees and bushes were growing along the riverbanks – weeping willows and alders and tall clumps of rhododendrons with their pink and red and mauve blossoms. In the meadows there were thousands of buttercups.

'*There!*' cried Mr Wonka, dancing up and down and pointing his gold-topped cane at the great brown river. 'It's *all* chocolate! Every drop of that river is hot melted chocolate of the finest quality. The *very* finest quality. There's enough chocolate in there to fill *every* bathtub in the *entire* country! *And* all the swimming pools as well! Isn't it *terrific*? And just look at my pipes! They suck up the chocolate and carry it away to all the other rooms in the factory where it is needed! Thousands of gallons an hour, my dear children! Thousands and thousands of gallons!'

The children and their parents were too flabbergasted to speak. They were staggered. They were dumbfounded. They were bewildered and dazzled. They were completely bowled over by the hugeness of the whole thing. They simply stood and stared.

'The waterfall is *most* important!' Mr Wonka went on. 'It mixes the chocolate! It churns it up! It pounds it and beats it! It makes it light and frothy! No other factory in the world mixes its chocolate by waterfall! But it's the *only* way to do it properly! The *only* way! And do you like my trees?' he cried, pointing with his stick. 'And my lovely bushes? Don't you think they look pretty? I told you I hated ugliness! And of course they are *all* eatable! All made of something different and delicious! And do you like my meadows? Do you like my grass and my buttercups? The grass you are standing on, my dear little ones, is made of a new kind of soft, minty sugar that I've just invented! I call it swudge! Try a blade! Please do! It's delectable!'

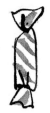

Automatically, everybody bent down and picked one blade of grass – everybody, that is, except Augustus Gloop, who took a big handful.

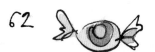

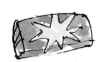

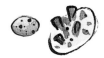
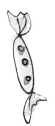

And Violet Beauregarde, before tasting her blade of grass, took the piece of world-record-breaking chewing-gum out of her mouth and stuck it carefully behind her ear.

'Isn't it *wonderful*!' whispered Charlie. 'Hasn't it got a wonderful taste, Grandpa?'

'I could eat the whole *field*!' said Grandpa Joe, grinning with delight. 'I could go around on all fours like a cow and eat every blade of grass in the field!'

'Try a buttercup!' cried Mr Wonka. 'They're even *nicer*!'

Suddenly, the air was filled with screams of excitement. The screams came from Veruca Salt. She was pointing frantically to the other side of the river. '*Look!* Look over there!' she screamed. 'What *is* it? He's moving! He's walking! It's a little *person*! It's a little *man*! Down there below the waterfall!'

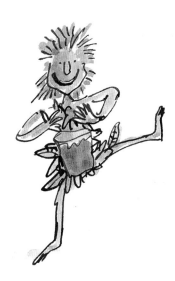

Everybody stopped picking buttercups and stared across the river.

'*She's right, Grandpa!*' cried Charlie. 'It *is* a little man! Can you *see* him?'

'I see him, Charlie!' said Grandpa Joe excitedly.

And now everybody started shouting at once.

'There's *two* of them!'

'My gosh, so there is!'

'There's more than two! There's one, two, three, four, five!'

'What are they *doing*?'

'Where do they *come* from?'

'Who *are* they?'

Children and parents alike rushed down to the edge of the river to get a closer look.

'Aren't they *fantastic*!'

'No higher than my knee!'

'Look at their funny long hair!'

The tiny men – they were no larger than medium-sized dolls – had stopped what they were doing, and now they were staring back across the river at the visitors. One of them pointed towards the children, and then he whispered something to the other four, and all five of them burst into peals of laughter.

'But they can't be *real* people,' Charlie said.

'Of course they're real people,' Mr Wonka answered. 'They're Oompa-Loompas.'

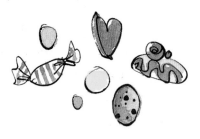

CHAPTER SIXTEEN

The Oompa-Loompas

'Oompa-Loompas!' everyone said at once. '*Oompa-Loompas!*'

'Imported direct from Loompaland,' said Mr Wonka proudly.

'There's no such place,' said Mrs Salt.

'Excuse me, dear lady, but . . .'

'*Mr Wonka*,' cried Mrs Salt. 'I'm a teacher of geography . . .'

'Then you'll know all about it,' said Mr Wonka. 'And oh, what a terrible country it is! Nothing but thick jungles infested by the most dangerous beasts in the world – hornswogglers and snozzwangers and those terrible wicked whangdoodles. A whangdoodle would eat ten Oompa-Loompas for breakfast and come galloping back for a second helping. When I went out there, I found the little Oompa-Loompas living in tree houses. They *had* to live in tree houses to escape from the whangdoodles and the hornswogglers and the snozzwangers. And they were living on green caterpillars, and the caterpillars tasted revolting, and the Oompa-Loompas spent every moment of their days climbing through the treetops looking for other things to mash up with the caterpillars to make them taste better – red beetles, for instance, and eucalyptus leaves, and the bark of the bong-bong tree, all of them beastly, but not quite so beastly as the caterpillars. Poor little Oompa-Loompas! The one food that they longed for more than any other was the cacao bean. But they couldn't get it. An Oompa-Loompa was lucky if he

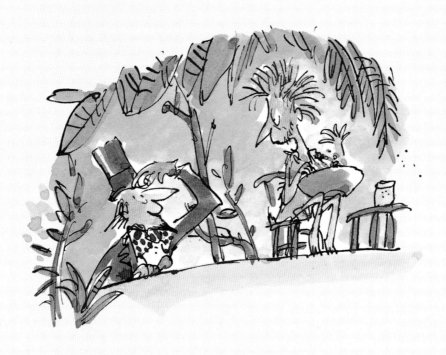

found three or four cacao beans a year. But oh, how they craved them.
They used to dream about cacao beans all night and talk about them all
day. You had only to *mention* the word "cacao" to an Oompa-Loompa
and he would start dribbling at the mouth. The cacao bean,' Mr Wonka
continued, 'which grows on the cacao tree, happens to be *the thing* from
which all chocolate is made. You cannot make chocolate without the
cacao bean. The cacao bean *is* chocolate. I myself use billions of cacao
beans every week in this factory. And so, my dear children, as soon as I
discovered that the Oompa-Loompas were crazy about this particular
food, I climbed up to their tree-house village and poked my head in
through the door of the tree house belonging to the leader of the tribe.
The poor little fellow, looking thin and starved, was sitting there trying
to eat a bowl full of mashed-up green caterpillars without being sick.
"Look here," I said (speaking not in English, of course, but in Oompa-
Loompish), "look here, if you and all your people will come back to my
country and live in my factory, you can have *all* the cacao beans you

want! I've got mountains of them in my storehouses! You can have cacao beans for every meal! You can gorge yourselves silly on them! I'll even pay your wages in cacao beans if you wish!"

' "You really mean it?" asked the Oompa-Loompa leader, leaping up from his chair.

' "Of course I mean it," I said. "And you can have chocolate as well. Chocolate tastes even better than cacao beans because it's got milk and sugar added."

'The little man gave a great whoop of joy and threw his bowl of mashed caterpillars right out of the tree-house window. "It's a deal!" he cried. "Come on! Let's go!"

'So I shipped them all over here, every man, woman, and child in the Oompa-Loompa tribe. It was easy. I smuggled them over in large packing cases with holes in them, and they all got here safely. They are wonderful workers. They all speak English now. They love dancing and music. They are always making up songs. I expect you will hear a good deal of singing today from time to time. I must warn you, though, that they are rather mischievous. They like jokes. They still wear the same kind of clothes they wore in the jungle. They insist upon that. The men, as you can see for yourselves across the river, wear only deerskins. The women wear leaves, and the children wear nothing at all. The women use fresh leaves every day . . .'

'*Daddy!*' shouted Veruca Salt (the girl who got everything she wanted). '*Daddy!* I want an Oompa-Loompa! I want you to get me an Oompa-Loompa! I want an Oompa-Loompa right away! I want to take it home with me! Go on, Daddy! Get me an Oompa-Loompa!'

'Now, now, my pet!' her father said to her, 'we mustn't interrupt Mr Wonka.'

'*But I want an Oompa-Loompa!*' screamed Veruca.

'All *right*, Veruca, all *right*. But I can't get it for you this second. Please be patient. I'll see you have one before the day is out.'

'Augustus!' shouted Mrs Gloop. 'Augustus, sweetheart, I don't think you had better do *that*.' Augustus Gloop, as you might have guessed, had quietly sneaked down to the edge of the river, and he was now kneeling on the riverbank, scooping hot melted chocolate into his mouth as fast as he could.

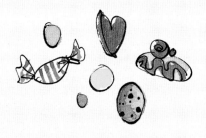

CHAPTER SEVENTEEN

Augustus Gloop Goes up the Pipe

When Mr Wonka turned round and saw what Augustus Gloop was doing, he cried out, 'Oh, no! *Please*, Augustus, *please*! I beg of you not to do that. My chocolate must be untouched by human hands!'

'Augustus!' called out Mrs Gloop. 'Didn't you hear what the man said? Come away from that river at once!'

'This stuff is fabulous!' said Augustus, taking not the slightest notice of his mother or Mr Wonka. 'Gosh, I need a bucket to drink it properly!'

'Augustus,' cried Mr Wonka, hopping up and down and waggling his stick in the air, 'you *must* come away. You are dirtying my chocolate!'

'Augustus!' cried Mrs Gloop.

'Augustus!' cried Mr Gloop.

But Augustus was deaf to everything except the call of his enormous stomach. He was now lying full length on the ground with his head far out over the river, lapping up the chocolate like a dog.

'Augustus!' shouted Mrs Gloop. 'You'll be giving that nasty cold of yours to about a million people all over the country!'

'Be careful, Augustus!' shouted Mr Gloop. 'You're leaning too far out!'

Mr Gloop was absolutely right. For suddenly there was a shriek, and then a splash, and into the river went Augustus Gloop, and in one second he had disappeared under the brown surface.

'Save him!' screamed Mrs Gloop, going white in the face, and waving

her umbrella about. 'He'll drown! He can't swim a yard! Save him!
Save him!'

'Good heavens, woman,' said Mr Gloop, 'I'm not diving in there!
I've got my best suit on!'

Augustus Gloop's face came up again to the surface, painted brown
with chocolate. 'Help! Help! Help!' he yelled. 'Fish me out!'

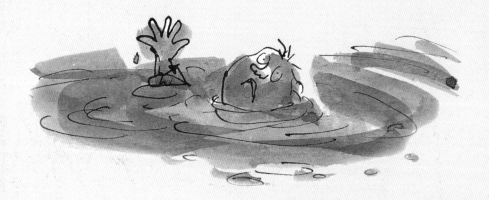

'Don't just *stand* there!' Mrs Gloop screamed at Mr Gloop. '*Do*
something!'

'I *am* doing something!' said Mr Gloop, who was now taking off his
jacket and getting ready to dive into the chocolate. But while he was
doing this, the wretched boy was being sucked closer and closer towards
the mouth of one of the great pipes that was dangling down into the
river. Then all at once, the powerful suction took hold of him
completely, and he was pulled under the surface and then into the mouth
of the pipe.

The crowd on the riverbank waited breathlessly to see where he
would come out.

'*There he goes!*' somebody shouted, pointing upwards.

And sure enough, because the pipe was made of glass, Augustus Gloop
could be clearly seen shooting up inside it, head first, like a torpedo.

'Help! Murder! Police!' screamed Mrs Gloop. 'Augustus, come back at once! Where are you going?'

'It's a wonder to me,' said Mr Gloop, 'how that pipe is big enough for him to go through it.'

'It *isn't* big enough!' said Charlie Bucket. 'Oh dear, look! He's slowing down!'

'So he is!' said Grandpa Joe.

'He's going to stick!' said Charlie.

'I think he is!' said Grandpa Joe.

'By golly, he *has* stuck!' said Charlie.

'It's his stomach that's done it!' said Mr Gloop.

'He's blocked the whole pipe!' said Grandpa Joe.

'Smash the pipe!' yelled Mrs Gloop, still waving her umbrella. 'Augustus, come out of there at once!'

The watchers below could see the chocolate swishing around the boy in the pipe, and they could see it building up behind him in a solid mass, pushing against the blockage. The pressure was terrific. Something had to give. Something did give, and that something was Augustus. *WHOOF!* Up he shot again like a bullet in the barrel of a gun.

'He's disappeared!' yelled Mrs Gloop. 'Where does that pipe go to? Quick! Call the fire brigade!'

'Keep calm!' cried Mr Wonka. 'Keep calm, my dear lady, keep calm. There is no danger! No danger whatsoever! Augustus has gone on a little journey, that's all. A most interesting little journey. But he'll come out of it just fine, you wait and see.'

'How can he possibly come out just fine!' snapped Mrs Gloop. 'He'll be made into marshmallows in five seconds!'

'Impossible!' cried Mr Wonka. 'Unthinkable! Inconceivable! Absurd! He could never be made into marshmallows!'

'And why not, may I ask?' shouted Mrs Gloop.

'Because that pipe doesn't go anywhere near it! That pipe – the one Augustus went up – happens to lead directly to the room where I make a most delicious kind of strawberry-flavoured chocolate-coated fudge . . .'

'Then he'll be made into strawberry-flavoured chocolate-coated fudge!' screamed Mrs Gloop. 'My poor Augustus! They'll be selling him by the pound all over the country tomorrow morning!'

'Quite right,' said Mr Gloop.

'I know I'm right,' said Mrs Gloop.

'It's beyond a joke,' said Mr Gloop.

'Mr Wonka doesn't seem to think so!' cried Mrs Gloop. 'Just look at him! He's laughing his head off! How *dare* you laugh like that when my boy's just gone up the pipe! You monster!' she shrieked, pointing her umbrella at Mr Wonka as though she were going to run him through. 'You think it's a joke, do you? You think that sucking my boy up into your Fudge Room like that is just one great big colossal joke?'

'He'll be perfectly safe,' said Mr Wonka, giggling slightly.

'He'll be chocolate fudge!' shrieked Mrs Gloop.

'Never!' cried Mr Wonka.

'Of course he will!' shrieked Mrs Gloop.

'I wouldn't allow it!' cried Mr Wonka.

'And why not?' shrieked Mrs Gloop.

'Because the taste would be terrible,' said Mr Wonka. 'Just imagine it! Augustus-flavoured chocolate-coated Gloop! No one would buy it.'

'They most certainly would!' cried Mr Gloop indignantly.

'I don't want to think about it!' shrieked Mrs Gloop.

'Nor do I,' said Mr Wonka. 'And I do promise you, madam, that your darling boy is perfectly safe.'

'If he's perfectly safe, then where is he?' snapped Mrs Gloop. 'Lead me to him this instant!'

Mr Wonka turned around and clicked his fingers sharply, *click, click, click*, three times. Immediately, an Oompa-Loompa appeared, as if from nowhere, and stood beside him.

The Oompa-Loompa bowed and smiled, showing beautiful white

teeth. His skin was rosy-white, his long hair was golden-brown, and the top of his head came just above the height of Mr Wonka's knee. He wore the usual deerskin slung over his shoulder.

'Now listen to me!' said Mr Wonka, looking down at the tiny man. 'I want you to take Mr and Mrs Gloop up to the Fudge Room and help them to find their son, Augustus. He's just gone up the pipe.'

The Oompa-Loompa took one look at Mrs Gloop and exploded into peals of laughter.

'Oh, do be quiet!' said Mr Wonka. 'Control yourself! Pull yourself together! Mrs Gloop doesn't think it's at all funny!'

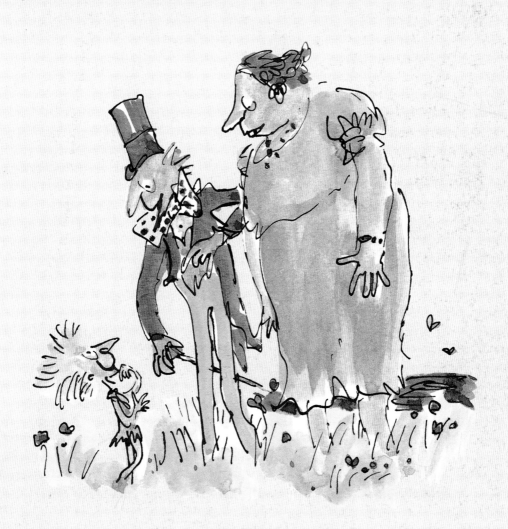

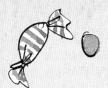

'You can say that again!' said Mrs Gloop.

'Go straight to the Fudge Room,' Mr Wonka said to the Oompa-Loompa, 'and when you get there, take a long stick and start poking around inside the big chocolate-mixing barrel. I'm almost certain you'll find him in there. But you'd better look sharp! You'll have to hurry! If you leave him in the chocolate-mixing barrel too long, he's liable to get poured out into the fudge boiler, and that really *would* be a disaster, wouldn't it? My fudge would become *quite* uneatable!'

Mrs Gloop let out a shriek of fury.

'I'm joking,' said Mr Wonka, giggling madly behind his beard. 'I didn't mean it. Forgive me. I'm so sorry. Goodbye, Mrs Gloop! And Mr Gloop! Goodbye! I'll see you later . . .'

As Mr and Mrs Gloop and their tiny escort hurried away, the five Oompa-Loompas on the far side of the river suddenly began hopping and dancing about and beating wildly upon a number of very small drums. 'Augustus Gloop!' they chanted. 'Augustus Gloop! Augustus Gloop! Augustus Gloop!'

'Grandpa!' cried Charlie. 'Listen to them, Grandpa! What *are* they doing?'

'Ssshh!' whispered Grandpa Joe. 'I think they're going to sing us a song!'

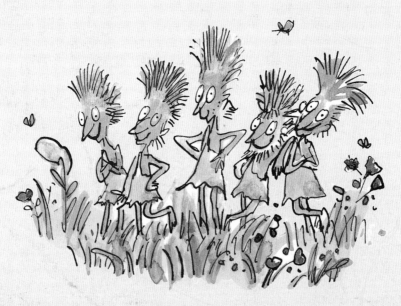

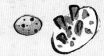

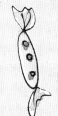

'Augustus Gloop!' chanted the Oompa-Loompas.
'Augustus Gloop! Augustus Gloop!
The great big greedy nincompoop!
How long could we allow this beast
To gorge and guzzle, feed and feast
On everything he wanted to?
Great Scott! It simply wouldn't do!
However long this pig might live,
We're positive he'd never give
Even the smallest bit of fun
Or happiness to anyone.
So what we do in cases such
As this, we use the gentle touch,
And carefully we take the brat
And turn him into something that
Will give great pleasure to us all –
A doll, for instance, or a ball,
Or marbles or a rocking horse.
But this revolting boy, of course,
Was so unutterably vile,
So greedy, foul, and infantile,
He left a most disgusting taste
Inside our mouths, and so in haste
We chose a thing that, come what may,
Would take the nasty taste away.
"Come on!" we cried. "The time is ripe
To send him shooting up the pipe!
He has to go! It has to be!"
And very soon, he's going to see
Inside the room to which he's gone
Some funny things are going on.

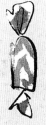

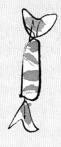

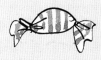

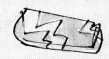

But don't, dear children, be alarmed;
Augustus Gloop will not be harmed,
Although, of course, we must admit
He will be altered quite a bit.
He'll be quite changed from what he's been,
When he goes through the fudge machine:
Slowly, the wheels go round and round,
The cogs begin to grind and pound;
A hundred knives go slice, slice, slice;
We add some sugar, cream, and spice;
We boil him for a minute more,
Until we're absolutely sure
That all the greed and all the gall
Is boiled away for once and all.
Then out he comes! And now! By grace!
A miracle has taken place!
This boy, who only just before
Was loathed by men from shore to shore,
This greedy brute, this louse's ear,
Is loved by people everywhere!
For who could hate or bear a grudge
Against a luscious bit of fudge?'

'I *told* you they loved singing!' cried Mr Wonka. 'Aren't they delightful? Aren't they charming? But you mustn't believe a word they said. It's all nonsense, every bit of it!'

'Are the Oompa-Loompas really joking, Grandpa?' asked Charlie.

'Of course they're joking,' answered Grandpa Joe. 'They *must* be joking. At least, I hope they're joking. Don't you?'

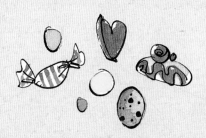

CHAPTER EIGHTEEN

Down the Chocolate River

'Off we go!' cried Mr Wonka. 'Hurry up, everybody! Follow me to the next room! And please don't worry about Augustus Gloop. He's bound to come out in the wash. They always do. We shall have to make the next part of the journey by boat! Here she comes! Look!'

A steamy mist was rising up now from the great warm chocolate river, and out of the mist there appeared suddenly a most fantastic pink boat. It was a large open row boat with a tall front and a tall back (like a Viking boat of old), and it was of such a shining sparkling glistening pink colour that the whole thing looked as though it were made of bright, pink glass. There were many oars on either side of it, and as the boat came closer, the watchers on the riverbank could see that the oars were being pulled by masses of Oompa-Loompas – at least ten of them to each oar.

'This is my private yacht!' cried Mr Wonka, beaming with pleasure. 'I made her by hollowing out an enormous boiled sweet! Isn't she beautiful! See how she comes cutting through the river!'

The gleaming pink boiled-sweet boat glided up to the riverbank. One hundred Oompa-Loompas rested on their oars and stared up at the visitors. Then suddenly, for some reason best known to themselves, they all burst into shrieks of laughter.

'What's so funny?' asked Violet Beauregarde.

'Oh, don't worry about *them*!' cried Mr Wonka. 'They're always laughing! They think everything's a colossal joke! Jump into the boat, all of you! Come on! Hurry up!'

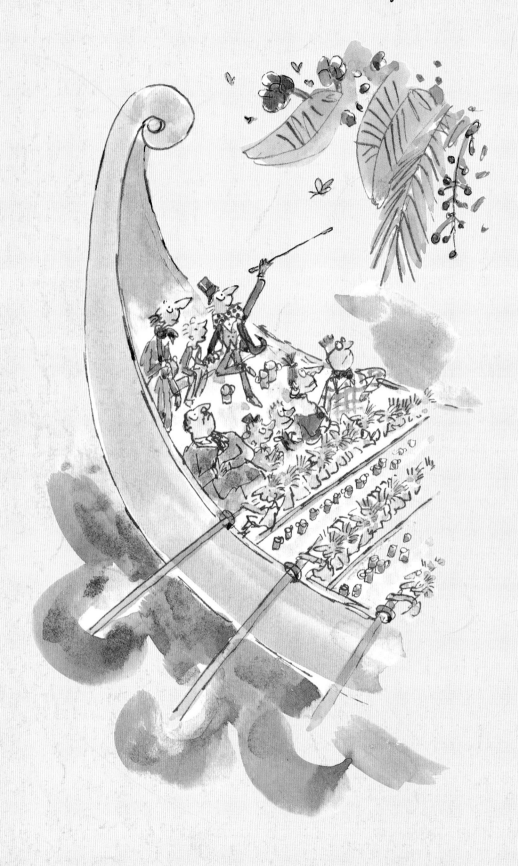

Down the Chocolate River

As soon as everyone was safely in, the Oompa-Loompas pushed the boat away from the bank and began to row swiftly downriver.

'Hey, there! Mike Teavee!' shouted Mr Wonka. 'Please do not lick the boat with your tongue! It'll only make it sticky!'

'Daddy,' said Veruca Salt, 'I want a boat like this! I want you to buy me a big pink boiled-sweet boat exactly like Mr Wonka's! And I want lots of Oompa-Loompas to row me about, and I want a chocolate river and I want . . . I want . . .'

'She wants a good kick in the pants,' whispered Grandpa Joe to Charlie. The old man was sitting in the back of the boat and little Charlie Bucket was right beside him. Charlie was holding tightly on to his grandfather's bony old hand. He was in a whirl of excitement. Everything that he had seen so far – the great chocolate river, the waterfall, the huge sucking pipes, the minty sugar meadows, the Oompa-Loompas, the beautiful pink boat, and most of all, Mr Willy Wonka himself – had been so astonishing that he began to wonder whether there could possibly be any more astonishments left. Where were they going now? What were they going to see? And what in the world was going to happen in the next room?

'Isn't it marvellous?' said Grandpa Joe, grinning at Charlie.

Charlie nodded and smiled up at the old man.

Suddenly, Mr Wonka, who was sitting on Charlie's other side, reached down into the bottom of the boat, picked up a large mug, dipped it into the river, filled it with chocolate, and handed it to Charlie. 'Drink this,' he said. 'It'll do you good! You look starved to death!'

Then Mr Wonka filled a second mug and gave it to Grandpa Joe. 'You, too,' he said. 'You look like a skeleton! What's the matter? Hasn't there been anything to eat in your house lately?'

'Not much,' said Grandpa Joe.

Charlie put the mug to his lips, and as the rich warm creamy

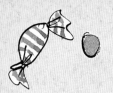
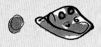

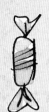

chocolate ran down his throat into his empty tummy, his whole body from head to toe began to tingle with pleasure, and a feeling of intense happiness spread over him.

'You like it?' asked Mr Wonka.

'Oh, it's wonderful!' Charlie said.

'The creamiest loveliest chocolate I've ever tasted!' said Grandpa Joe, smacking his lips.

'That's because it's been mixed by waterfall,' Mr Wonka told him.

The boat sped on down the river. The river was getting narrower. There was some kind of a dark tunnel ahead – a great round tunnel that looked like an enormous pipe – and the river was running right into the tunnel. And so was the boat! 'Row on!' shouted Mr Wonka, jumping up and waving his stick in the air. 'Full speed ahead!' And with the Oompa-Loompas rowing faster than ever, the boat shot into the pitch-dark tunnel, and all the passengers screamed with excitement.

'How can they see where they're going?' shrieked Violet Beauregarde in the darkness.

'There's no knowing where they're going!' cried Mr Wonka, hooting with laughter.

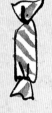

> 'There's no earthly way of knowing
> Which direction they are going!
> There's no knowing where they're rowing,
> Or which way the river's flowing!
> Not a speck of light is showing,
> So the danger must be growing,
> For the rowers keep on rowing,
> And they're certainly not showing
> Any signs that they are slowing . . .'

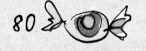

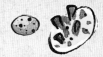

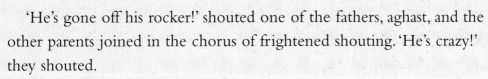

'He's gone off his rocker!' shouted one of the fathers, aghast, and the other parents joined in the chorus of frightened shouting. 'He's crazy!' they shouted.

'He's balmy!'

'He's nutty!'

'He's screwy!'

'He's batty!'

'He's dippy!'

'He's dotty!'

'He's daffy!'

'He's goofy!'

'He's beany!'

'He's buggy!'

'He's wacky!'

'He's loony!'

'No, he is *not*!' said Grandpa Joe.

'Switch on the lights!' shouted Mr Wonka. And suddenly, on came the lights and the whole tunnel was brilliantly lit up, and Charlie could see that they were indeed inside a gigantic pipe, and the great upward-curving walls of the pipe were pure white and spotlessly clean. The river of chocolate was flowing very fast inside the pipe, and the Oompa-Loompas were all rowing like mad, and the boat was rocketing along at a furious pace. Mr Wonka was jumping up and down in the back of the boat and calling to the rowers to row faster and faster still. He seemed to love the sensation of whizzing through a white tunnel in a pink boat on a chocolate river, and he clapped his hands and laughed and kept glancing at his passengers to see if they were enjoying it as much as he.

'Look, Grandpa!' cried Charlie. 'There's a door in the wall!' It was a green door and it was set into the wall of the tunnel just above the level of the river. As they flashed past it there was just enough time to read the writing on the door:

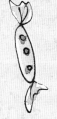

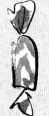

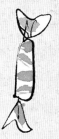

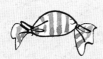

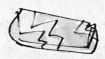

STOREROOM NUMBER 54, it said. ALL THE CREAMS – DAIRY CREAM, WHIPPED CREAM, VIOLET CREAM, COFFEE CREAM, PINEAPPLE CREAM, VANILLA CREAM AND HAIR CREAM.

'Hair cream?' cried Mike Teavee. 'You don't use *hair cream*?'

'Row on!' shouted Mr Wonka. 'There's no time to answer silly questions!'

They streaked past a black door. STOREROOM NUMBER 71, it said on it. WHIPS – ALL SHAPES AND SIZES.

'*Whips!*' cried Veruca Salt. 'What on earth do you use whips for?'

'For whipping cream, of course,' said Mr Wonka. 'How can you whip cream without whips? Whipped cream isn't whipped cream at all unless it's been whipped with whips. Just as a poached egg isn't a poached egg unless it's been stolen from the woods in the dead of night! Row on, please!'

They passed a yellow door on which it said: STOREROOM NUMBER 77, ALL THE BEANS – CACAO BEANS, COFFEE BEANS, JELLY BEANS AND HAS BEANS.

'*Has beans?*' cried Violet Beauregarde.

'You're one yourself!' said Mr Wonka. 'There's no time for arguing! Press on, press on!' But five seconds later, when a bright red door came into sight ahead, he suddenly waved his gold-topped cane in the air and shouted, 'Stop the boat!'

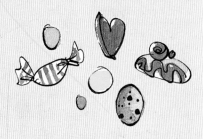

CHAPTER NINETEEN

The Inventing Room – Everlasting Gobstoppers and Hair Toffee

When Mr Wonka shouted 'Stop the boat!' the Oompa-Loompas jammed their oars into the river and backed water furiously. The boat stopped.

The Oompa-Loompas guided the boat alongside the red door. On the door it said, INVENTING ROOM – PRIVATE – KEEP OUT. Mr Wonka took a key from his pocket, leaned over the side of the boat, and put the key in the keyhole.

'*This* is the most important room in the entire factory!' he said. 'All my most secret new inventions are cooking and simmering in here! Old Fickelgruber would give his front teeth to be allowed inside just for three minutes! So would Prodnose and Slugworth and all the other rotten chocolate makers! But now, listen to me! I want no messing about when you go in! No touching, no meddling, and no tasting! Is that agreed?'

'Yes, yes!' the children cried. 'We won't touch a thing!'

'Up to now,' Mr Wonka said, 'nobody else, not even an Oompa-Loompa, has ever been allowed in here!' He opened the door and stepped out of the boat into the room. The four children and their parents all scrambled after him.

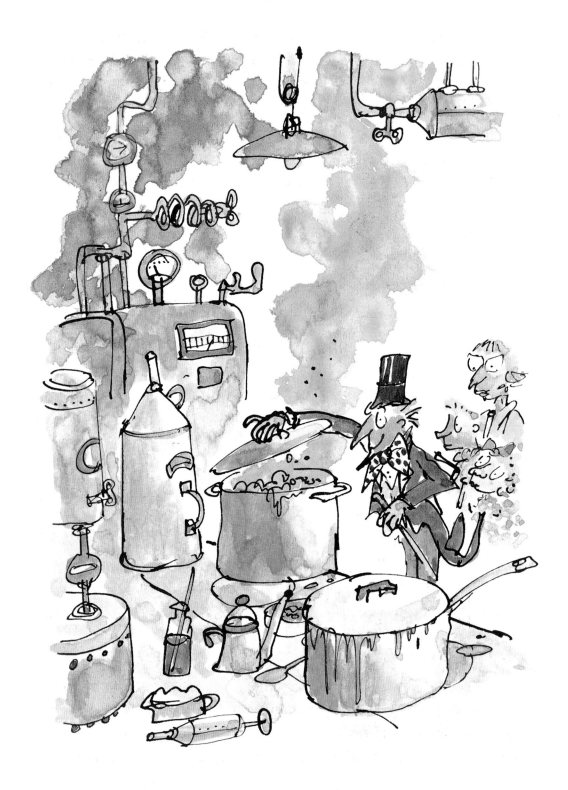

'Don't touch!' shouted Mr Wonka. 'And don't knock anything over!'

Charlie Bucket stared around the gigantic room in which he now found himself. The place was like a witch's kitchen! All about him black metal pots were boiling and bubbling on huge stoves, and kettles were hissing and pans were sizzling, and strange iron machines were clanking and spluttering, and there were pipes running all over the ceiling and walls, and the whole place was filled with smoke and steam and delicious rich smells.

Mr Wonka himself had suddenly become even more excited than usual, and anyone could see that this was the room he loved best of all. He was hopping about among the saucepans and the machines like a child among his Christmas presents, not knowing which thing to look at first. He lifted the lid from a huge pot and took a sniff; then he rushed over and dipped a finger into a barrel of sticky yellow stuff and had a taste; then he skipped across to one of the machines and turned half a dozen knobs this way and that; then he peered anxiously through the glass door of a gigantic oven, rubbing his hands and cackling with delight at what he saw inside. Then he ran over to another machine, a small shiny affair that kept going *phut-phut-phut-phut-phut*, and every time it went *phut*, a large green marble dropped out of it into a basket on the floor. At least it looked like a marble.

'Everlasting Gobstoppers!' cried Mr Wonka proudly. 'They're completely new! I am inventing them for children who are given very little pocket money. You can put an Everlasting Gobstopper in your mouth and you can suck it and suck it and suck it and suck it and it will *never* get any smaller!'

'It's like gum!' cried Violet Beauregarde.

'It is *not* like gum,' Mr Wonka said. 'Gum is for chewing, and if you tried chewing one of these Gobstoppers here you'd break your teeth off! And they *never* get any smaller! They *never* disappear! *NEVER!* At least I don't think they do. There's one of them being tested this very moment in the Testing Room next door. An Oompa-Loompa is sucking it. He's been sucking it for very nearly a year now without stopping, and it's still just as good as ever!

'Now, over here,' Mr Wonka went on, skipping excitedly across the room to the opposite wall, 'over here I am inventing a completely new line in toffees!' He stopped beside a large saucepan. The saucepan was full of a thick gooey purplish treacle, boiling and bubbling. By standing on his toes, little Charlie could just see inside it.

'That's Hair Toffee!' cried Mr Wonka. 'You eat just one tiny bit of that, and in exactly half an hour a brand-new luscious thick silky beautiful crop of hair will start growing out all over the top of your head! And a moustache! And a beard!'

'A beard!' cried Veruca Salt. 'Who wants a beard, for heaven's sake?'

'It would suit you very well,' said Mr Wonka, 'but unfortunately the mixture is not quite right yet. I've got it too strong. It works too well. I tried it on an Oompa-Loompa yesterday in the Testing Room and immediately a huge black beard started shooting out of his chin, and the beard grew so fast that soon it was trailing all over the floor in a thick hairy carpet. It was growing faster than we could cut it! In the end we had to use a lawn mower to keep it in check! But I'll get the mixture right soon! And when I do, then there'll be no excuse any more for little boys and girls going about with bald heads!'

'But Mr Wonka,' said Mike Teavee, 'little boys and girls never *do* go about with . . .'

'Don't argue, my dear child, *please* don't argue!' cried Mr Wonka. 'It's such a waste of precious time! Now, over *here*, if you will all step this way, I will show you something that I am terrifically proud of. Oh, do be careful! Don't knock anything over! Stand back!'

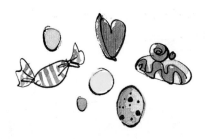

CHAPTER TWENTY

The Great Gum Machine

Mr Wonka led the party over to a gigantic machine that stood in the very centre of the Inventing Room. It was a mountain of gleaming metal that towered high above the children and their parents. Out of the very top of it there sprouted hundreds and hundreds of thin glass tubes, and the glass tubes all curled downwards and came together in a bunch and hung suspended over an enormous round tub as big as a bath.

'Here we go!' cried Mr Wonka, and he pressed three different buttons on the side of the machine. A second later, a mighty rumbling sound came from inside it, and the whole machine began to shake most frighteningly, and steam began hissing out of it all over, and then suddenly the watchers noticed that runny stuff was pouring down the insides of all the hundreds of little glass tubes and squirting out into the great tub below. And in every single tube the runny stuff was of a different colour, so that all the colours of the rainbow (and many others as well) came sloshing and splashing into the tub. It was a lovely sight. And when the tub was nearly full, Mr Wonka pressed another button, and immediately the runny stuff disappeared, and a whizzing whirring noise took its place; and then a giant whizzer started whizzing round inside the enormous tub, mixing up all the different coloured liquids like an ice-cream soda. Gradually, the mixture began to froth. It became frothier and frothier, and it turned from blue to white to green to brown to yellow, then back to blue again.

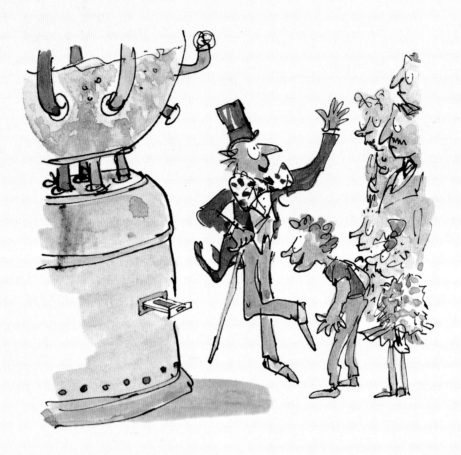

'Watch!' said Mr Wonka.

Click went the machine, and the whizzer stopped whizzing. And now there came a sort of sucking noise, and very quickly all the blue frothy mixture in the huge basin was sucked back into the stomach of the machine. There was a moment of silence. Then a few queer rumblings were heard. Then silence again. Then suddenly, the machine let out a monstrous mighty groan, and at the same moment a tiny drawer (no bigger than the drawer in a slot machine) popped out of the side of the machine, and in the drawer there lay something so small and thin and grey that everyone thought it must be a mistake. The thing looked like a little strip of grey cardboard.

The children and their parents stared at the little grey strip lying in the drawer.

'You mean that's *all*?' said Mike Teavee, disgusted.

'That's all,' answered Mr Wonka, gazing proudly at the result. 'Don't you know what it is?'

There was a pause. Then suddenly, Violet Beauregarde, the silly gum-chewing girl, let out a yell of excitement. 'By gum, it's *gum*!' she shrieked. 'It's a stick of chewing-gum!'

'Right you are!' cried Mr Wonka, slapping Violet hard on the back. 'It's a stick of gum! It's a stick of the most *amazing* and *fabulous* and *sensational* gum in the world!'

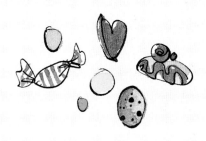

CHAPTER TWENTY-ONE
Goodbye Violet

'This gum,' Mr Wonka went on, 'is my latest, my greatest, my most fascinating invention! It's a chewing-gum meal! It's . . . it's . . . it's . . . That tiny little strip of gum lying there is a whole three-course dinner all by itself!'

'What sort of nonsense is this?' said one of the fathers.

'My dear sir!' cried Mr Wonka, 'when I start selling this gum in the shops it will change *everything*! It will be the end of all kitchens and all cooking! There will be no more shopping to do! No more buying of meat and groceries! There'll be no knives and forks at mealtimes! No plates! No washing up! No rubbish! No mess! Just a little strip of Wonka's magic chewing-gum – and that's all you'll ever need at breakfast, lunch, and supper! This piece of gum I've just made happens to be tomato soup, roast beef, and blueberry pie, but you can have almost anything you want!'

'What *do* you mean, it's tomato soup, roast beef, and blueberry pie?' said Violet Beauregarde.

'If you were to start chewing it,' said Mr Wonka, 'then that is exactly what you would get on the menu. It's absolutely amazing! You can actually *feel* the food going down your throat and into your tummy! And you can taste it perfectly! And it fills you up! It satisfies you! It's terrific!'

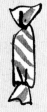

'It's utterly impossible,' said Veruca Salt.

'Just so long as it's gum,' shouted Violet Beauregarde, 'just so long as it's a piece of gum and I can chew it, then *that's* for me!' And quickly she

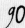
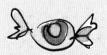

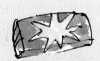

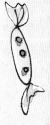

took her own world-record piece of chewing-gum out of her mouth and stuck it behind her left ear. 'Come on, Mr Wonka,' she said, 'hand over this magic gum of yours and we'll see if the thing works.'

'Now, Violet,' said Mrs Beauregarde, her mother, 'don't let's do anything silly, Violet.'

'I want the gum!' Violet said obstinately. 'What's so silly?'

'I would rather you didn't take it,' Mr Wonka told her gently. 'You see, I haven't got it *quite right* yet. There are still one or two things . . .'

'Oh, to blazes with that!' said Violet, and suddenly, before Mr Wonka could stop her, she shot out a fat hand and grabbed the stick of gum out of the little drawer and popped it into her mouth. At once, her huge, well-trained jaws started chewing away on it like a pair of tongs.

'Don't!' said Mr Wonka.

'Fabulous!' shouted Violet. 'It's tomato soup! It's hot and creamy and delicious! I can feel it running down my throat!'

'Stop!' said Mr Wonka. 'The gum isn't ready yet! It's not right!'

'Of course it's right!' said Violet. 'It's working beautifully! Oh my, what lovely soup this is!'

'Spit it out!' said Mr Wonka.

'It's changing!' shouted Violet, chewing and grinning both at the same time. 'The second course is coming up! It's roast beef! It's tender and juicy! Oh boy, what a flavour! The baked potato is marvellous, too! It's got a crispy skin and it's all filled with butter inside!'

'But how *in*-teresting, Violet,' said Mrs Beauregarde. 'You are a clever girl.'

'Keep chewing, baby!' said Mr Beauregarde. 'Keep right on chewing! This is a great day for the Beauregardes! Our little girl is the first person in the world to have a chewing-gum meal!'

Everybody was watching Violet Beauregarde as she stood there chewing this extraordinary gum. Little Charlie Bucket was staring at her absolutely spellbound, watching her huge rubbery lips as they pressed

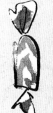

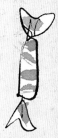

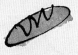
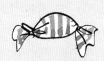

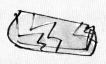

and unpressed with the chewing, and Grandpa Joe stood beside him, gaping at the girl. Mr Wonka was wringing his hands and saying, 'No, no, no, no, no! It isn't ready for eating! It isn't right! You mustn't do it!'

'Blueberry pie and cream!' shouted Violet. 'Here it comes! Oh my, it's perfect! It's beautiful! It's . . . it's exactly as though I'm swallowing it! It's as though I'm chewing and swallowing great big spoonfuls of the most marvellous blueberry pie in the world!'

'Good heavens, girl!' shrieked Mrs Beauregarde suddenly, staring at Violet, 'what's happening to your nose!'

'Oh, be quiet, mother, and let me finish!' said Violet.

'It's turning blue!' screamed Mrs Beauregarde. 'Your nose is turning blue as a blueberry!'

'Your mother is right!' shouted Mr Beauregarde. 'Your whole nose has gone purple!'

'What *do* you mean?' said Violet, still chewing away.

'Your cheeks!' screamed Mrs Beauregarde. 'They're turning blue as well! So is your chin! Your whole face is turning blue!'

'Spit that gum out at once!' ordered Mr Beauregarde.

'Mercy! Save us!' yelled Mrs Beauregarde. 'The girl's going blue and purple all over! Even her hair is changing colour! Violet, you're turning violet, Violet! What *is* happening to you?'

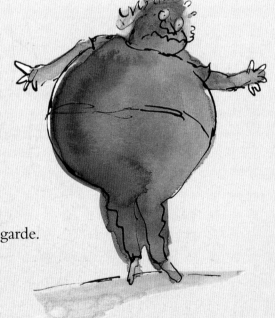

'I *told* you I hadn't got it quite right,' sighed Mr Wonka, shaking his head sadly.

'I'll say you haven't!' cried Mrs Beauregarde. 'Just look at the girl now!'

Everybody was staring at Violet. And what a terrible, peculiar sight she was!

Goodbye Violet

Her face and hands and legs and neck, in fact the skin all over her body, as well as her great big mop of curly hair, had turned a brilliant, purplish-blue, the colour of blueberry juice!

'It always goes wrong when we come to the dessert,' sighed Mr Wonka. 'It's the blueberry pie that does it. But I'll get it right one day, you wait and see.'

'Violet,' screamed Mrs Beauregarde, 'you're swelling up!'

'I feel sick,' Violet said.

'You're swelling up!' screamed Mrs Beauregarde again.

'I feel most peculiar!' gasped Violet.

'I'm not surprised!' said Mr Beauregarde.

'Great heavens, girl!' screeched Mrs Beauregarde. 'You're blowing up like a balloon!'

'Like a blueberry,' said Mr Wonka.

'Call a doctor!' shouted Mr Beauregarde.

'Prick her with a pin!' said one of the other fathers.

'Save her!' cried Mrs Beauregarde, wringing her hands.

But there was no saving her now. Her body was swelling up and changing shape at such a rate that within a minute it had turned into nothing less than an enormous round blue ball – a gigantic blueberry, in fact – and all that remained of Violet Beauregarde herself was a tiny pair of legs and a tiny pair of arms sticking out of the great round fruit and little head on top.

'It *always* happens like that,' sighed Mr Wonka. 'I've tried it twenty times in the Testing Room on twenty Oompa-Loompas, and every one of them finished up as a blueberry. It's most annoying. I just can't understand it.'

'But I don't want a blueberry for a daughter!' yelled Mrs Beauregarde. 'Put her back to what she was this instant!'

Mr Wonka clicked his fingers, and ten Oompa-Loompas appeared immediately at his side.

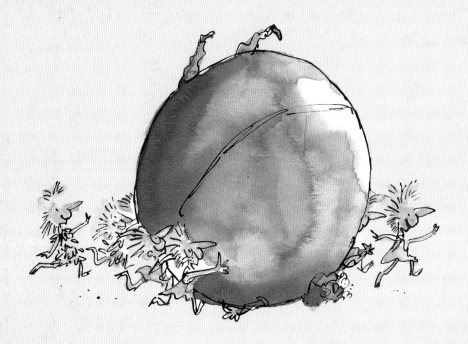

'Roll Miss Beauregarde into the boat,' he said to them, 'and take her along to the Juicing Room at once.'

'The *Juicing Room*?' cried Mrs Beauregarde. 'What are they going to do to her there?'

'Squeeze her,' said Mr Wonka. 'We've got to squeeze the juice out of her immediately. After that, we'll just have to see how she comes out. But don't worry, my dear Mrs Beauregarde. We'll get her repaired if it's the last thing we do. I am sorry about it all, I really am . . .'

Already the ten Oompa-Loompas were rolling the enormous blueberry across the floor of the Inventing Room towards the door that led to the chocolate river where the boat was waiting. Mr and Mrs Beauregarde hurried after them. The rest of the party, including little Charlie Bucket and Grandpa Joe, stood absolutely still and watched them go.

'Listen!' whispered Charlie. 'Listen, Grandpa! The Oompa-Loompas in the boat outside are starting to sing!'

Goodbye Violet

The voices, one hundred of them singing together, came loud and clear into the room:

'Dear friends, we surely all agree
There's almost nothing worse to see
Than some repulsive little bum
Who's always chewing chewing-gum.
(It's very near as bad as those
Who sit around and pick the nose.)
So please believe us when we say
That chewing gum will never pay;
This sticky habit's bound to send
The chewer to a sticky end.
Did any of you ever know
A person called Miss Bigelow?
This dreadful woman saw no wrong
In chewing, chewing all day long.
She chewed while bathing in the tub,
She chewed while dancing at her club,
She chewed in church and on the bus;
It really was quite ludicrous!
And when she couldn't find her gum,
She'd chew up the linoleum,
Or anything that happened near –
A pair of boots, the postman's ear,
Or other people's underclothes,
And once she chewed her boyfriend's nose.
She went on chewing till, at last,
Her chewing muscles grew so vast
That from her face her giant chin
Stuck out just like a violin.
For years and years she chewed away,

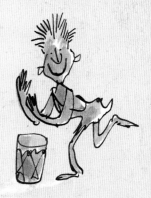

95

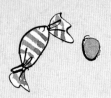

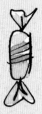

Consuming fifty bits a day,
Until one summer's eve, alas,
A horrid business came to pass.
Miss Bigelow went late to bed,
For half an hour she lay and read,
Chewing and chewing all the while
Like some great clockwork crocodile.
At last, she put her gum away
Upon a special little tray,

And settled back and went to sleep –
(She managed this by counting sheep).
But now, how strange! Although she slept,
Those massive jaws of hers still kept
On chewing, chewing through the night,
Even with nothing there to bite.

They were, you see, in such a groove
They positively had to move.
And very grim it was to hear

In pitchy darkness, loud and clear,
This sleeping woman's great big trap
Opening and shutting, snap-snap-snap!
Faster and faster, chop-chop-chop,
The noise went on, it wouldn't stop.
Until at last her jaws decide
To pause and open extra wide,
And with the most tremendous chew
They bit the lady's tongue in two.
Thereafter, just from chewing gum,
Miss Bigelow was always dumb,
And spent her life shut up in some
Disgusting sanatorium.

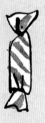

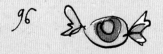

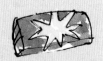

Goodbye Violet

And that is why we'll try so hard
To save Miss Violet Beauregarde
From suffering an equal fate.
She's still quite young. It's not too late,
Provided she survives the cure.
We hope she does. We can't be sure.'

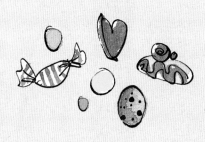

CHAPTER TWENTY-TWO

Along the Corridor

'Well, well, well,' sighed Mr Willy Wonka, 'two naughty little children gone. Three good little children left. I think we'd better get out of this room quickly before we lose anyone else!'

'But Mr Wonka,' said Charlie Bucket anxiously, 'will Violet Beauregarde *ever* be all right again or will she always be a blueberry?'

'They'll de-juice her in no time flat!' declared Mr Wonka. 'They'll roll her into the de-juicing machine, and she'll come out just as thin as a whistle!'

'But will she still be blue all over?' asked Charlie.

'She'll be *purple*!' cried Mr Wonka. 'A fine rich purple from head to toe! But there you are! That's what comes from chewing disgusting gum all day long!'

'If you think gum is so disgusting,' said Mike Teavee, 'then why do you make it in your factory?'

'I do wish you wouldn't mumble,' said Mr Wonka. 'I can't hear a word you're saying. Come on! Off we go! Hurry up! Follow me! We're going into the corridors again!' And so saying, Mr Wonka scuttled across to the far end of the Inventing Room and went out through a small secret door hidden behind a lot of pipes and stoves. The three remaining children – Veruca Salt, Mike Teavee, and Charlie Bucket – together with the five remaining grown-ups, followed after him.

Charlie Bucket saw that they were now back in one of those long pink corridors with many other pink corridors leading out of it. Mr

Along the Corridor

Wonka was rushing along in front, turning left and right and right and left, and Grandpa Joe was saying, 'Keep a good hold of my hand, Charlie. It would be terrible to get lost in here.'

Mr Wonka was saying, 'No time for any more messing about! We'll never get *anywhere* at the rate we've been going!' And on he rushed, down the endless pink corridors, with his black top hat perched on the top of his head and his plum-coloured velvet coat-tails flying out behind him like a flag in the wind.

They passed a door in the wall. 'No time to go in!' shouted Mr Wonka. 'Press on! Press on!'

They passed another door, then another and another. There were doors every twenty paces or so along the corridor now, and they all had something written on them, and strange clanking noises were coming from behind several of them, and delicious smells came wafting through the keyholes, and sometimes little jets of coloured steam shot out from the cracks underneath.

Grandpa Joe and Charlie were half running and half walking to keep

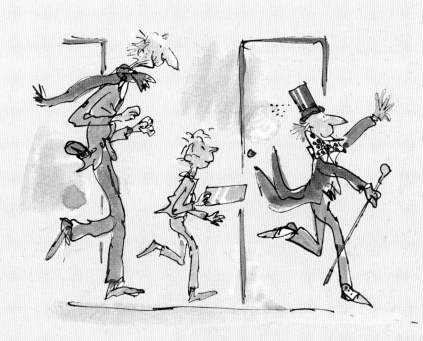

up with Mr Wonka, but they were able to read what it said on quite a few of the doors as they hurried by. EATABLE MARSHMALLOW PILLOWS, it said on one.

'Marshmallow pillows are terrific!' shouted Mr Wonka as he dashed by. 'They'll be all the rage when I get them into the shops! No time to go in, though! No time to go in!'

LICKABLE WALLPAPER FOR NURSERIES, it said on the next door.

'Lovely stuff, lickable wallpaper!' cried Mr Wonka, rushing past. 'It has pictures of fruits on it – bananas, apples, oranges, grapes, pineapples, strawberries and snozzberries . . .'

'*Snozzberries?*' said Mike Teavee.

'Don't interrupt!' said Mr Wonka. 'The wallpaper has pictures of all these fruits printed on it, and when you lick the picture of a banana, it tastes of banana. When you lick a strawberry, it tastes of strawberry. And when you lick a snozzberry, it tastes just exactly like a snozzberry . . .'

'But what *does* a snozzberry taste like?'

'You're mumbling again,' said Mr Wonka. 'Speak louder next time. On we go! Hurry up!'

HOT ICE CREAMS FOR COLD DAYS, it said on the next door.

'*Extremely* useful in the winter,' said Mr Wonka, rushing on. 'Hot ice cream warms you up no end in freezing weather. I also make hot ice cubes for putting in hot drinks. Hot ice cubes make hot drinks hotter.'

COWS THAT GIVE CHOCOLATE MILK, it said on the next door.

'Ah, my pretty little cows!' cried Mr Wonka. 'How I love those cows!'

'But why can't we *see* them?' asked Veruca Salt. 'Why do we have to go rushing on past all these lovely rooms?'

'We shall stop in time!' called out Mr Wonka. 'Don't be so madly impatient!'

FIZZY LIFTING DRINKS, it said on the next door.

'Oh, those are fabulous!' cried Mr Wonka. 'They fill you with bubbles, and the bubbles are full of a special kind of gas, and this gas is so terrifically *lifting* that it lifts you right off the ground just like a balloon, and up you go until your head hits the ceiling – and there you stay.'

'But how do you come down again?' asked little Charlie.

'You do a burp, of course,' said Mr Wonka. 'You do a great big long rude burp, and *up* comes the gas and down comes you! But don't drink it outdoors! There's no knowing how high up you'll be carried if you do that. I gave some to an old Oompa-Loompa once out in the back yard and he went up and up and disappeared out of sight! It was very sad. I never saw him again.'

'He should have burped,' Charlie said.

'Of course he should have burped,' said Mr Wonka. 'I stood there shouting, "Burp, you silly ass, burp, or you'll never come down again!" But he didn't or couldn't or wouldn't, I don't know which. Maybe he was too polite. He must be on the moon by now.'

On the next door, it said, SQUARE SWEETS THAT LOOK ROUND.

'Wait!' cried Mr Wonka, skidding suddenly to a halt. 'I am very proud of my square sweets that look round. Let's take a peek.'

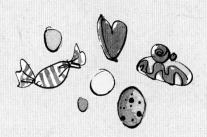

CHAPTER TWENTY-THREE

Square Sweets That Look Round

Everybody stopped and crowded to the door. The top half of the door was made of glass. Grandpa Joe lifted Charlie up so that he could get a better view, and looking in, Charlie saw a long table, and on the table there were rows and rows of small white square-shaped sweets. The sweets looked very much like square sugar lumps – except that each of them had a funny little pink face painted on one side. At the end of the table, a number of Oompa-Loompas were busily painting more faces on more sweets.

'There you are!' cried Mr Wonka. 'Square sweets that look round!'

'They don't look round to me,' said Mike Teavee.

'They look square,' said Veruca Salt. 'They look completely square.'

'But they *are* square,' said Mr Wonka. 'I never said they weren't.'

'You said they were *round*!' said Veruca Salt.

'I never said anything of the sort,' said Mr Wonka. 'I said they *looked* round.'

'But they *don't* look round!' said Veruca Salt. 'They look square!'

'They look round,' insisted Mr Wonka.

'They most certainly do not look round!' cried Veruca Salt.

'Veruca, darling,' said Mrs Salt, 'pay no attention to Mr Wonka! He's lying to you!'

'My dear old fish,' said Mr Wonka, 'go and boil your head!'

'How dare you speak to me like that!' shouted Mrs Salt.

'Oh, do shut up,' said Mr Wonka. 'Now watch this!'

He took a key from his pocket, and unlocked the door, and flung it open . . . and suddenly . . . at the sound of the door opening, all the rows of little square sweets looked quickly round to see who was coming in. The tiny faces actually turned towards the door and stared at Mr Wonka.

'There you are!' he cried triumphantly. 'They're looking round! There's no argument about it! They are square sweets that look round!'

'By golly, he's right!' said Grandpa Joe.

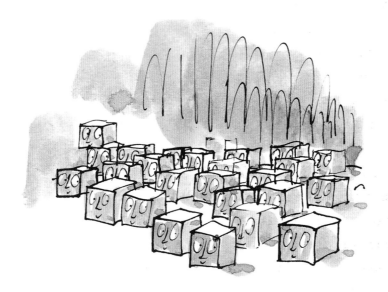

'Come on!' said Mr Wonka, starting off down the corridor again. 'On we go! We mustn't dawdle!'

BUTTERSCOTCH AND BUTTERGIN, it said on the next door they passed.

'Now *that* sounds a bit more interesting,' said Mr Salt, Veruca's father.

'Glorious stuff!' said Mr Wonka. 'The Oompa-Loompas all adore it. It makes them tiddly. Listen! You can hear them in there now, whooping it up.'

Shrieks of laughter and snatches of singing could be heard coming through the closed door.

'They're drunk as lords,' said Mr Wonka. 'They're drinking butterscotch and soda. They like that best of all. Buttergin and tonic is also very popular. Follow me, please! We really mustn't keep stopping like this.' He turned left. He turned right. They came to a long flight of stairs. Mr Wonka slid down the banisters. The three children did the same. Mrs Salt and Mrs Teavee, the only women now left in the party, were getting very out of breath. Mrs Salt was a great fat creature with short legs, and she was blowing like a rhinoceros. 'This way!' cried Mr Wonka, turning left at the bottom of the stairs.

'Go *slower*!' panted Mrs Salt.

'Impossible,' said Mr Wonka. 'We should never get there in time if I did.'

'Get where?' asked Veruca Salt.

'Never you mind,' said Mr Wonka. 'You just wait and see.'

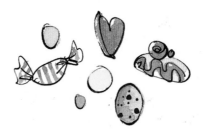

CHAPTER TWENTY-FOUR

Veruca in the Nut Room

Mr Wonka rushed on down the corridor. **THE NUT ROOM**, it said on the next door they came to.

'All right,' said Mr Wonka, 'stop here for a moment and catch your breath, and take a peek through the glass panel of this door. But don't go in! Whatever you do, don't go into **THE NUT ROOM**! If you go in, you'll disturb the squirrels!'

Everyone crowded around the door.

'Oh look, Grandpa, look!' cried Charlie.

'Squirrels!' shouted Veruca Salt.

'Crikey!' said Mike Teavee.

It was an amazing sight. One hundred squirrels were seated upon high stools around a large table. On the table, there were mounds and mounds of walnuts, and the squirrels were all working away like mad, shelling the walnuts at a tremendous speed.

'These squirrels are specially trained for getting the nuts out of walnuts,' Mr Wonka explained.

'Why use squirrels?' Mike Teavee asked. 'Why not use Oompa-Loompas?'

'Because,' said Mr Wonka, 'Oompa-Loompas can't get walnuts out of walnut shells in one piece. They always break them in two. Nobody except squirrels can get walnuts *whole* out of walnut shells every time.

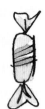

It is extremely difficult. But in my factory, I insist upon only whole walnuts. Therefore I have to have squirrels to do the job. Aren't they wonderful, the way they get those nuts out! And see how they first tap each walnut with their knuckles to be sure it's not a bad one! If it's bad, it makes a hollow sound, and they don't bother to open it. They just throw it down the rubbish chute. There! Look! Watch that squirrel nearest to us! I think he's got a bad one now!'

They watched the little squirrel as he tapped the walnut shell with his knuckles. He cocked his head to one side, listening intently, then suddenly he threw the nut over his shoulder into a large hole in the floor.

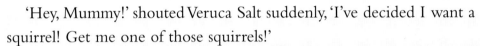
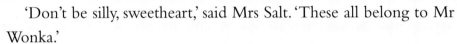

'Hey, Mummy!' shouted Veruca Salt suddenly, 'I've decided I want a squirrel! Get me one of those squirrels!'

'Don't be silly, sweetheart,' said Mrs Salt. 'These all belong to Mr Wonka.'

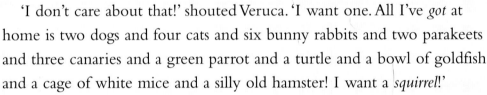

'I don't care about that!' shouted Veruca. 'I want one. All I've *got* at home is two dogs and four cats and six bunny rabbits and two parakeets and three canaries and a green parrot and a turtle and a bowl of goldfish and a cage of white mice and a silly old hamster! I want a *squirrel*!'

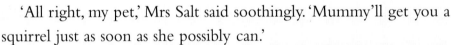

'All right, my pet,' Mrs Salt said soothingly. 'Mummy'll get you a squirrel just as soon as she possibly can.'

'But I don't want *any* old squirrel!' Veruca shouted. 'I want a *trained* squirrel!'

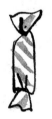

At this point, Mr Salt, Veruca's father, stepped forward. 'Very well, Wonka,' he said importantly, taking out a wallet full of money, 'how much d'you want for one of these squirrels? Name your price.'

'They're not for sale,' Mr Wonka answered. 'She can't have one.'

'Who says I can't!' shouted Veruca. 'I'm going in to get myself one this very minute!'

'Don't!' said Mr Wonka quickly, but he was too late. The girl had already thrown open the door and rushed in.

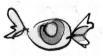

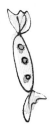

The moment she entered the room, one hundred squirrels stopped what they were doing and turned their heads and stared at her with small black beady eyes.

Veruca Salt stopped also, and stared back at them. Then her gaze fell upon a pretty little squirrel sitting nearest to her at the end of the table. The squirrel was holding a walnut in its paws.

'All right,' Veruca said, 'I'll have *you*!'

She reached out her hands to grab the squirrel . . . but as she did so . . . in that first split second when her hands started to go forward, there was a sudden flash of movement in the room, like a flash of brown lightning, and every single squirrel around the table took a flying leap towards her and landed on her body.

Twenty-five of them caught hold of her right arm, and pinned it down.

Twenty-five more caught hold of her left arm, and pinned that down.

Twenty-five caught hold of her right leg and anchored it to the ground.

Twenty-*four* caught hold of her left leg.

And the one remaining squirrel (obviously the leader of them all) climbed up on to her shoulder and started tap-tap-tapping the wretched girl's head with its knuckles.

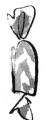

'Save her!' screamed Mrs Salt. 'Veruca! Come back! What are they *doing* to her?'

'They're testing her to see if she's a bad nut,' said Mr Wonka. 'You watch.'

Veruca struggled furiously, but the squirrels held her tight and she couldn't move. The squirrel on her shoulder went tap-tap-tapping the side of her head with his knuckles.

Then all at once, the squirrels pulled Veruca to the ground and started carrying her across the floor.

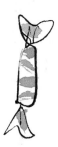

'My goodness, she *is* a bad nut after all,' said Mr Wonka. 'Her head

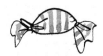

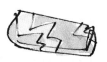

must have sounded quite hollow.'

Veruca kicked and screamed, but it was no use. The tiny strong paws held her tightly and she couldn't escape.

'Where are they taking her?' shrieked Mrs Salt.

'She's going where all the other bad nuts go,' said Mr Willy Wonka. 'Down the rubbish chute.'

'By golly, she *is* going down the chute!' said Mr Salt, staring through the glass door at his daughter.

'Then save her!' cried Mrs Salt.

'Too late,' said Mr Wonka. 'She's gone!'

And indeed she had.

'But where?' shrieked Mrs Salt, flapping her arms. 'What happens to the bad nuts? Where does the chute go to?'

'That *particular* chute,' Mr Wonka told her, 'runs directly into the great big main rubbish pipe which carries away all the rubbish from every part of the factory – all the floor sweepings and potato peelings and rotten cabbages and fish heads and stuff like that.'

'Who eats fish and cabbage and potatoes in *this* factory, I'd like to know?' said Mike Teavee.

'I do, of course,' answered Mr Wonka. 'You don't think I live on cacao beans, do you?'

'But . . . but . . . but . . .' shrieked Mrs Salt, 'where does the great big pipe go to in the end?'

'Why, to the furnace, of course,' Mr Wonka said calmly. 'To the incinerator.'

Mrs Salt opened her huge red mouth and started to scream.

'Don't worry,' said Mr Wonka, 'there's always a chance that they've decided not to light it today.'

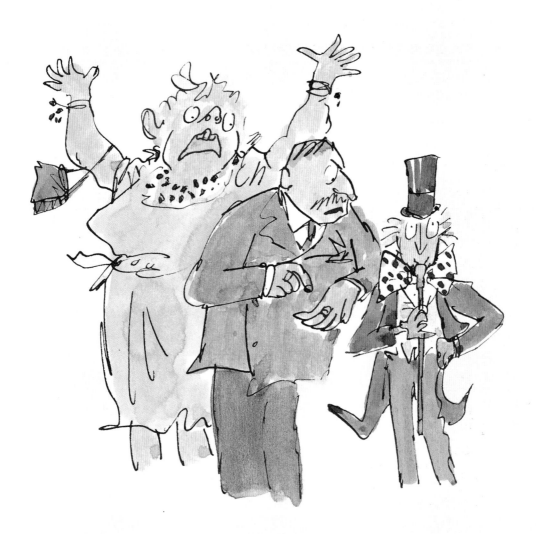

'A *chance*!' yelled Mrs Salt. 'My darling Veruca! She'll . . . she'll . . . she'll be sizzled like a sausage!'

'Quite right, my dear,' said Mr Salt. 'Now see here, Wonka,' he added, 'I think you've gone *just* a shade too far this time, I do indeed. My daughter may be a bit of a frump – I don't mind admitting it – but that doesn't mean you can roast her to a crisp. I'll have you know I'm extremely cross about this, I really am.'

'Oh, don't be cross, my dear sir!' said Mr Wonka. 'I expect she'll turn up again sooner or later. She may not even have gone down at all. She may be stuck in the chute just below the entrance hole, and if *that's* the case, all you'll have to do is go in and pull her up again.'

Hearing this, both Mr and Mrs Salt dashed into the Nut Room and ran over to the hole in the floor and peered in.

'Veruca!' shouted Mrs Salt. 'Are you down there!'

There was no answer.

Mrs Salt bent further forward to get a closer look. She was now kneeling right on the edge of the hole with her head down and her enormous behind sticking up in the air like a giant mushroom. It was a dangerous position to be in. She needed only one tiny little push . . . one gentle nudge in the right place . . . and *that* is exactly what the squirrels gave her! Over she toppled, into the hole head first, screeching like a parrot.

'Good gracious me!' said Mr Salt, as he watched his fat wife go tumbling down the hole, 'what a lot of rubbish there's going to be today!' He saw her disappearing into the darkness. 'What's it like down there, Angina?' he called out. He leaned further forward.

The squirrels rushed up behind him . . .

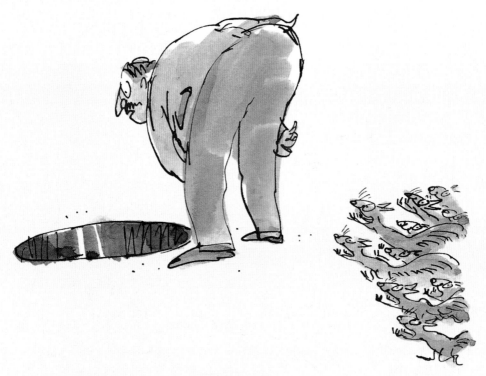

'Help!' he shouted.

But he was already toppling forward, and down the chute he went, just as his wife had done before him – and his daughter.

'Oh *dear*!' cried Charlie, who was watching with the others through the door, 'what on earth's going to happen to them now?'

'I expect someone will catch them at the bottom of the chute,' said Mr Wonka.

'But what about the great fiery incinerator?' asked Charlie.

'They only light it every other day,' said Mr Wonka. 'Perhaps this is one of the days when they let it go out. You never know . . . they might be lucky . . .'

'Ssshh!' said Grandpa Joe. 'Listen! Here comes another song!'

From far away down the corridor came the beating of drums. Then the singing began.

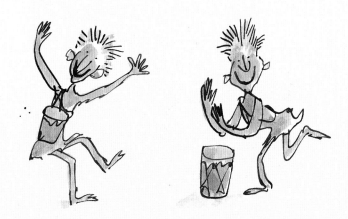

'*Veruca Salt!*' sang the Oompa-Loompas.
'*Veruca Salt, the little brute,*
Has just gone down the rubbish chute
(And as we very rightly thought
That in a case like this we ought
To see the thing completely through,
We've polished off her parents, too).
Down goes Veruca! Down the drain!
And here, perhaps, we should explain
That she will meet, as she descends,
A rather different set of friends
To those that she has left behind –
These won't be nearly so refined.
A fish head, for example, cut
This morning from a halibut.
"Hello! Good morning! How d'you do?
How nice to meet you! How are you?"
And then a little further down
A mass of others gather round:
A bacon rind, some rancid lard,
A loaf of bread gone stale and hard,
A steak that nobody could chew,
An oyster from an oyster stew,
Some liverwurst so old and grey
One smelled it from a mile away,
A rotten nut, a reeky pear,
A thing the cat left on the stair,
And lots of other things as well,
Each with a rather horrid smell.
These are Veruca's new-found friends
That she will meet as she descends,

Veruca in the Nut Room

And this *is the price she has to pay*
For going so very far astray.
But now, my dears, we think you might
Be wondering — is it really right
That every single bit of blame
And all the scolding and the shame
Should fall upon Veruca Salt?
Is she *the only one at fault?*
For though she's spoiled, and dreadfully so,
A girl can't spoil herself, you know.
Who spoiled *her, then? Ah, who indeed?*
Who pandered *to her every need?*
Who turned *her into such a brat?*
Who are *the culprits? Who* did *that?*
Alas! You needn't look so far
To find out who these sinners are.
They are (and this is very sad)
Her loving parents, MUM and DAD.
And that is why we're glad they fell
Into the rubbish chute as well.'

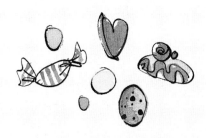

CHAPTER TWENTY-FIVE

The Great Glass Lift

'I've never seen anything like it!' cried Mr Wonka. 'The children are disappearing like rabbits! But you mustn't worry about it! They'll *all* come out in the wash!'

Mr Wonka looked at the little group that stood beside him in the corridor. There were only two children left now – Mike Teavee and Charlie Bucket. And there were three grown-ups, Mr and Mrs Teavee and Grandpa Joe. 'Shall we move on?' Mr Wonka asked.

'Oh, yes!' cried Charlie and Grandpa Joe, both together.

'My feet are getting tired,' said Mike Teavee. 'I want to watch television.'

'If you're tired then we'd better take the lift,' said Mr Wonka. 'It's over here. Come on! In we go!' He skipped across the passage to a pair of double doors. The doors slid open. The two children and the grown-ups went in.

'Now then,' cried Mr Wonka, 'which button shall we press first? Take your pick!'

Charlie Bucket stared around him in astonishment. This was the craziest lift he had ever seen. There were buttons everywhere! The walls, and even the *ceiling*, were covered all over with rows and rows and rows of small, black push buttons! There must have been a thousand of them on each wall, and another thousand on the ceiling! And now Charlie noticed that every single button had a tiny printed label beside it telling

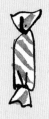

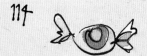

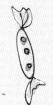

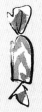

you which room you would be taken to if you pressed it.

'This isn't just an ordinary up-and-down lift!' announced Mr Wonka proudly. 'This lift can go sideways and longways and slantways and any other way you can think of! It can visit any single room in the whole factory, no matter where it is! You simply press the button . . . and *zing*! . . . you're off!'

'*Fantastic!*' murmured Grandpa Joe. His eyes were shining with excitement as he stared at the rows of buttons.

'The whole lift is made of thick, clear glass!' Mr Wonka declared. 'Walls, doors, ceiling, floor, everything is made of glass so that you can see out!'

'But there's nothing to see,' said Mike Teavee.

'Choose a button!' said Mr Wonka. 'The two children may press one button each. So take your pick! Hurry up! In every room, something delicious and wonderful is being made.'

Quickly, Charlie started reading some of the labels alongside the buttons.

THE ROCK-CANDY MINE – 10,000 FEET DEEP. , it said on one.

COKERNUT-ICE SKATING RINKS. , it said on another.

Then . . . STRAWBERRY-JUICE WATER PISTOLS.

TOFFEE-APPLE TREES FOR PLANTING OUT IN YOUR GARDEN – ALL SIZES.

EXPLODING SWEETS FOR YOUR ENEMIES.

LUMINOUS LOLLIES FOR EATING IN BED AT NIGHT.

MINT JUJUBES FOR THE BOY NEXT DOOR – THEY'LL GIVE HIM GREEN TEETH FOR A MONTH.

CAVITY-FILLING CARAMELS – NO MORE DENTISTS.

STICKJAW FOR TALKATIVE PARENTS.

WRIGGLE-SWEETS THAT WRIGGLE DELIGHTFULLY IN YOUR TUMMY AFTER SWALLOWING.

INVISIBLE CHOCOLATE BARS FOR EATING IN CLASS.

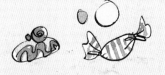

SUGAR-COATED PENCILS FOR SUCKING.

FIZZY LEMONADE SWIMMING POOLS.

MAGIC HAND-FUDGE – WHEN YOU HOLD IT IN YOUR HAND, YOU TASTE IT IN YOUR MOUTH.

RAINBOW DROPS – SUCK THEM AND YOU CAN SPIT IN SIX DIFFERENT COLOURS.

'Come on, come on!' cried Mr Wonka. 'We can't wait all day!'

'Isn't there a *Television Room* in all this lot?' asked Mike Teavee.

'Certainly there's a television room,' Mr Wonka said. 'That button over there.' He pointed with his finger. Everybody looked.

TELEVISION CHOCOLATE. , it said on the tiny label beside the button.

'*Whoopee!*' shouted Mike Teavee. 'That's for me!' He stuck out his thumb and pressed the button. Instantly, there was a tremendous whizzing noise. The doors clanged shut and the lift leaped away as though it had been stung by a wasp. But it leapt *sideways*! And all the passengers (except Mr Wonka, who was holding on to a strap from the ceiling) were flung off their feet on to the floor.

'Get up, get up!' cried Mr Wonka, roaring with laughter. But just as they were staggering to their feet, the lift changed direction and swerved violently round a corner. And over they went once more.

'Help!' shouted Mrs Teavee.

'Take my hand, madam,' said Mr Wonka gallantly. 'There you are! Now grab this strap! Everybody grab a strap. The journey's not over yet!'

Old Grandpa Joe staggered to his feet and caught hold of a strap. Little Charlie, who couldn't possibly reach as high as that, put his arms around Grandpa Joe's legs and hung on tight.

The lift rushed on at the speed of a rocket. Now it was beginning to climb. It was shooting up and up and up on a steep slanty course as if it were climbing a very steep hill. Then suddenly, as though it had come to the top of the hill and gone over a precipice, it dropped like a stone and

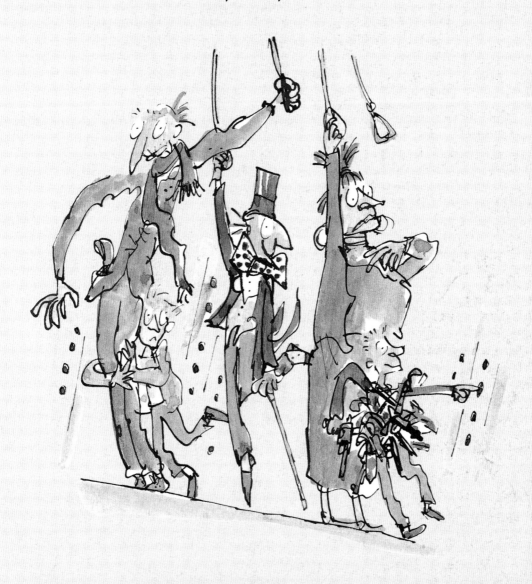

Charlie felt his tummy coming right up into his throat, and Grandpa Joe shouted, 'Yippee! Here we go!' and Mrs Teavee cried out, 'The rope has broken! We're going to crash!' And Mr Wonka said, 'Calm yourself, my dear lady,' and patted her comfortingly on the arm. And then Grandpa Joe looked down at Charlie who was clinging to his legs, and he said, 'Are you all right, Charlie?' Charlie shouted, 'I love it! It's like being on a roller coaster!' And through the glass walls of the lift, as it rushed along,

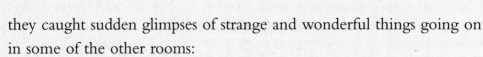

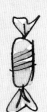

they caught sudden glimpses of strange and wonderful things going on in some of the other rooms:

An enormous spout with brown sticky stuff oozing out of it on to the floor . . .

A great, craggy mountain made entirely of fudge, with Oompa-Loompas (all roped together for safety) hacking huge hunks of fudge out of its sides . . .

A machine with white powder spraying out of it like a snowstorm . . .

A lake of hot caramel with steam coming off it . . .

A village of Oompa-Loompas, with tiny houses and streets and hundreds of Oompa-Loompa children no more than four inches high playing in the streets . . .

And now the lift began flattening out again, but it seemed to be going faster than ever, and Charlie could hear the scream of the wind outside as it hurtled forward . . . and it twisted . . . and it turned . . . and it went up . . . and it went down . . . and . . .

'I'm going to be sick!' yelled Mrs Teavee, turning green in the face.

'Please don't be sick,' said Mr Wonka.

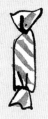

'Try and stop me!' said Mrs Teavee.

'Then you'd better take this,' said Mr Wonka, and he swept his magnificent black top hat off his head, and held it out, upside down, in front of Mrs Teavee's mouth.

'Make this awful thing stop!' ordered Mr Teavee.

'Can't do that,' said Mr Wonka. 'It won't stop till we get there. I only hope no one's using the *other* lift at this moment.'

'What other lift?' screamed Mrs Teavee.

'The one that goes the opposite way on the same track as this one,' said Mr Wonka.

'Holy mackerel!' cried Mr Teavee. 'You mean we might have a collision?'

'I've always been lucky so far,' said Mr Wonka.

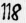

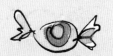

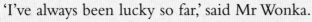

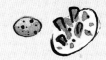

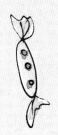

'Now I *am* going to be sick!' yelled Mrs Teavee.

'No, no!' said Mr Wonka. 'Not now! We're nearly there! Don't spoil my hat!'

The next moment, there was a screaming of brakes, and the lift began to slow down. Then it stopped altogether.

'Some ride!' said Mr Teavee, wiping his great sweaty face with a handkerchief.

'Never again!' gasped Mrs Teavee. And then the doors of the lift slid open and Mr Wonka said, 'Just a minute now! Listen to me! I want everybody to be very careful in this room. There is dangerous stuff around in here and you *must not* tamper with it.'

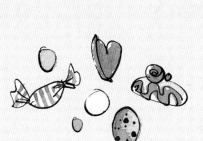

CHAPTER TWENTY-SIX

The Television-Chocolate Room

The Teavee family, together with Charlie and Grandpa Joe, stepped out of the lift into a room so dazzlingly bright and dazzlingly white that they screwed up their eyes in pain and stopped walking. Mr Wonka handed each of them a pair of dark glasses and said, 'Put these on quick! And don't take them off in here whatever you do! This light could blind you!'

As soon as Charlie had his dark glasses on, he was able to look around him in comfort. He saw a long narrow room. The room was painted white all over. Even the floor was white, and there wasn't a speck of dust anywhere. From the ceiling, huge lamps hung down and bathed the room in a brilliant blue-white light. The room was completely bare except at the far ends. At one of these ends there was an enormous camera on wheels, and a whole army of Oompa-Loompas was clustering around it, oiling its joints and adjusting its knobs and polishing its great glass lens. The Oompa-Loompas were all dressed in the most extraordinary way. They were wearing bright-red space suits, complete with helmets and goggles – at least they looked like space suits – and they were working in complete silence. Watching them, Charlie experienced a queer sense of danger. There was something dangerous about this whole business, and the Oompa-Loompas knew it. There was no chattering or singing among them here, and they moved about over the huge black camera slowly and carefully in their scarlet space suits.

At the other end of the room, about fifty paces away from the camera, a single Oompa-Loompa (also wearing a space suit) was sitting at a black table gazing at the screen of a very large television set.

'Here we go!' cried Mr Wonka, hopping up and down with excitement. 'This is the Testing Room for my very latest and greatest invention – Television Chocolate!'

'But what *is* Television Chocolate?' asked Mike Teavee.

'Good heavens, child, stop interrupting me!' said Mr Wonka. 'It works by television. I don't like television myself. I suppose it's all right in small doses, but children never seem to be able to take it in small doses. They want to sit there all day long staring and staring at the screen . . .'

'That's me!' said Mike Teavee.

'Shut up!' said Mr Teavee.

'Thank you,' said Mr Wonka. 'I shall now tell you how this amazing television set of mine works. But first of all, do you know how ordinary television works? It is very simple. At one end, where the picture is being taken, you have a large ciné camera and you start photographing something. The photographs are then split up into millions of tiny little pieces which are so small that you can't see them, and these little pieces are shot out into the sky by electricity. In the sky, they go whizzing around all over the place until suddenly they hit the antenna on the roof of somebody's house. They then go flashing down the wire that leads right into the back of the television set, and in there they get jiggled and joggled around until at last every single one of those millions of tiny pieces is fitted back into its right place (just like a jigsaw puzzle), and presto! – the photograph appears on the screen . . .'

'That isn't *exactly* how it works,' Mike Teavee said.

'I am a little deaf in my left ear,' Mr Wonka said. 'You must forgive me if I don't hear everything you say.'

'I said, that isn't *exactly* how it works!' shouted Mike Teavee.

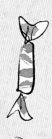

'You're a nice boy,' Mr Wonka said, 'but you talk too much. Now then! The very first time I saw ordinary television working, I was struck by a tremendous idea. "Look here!" I shouted. "If these people can break up a *photograph* into millions of pieces and send the pieces whizzing through the air and then put them together again at the other end, why can't I do the same thing with a bar of chocolate? Why can't *I* send a real bar of chocolate whizzing through the air in tiny pieces and then put the pieces together at the other end, all ready to be eaten?" '

'Impossible!' said Mike Teavee.

'You think so?' cried Mr Wonka. 'Well, watch this! I shall now send a bar of my very best chocolate from one end of this room to the other – by television! Get ready, there! Bring in the chocolate!'

Immediately, six Oompa-Loompas marched forward carrying on their shoulders the most enormous bar of chocolate Charlie had ever seen. It was about the size of the mattress he slept on at home.

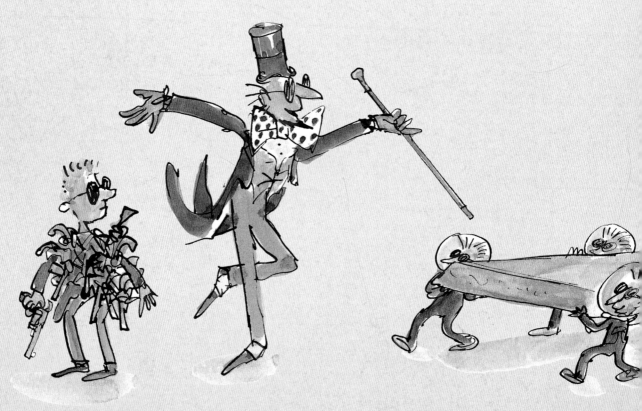

The Television-Chocolate Room

'It has to be big,' Mr Wonka explained, 'because whenever you send something by television, it always comes out much smaller than it was when it went in. Even with *ordinary* television, when you photograph a big man, he never comes out on your screen any taller than a pencil, does he? Here we go, then! Get ready! *No, no! Stop! Hold everything!* You there! Mike Teavee! Stand back! You're too close to the camera! There are dangerous rays coming out of that thing! They could break you up into a million tiny pieces in one second! That's why the Oompa-Loompas are wearing space suits! The suits protect them! All right! That's better! Now, then! *Switch on!*'

One of the Oompa-Loompas caught hold of a large switch and pulled it down.

There was a blinding flash.

'The chocolate's gone!' shouted Grandpa Joe, waving his arms.

He was quite right! The whole enormous bar of chocolate had disappeared completely into thin air!

'It's on its way!' cried Mr Wonka. 'It is now rushing through the air above our heads in a million tiny pieces. Quick! Come over here!' He dashed over to the other end of the room where the large television set was standing, and the others followed him. 'Watch the screen!' he cried. 'Here it comes! Look!'

The screen flickered and lit up. Then suddenly, a small bar of chocolate appeared in the middle of the screen.

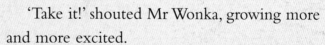

'Take it!' shouted Mr Wonka, growing more and more excited.

'How can you take it?' asked Mike Teavee, laughing. 'It's just a picture on a television screen!'

'Charlie Bucket!' cried Mr Wonka. '*You* take it! Reach out and grab it!'

Charlie put out his hand and touched the screen,

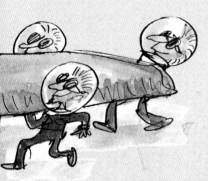

and suddenly, miraculously, the bar of chocolate came away in his fingers. He was so surprised he nearly dropped it.

'Eat it!' shouted Mr Wonka. 'Go on and eat it! It'll be delicious! It's the same bar! It's got smaller on the journey, that's all!'

'It's absolutely fantastic!' gasped Grandpa Joe. 'It's . . . it's . . . it's a miracle!'

'Just imagine,' cried Mr Wonka, 'when I start using this across the country . . . you'll be sitting at home watching television and suddenly a commercial will flash on to the screen and a voice will say, "EAT WONKA'S CHOCOLATES! THEY'RE THE BEST IN THE WORLD! IF YOU DON'T BELIEVE US, TRY ONE FOR YOURSELF – *NOW*!" And you simply reach out and take one! How about that, eh?'

'Terrific!' cried Grandpa Joe. 'It will change the world!'

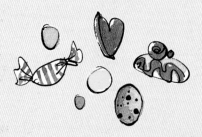

CHAPTER TWENTY-SEVEN

Mike Teavee is Sent by Television

Mike Teavee was even more excited than Grandpa Joe at seeing a bar of chocolate being sent by television. 'But Mr Wonka,' he shouted, 'can you send *other things* through the air in the same way? Breakfast cereal, for instance?'

'Oh, my sainted aunt!' cried Mr Wonka. 'Don't mention that disgusting stuff in front of me! Do you know what breakfast cereal is made of? It's made of all those little curly wooden shavings you find in pencil sharpeners!'

'But could you send it by television if you wanted to, as you do chocolate?' asked Mike Teavee.

'Of course I could!'

'And what about people?' asked Mike Teavee. 'Could you send a real live person from one place to another in the same way?'

'A *person*!' cried Mr Wonka. 'Are you off your rocker?'

'But *could* it be done?'

'Good heavens, child, I really don't know . . . I suppose it *could* . . . yes. I'm pretty sure it could . . . of course it could . . . I wouldn't like to risk it, though . . . it might have some very nasty results . . .'

But Mike Teavee was already off and running. The moment he heard Mr Wonka saying, 'I'm pretty sure it could . . . of course it could,' he turned away and started running as fast as he could towards the other end of the room where the great camera was standing. 'Look at me!' he shouted as he ran. 'I'm going to be the first person in the world to be sent by television!'

'*No, no, no, no!*' cried Mr Wonka.

'Mike!' screamed Mrs Teavee. 'Stop! Come back! You'll be turned into a million tiny pieces!'

But there was no stopping Mike Teavee now. The crazy boy rushed on, and when he reached the enormous camera, he jumped straight for the switch, scattering Oompa-Loompas right and left as he went.

'See you later, alligator!' he shouted, and he pulled down the switch, and as he did so, he leaped out into the full glare of the mighty lens.

There was a blinding flash.

Then there was silence.

Then Mrs Teavee ran forward . . . but she stopped dead in the middle of the room . . . and she stood there . . . she stood staring at the place where her son had been . . . and her great red mouth opened wide and she screamed, 'He's gone! He's gone!'

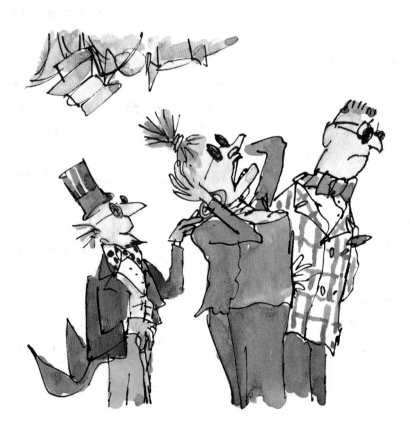

Mike Teavee is Sent by Television

'Great heavens, he *has* gone!' shouted Mr Teavee.

Mr Wonka hurried forward and placed a hand gently on Mrs Teavee's shoulder. 'We shall have to hope for the best,' he said. 'We must pray that your little boy will come out unharmed at the other end.'

'Mike!' screamed Mrs Teavee, clasping her head in her hands. 'Where are you?'

'I'll tell you where he is,' said Mr Teavee, 'he's whizzing around above our heads in a million tiny pieces!'

'Don't talk about it!' wailed Mrs Teavee.

'We must watch the television set,' said Mr Wonka. 'He may come through any moment.'

Mr and Mrs Teavee and Grandpa Joe and little Charlie and Mr Wonka all gathered round the television and stared tensely at the screen. The screen was quite blank.

'He's taking a heck of a long time to come across,' said Mr Teavee, wiping his brow.

'Oh dear, oh dear,' said Mr Wonka, 'I do hope that no part of him gets left behind.'

'What on earth do you mean?' asked Mr Teavee sharply.

'I don't wish to alarm you,' said Mr Wonka, 'but it does sometimes happen that only about half the little pieces find their way into the television set. It happened last week. I don't know why, but the result was that only half a bar of chocolate came through.'

Mrs Teavee let out a scream of horror. 'You mean only a half of Mike is coming back to us?' she cried.

'Let's hope it's the top half,' said Mr Teavee.

'Hold everything!' said Mr Wonka. 'Watch the screen! Something's happening!'

The screen had suddenly begun to flicker.

Then some wavy lines appeared.

Mr Wonka adjusted one of the knobs and the wavy lines went away.

And now, very slowly, the screen began to get brighter and brighter.

'Here he comes!' yelled Mr Wonka. 'Yes, that's him all right!'

'Is he all in one piece?' cried Mrs Teavee.

'I'm not sure,' said Mr Wonka. 'It's too early to tell.'

Faintly at first, but becoming clearer and clearer every second, the picture of Mike Teavee appeared on the screen. He was standing up and waving at the audience and grinning from ear to ear.

'But he's a midget!' shouted Mr Teavee.

'Mike,' cried Mrs Teavee, 'are you all right? Are there any bits of you missing?'

'Isn't he going to get any bigger?' shouted Mr Teavee.

'Talk to me, Mike!' cried Mrs Teavee. 'Say something! Tell me you're all right!'

A tiny little voice, no louder than the squeaking of a mouse, came out of the television set. 'Hi, Mum!' it said. 'Hi, Pop! Look at *me*! I'm the first person ever to be sent by television!'

'Grab him!' ordered Mr Wonka. 'Quick!'

Mrs Teavee shot out a hand and picked the tiny figure of Mike Teavee out of the screen.

'Hooray!' cried Mr Wonka. 'He's all in one piece! He's completely unharmed!'

'You call *that* unharmed?' snapped Mrs Teavee, peering at the little speck of a boy who was now running to and fro across the palm of her hand, waving his pistols in the air.

He was certainly not more than an inch tall.

'He's *shrunk*!' said Mr Teavee.

'Of course he's shrunk,' said Mr Wonka. 'What did you expect?'

'This is terrible!' wailed Mrs Teavee. 'What *are* we going to do?'

And Mr Teavee said, 'We can't send him back to school like this! He'll get trodden on! He'll get squashed!'

'He won't be able to do *anything*!' cried Mrs Teavee.

Mike Teavee is Sent by Television

'Oh, yes I will!' squeaked the tiny voice of Mike Teavee. 'I'll still be able to watch television!'

'*Never again!*' shouted Mr Teavee. 'I'm throwing the television set right out the window the moment we get home. I've had enough of television!'

When he heard this, Mike Teavee flew into a terrible tantrum. He started jumping up and down on the palm of his mother's hand, screaming and yelling and trying to bite her fingers. 'I want to watch television!' he squeaked. 'I want to watch television! I want to watch television! I want to watch television!'

'Here! Give him to me!' said Mr Teavee, and he took the tiny boy and shoved him into the breast pocket of his jacket and stuffed a handkerchief on top. Squeals and yells came from inside the pocket, and the pocket shook as the furious little prisoner fought to get out.

'Oh, Mr Wonka,' wailed Mrs Teavee, 'how can we make him grow?'

'Well,' said Mr Wonka, stroking his beard and gazing thoughtfully at the ceiling, 'I must say that's a wee bit tricky. But small boys are extremely springy and elastic. They stretch like mad. So what we'll do, we'll put him in a special machine I have for testing the stretchiness of chewing-gum! Maybe that will bring him back to what he was.'

'Oh, thank you!' said Mrs Teavee.

'Don't mention it, dear lady.'

'How far d'you think he'll stretch?' asked Mr Teavee.

'Maybe miles,' said Mr Wonka. 'Who knows? But he's going to be awfully thin.

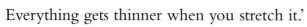

Everything gets thinner when you stretch it.'

'You mean like chewing-gum?' asked Mr Teavee.

'Exactly.'

'How thin will he be?' asked Mrs Teavee anxiously.

'I haven't the foggiest idea,' said Mr Wonka. 'And it doesn't really matter, anyway, because we'll soon fatten him up again. All we'll have to do is give him a triple overdose of my wonderful Supervitamin Chocolate. Supervitamin Chocolate contains huge amounts of vitamin A and vitamin B. It also contains vitamin C, vitamin D, vitamin E, vitamin F, vitamin G, vitamin I, vitamin J, vitamin K, vitamin L, vitamin M, vitamin N, vitamin O, vitamin P, vitamin Q, vitamin R, vitamin T, vitamin U, vitamin V, vitamin W, vitamin X, vitamin Y, *and*, believe it or not, vitamin Z! The only two vitamins it doesn't have in it are vitamin S, because it makes you sick, and vitamin H, because it makes you grow horns on the top of your head, like a bull. But it *does* have in it a very small amount of the rarest and most magical vitamin of them all – vitamin Wonka.'

'And what will *that* do to him?' asked Mr Teavee anxiously.

'It'll make his toes grow out until they're as long as his fingers . . .'

'Oh, no!' cried Mrs Teavee.

'Don't be silly,' said Mr Wonka. 'It's most useful. He'll be able to play the piano with his feet.'

'But Mr Wonka . . .'

'No arguments, *please*!' said Mr Wonka. He turned away and clicked his fingers three times in the air. An Oompa-Loompa appeared immediately and stood beside him. 'Follow these orders,' said Mr Wonka, handing the Oompa-Loompa a piece of paper on which he had written full instructions. 'And you'll find the boy in his father's pocket. Off you go! Goodbye, Mr Teavee! Goodbye, Mrs Teavee! And please don't look so worried! They all come out in the wash, you know; every one of them . . .'

Mike Teavee is Sent by Television

At the end of the room, the Oompa-Loompas around the giant camera were already beating their tiny drums and beginning to jog up and down to the rhythm.

'There they go again!' said Mr Wonka. 'I'm afraid you can't stop them singing.'

Little Charlie caught Grandpa Joe's hand, and the two of them stood beside Mr Wonka in the middle of the long bright room, listening to the Oompa-Loompas. And this is what they sang:

'The most important thing we've learned,
So far as children are concerned,
Is never, NEVER, NEVER let
Them near your television set —
Or better still, just don't install
The idiotic thing at all.
In almost every house we've been,
We've watched them gaping at the screen.
They loll and slop and lounge about,
And stare until their eyes pop out.
(Last week in someone's place we saw
A dozen eyeballs on the floor.)
They sit and stare and stare and sit
Until they're hypnotized by it,
Until they're absolutely drunk
With all that shocking ghastly junk.
Oh yes, we know it keeps them still,
They don't climb out the window sill,
They never fight or kick or punch,
They leave you free to cook the lunch
And wash the dishes in the sink —
But did you ever stop to think,

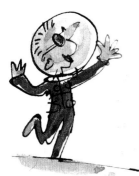

Charlie and the Chocolate Factory

To wonder just exactly what
This does to your beloved tot?
IT ROTS THE SENSES IN THE HEAD!
IT KILLS IMAGINATION DEAD!
IT CLOGS AND CLUTTERS UP THE MIND!
IT MAKES A CHILD SO DULL AND BLIND
HE CAN NO LONGER UNDERSTAND
A FANTASY, A FAIRYLAND!
HIS BRAIN BECOMES AS SOFT AS CHEESE!
HIS POWERS OF THINKING RUST AND FREEZE!
HE CANNOT THINK – HE ONLY SEES!
"All right!" you'll cry. "All right!" you'll say,
"But if we take the set away,
What shall we do to entertain
Our darling children! Please explain!"
We'll answer this by asking you,

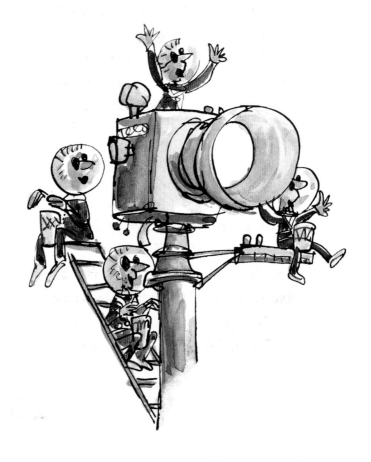

Mike Teavee is Sent by Television

"What used the darling ones to do?
How used they keep themselves contented
Before this monster was invented?"
Have you forgotten? Don't you know?
We'll say it very loud and slow:
THEY . . . USED . . . TO . . . READ! They'd READ and READ,
AND READ and READ, and then proceed
TO READ some more. Great Scott! Gadzooks!
One half their lives was reading books!
The nursery shelves held books galore!
Books cluttered up the nursery floor!
And in the bedroom, by the bed,
More books were waiting to be read!
Such wondrous, fine, fantastic tales
Of dragons, gypsies, queens, and whales
And treasure isles, and distant shores
Where smugglers rowed with muffled oars,
And pirates wearing purple pants,
And sailing ships and elephants,
And cannibals crouching round the pot,
Stirring away at something hot.
(It smells so good, what can it be?
Good gracious, it's Penelope.)
The younger ones had Beatrix Potter
With Mr Tod, the dirty rotter,
And Squirrel Nutkin, Pigling Bland,
And Mrs Tiggy-Winkle and –
Just How The Camel Got His Hump,
And How The Monkey Lost His Rump,
And Mr Toad, and bless my soul,
There's Mr Rat and Mr Mole –

Charlie and the Chocolate Factory

Oh, books, what books they used to know,
Those children living long ago!
So please, oh please, we beg, we pray,
Go throw your TV set away,
And in its place you can install
A lovely bookshelf on the wall.
Then fill the shelves with lots of books,
Ignoring all the dirty looks,
The screams and yells, the bites and kicks,
And children hitting you with sticks —
Fear not, because we promise you
That, in about a week or two
Of having nothing else to do,
They'll now begin to feel the need
Of having something good to read.
And once they start — oh boy, oh boy!
You watch the slowly growing joy
That fills their hearts. They'll grow so keen
They'll wonder what they'd ever seen
In that ridiculous machine,
That nauseating, foul, unclean,
Repulsive television screen!
And later, each and every kid
Will love you more for what you did.
P.S. Regarding Mike Teavee,
We very much regret that we
Shall simply have to wait and see
If we can get him back his height.
But if we can't — it serves him right.'

CHAPTER TWENTY-EIGHT

Only Charlie Left

'Which room shall it be next?' said Mr Wonka as he turned away and darted into the lift. 'Come on! Hurry up! We *must* get going! And how many children are there left now?'

Little Charlie looked at Grandpa Joe, and Grandpa Joe looked back at little Charlie.

'But Mr Wonka,' Grandpa Joe called after him, 'there's . . . there's only Charlie left now.'

Mr Wonka swung round and stared at Charlie.

There was a silence. Charlie stood there holding tightly on to Grandpa Joe's hand.

'You mean you're the *only* one left?' Mr Wonka said, pretending to be surprised.

'Why, yes,' whispered Charlie. 'Yes.'

Mr Wonka suddenly exploded with excitement. 'But my *dear boy*,' he cried out, '*that means you've won!*' He rushed out of the lift and started shaking Charlie's hand so furiously it nearly came off. 'Oh, I do congratulate you!' he cried. 'I really do! I'm absolutely delighted! It couldn't be better! How wonderful this is! I had a hunch, you know, right from the beginning, that it was going to be you! Well *done*, Charlie, well *done*! This is terrific! Now the fun is really going to start! But we mustn't dilly! We mustn't dally! There's even less time to lose now than there was before! We have an *enormous* number of things to do before the day is out! Just think of the *arrangements* that have to be made! And the

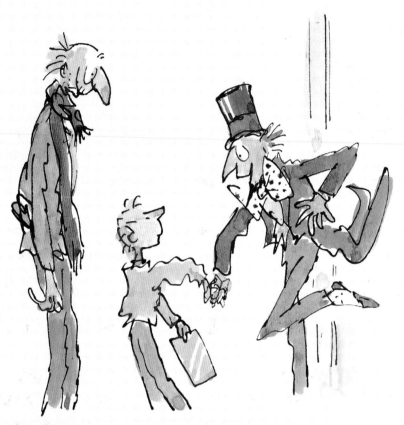

people we have to fetch! But luckily for us, we have the great glass lift to speed things up! Jump in, my dear Charlie, jump in! You too, Grandpa Joe, sir! No, no, *after* you! That's the way! Now then! This time *I* shall choose the button we are going to press!' Mr Wonka's bright twinkling blue eyes rested for a moment on Charlie's face.

Something crazy is going to happen now, Charlie thought. But he wasn't frightened. He wasn't even nervous. He was just terrifically excited. And so was Grandpa Joe. The old man's face was shining with excitement as he watched every move that Mr Wonka made. Mr Wonka was reaching for a button high up on the glass ceiling of the lift. Charlie and Grandpa Joe both craned their necks to read what it said on the little label beside the button.

Only Charlie Left

It said . . . UP AND OUT.

'*Up* and *out*,' thought Charlie. 'What sort of a room is that?'

Mr Wonka pressed the button.

The glass doors closed.

'Hold on!' cried Mr Wonka.

Then *WHAM!* The lift shot straight up like a rocket! 'Yippee!' shouted Grandpa Joe. Charlie was clinging to Grandpa Joe's legs and Mr Wonka was holding on to a strap from the ceiling, and up they went, up, up, up, straight up this time, with no twistings or turnings, and Charlie could hear the whistling of the air outside as the lift went faster and faster. 'Yippee!' shouted Grandpa Joe again. 'Yippee! Here we go!'

'Faster!' cried Mr Wonka, banging the wall of the lift with his hand. 'Faster! Faster! If we don't go any faster than this, we shall never get through!'

'Through what?' shouted Grandpa Joe. 'What have we got to get through?'

'Ah-ha!' cried Mr Wonka, 'you wait and see! I've been *longing* to press this button for years! But I've never done it until now! I was tempted many times! Oh, yes, I was tempted! But I couldn't bear the thought of making a great big hole in the roof of the factory! Here we go, boys! Up and out!'

'But you don't mean . . .' shouted Grandpa Joe, '. . . you don't *really* mean that this lift . . .'

'Oh yes, I do!' answered Mr Wonka. 'You wait and see! Up and out!'

'But . . . but . . . but . . . it's made of glass!' shouted Grandpa Joe. 'It'll break into a million pieces!'

'I suppose it might,' said Mr Wonka, cheerful as ever, 'but it's pretty thick glass, all the same.'

The lift rushed on, going up and up and up, faster and faster and faster . . .

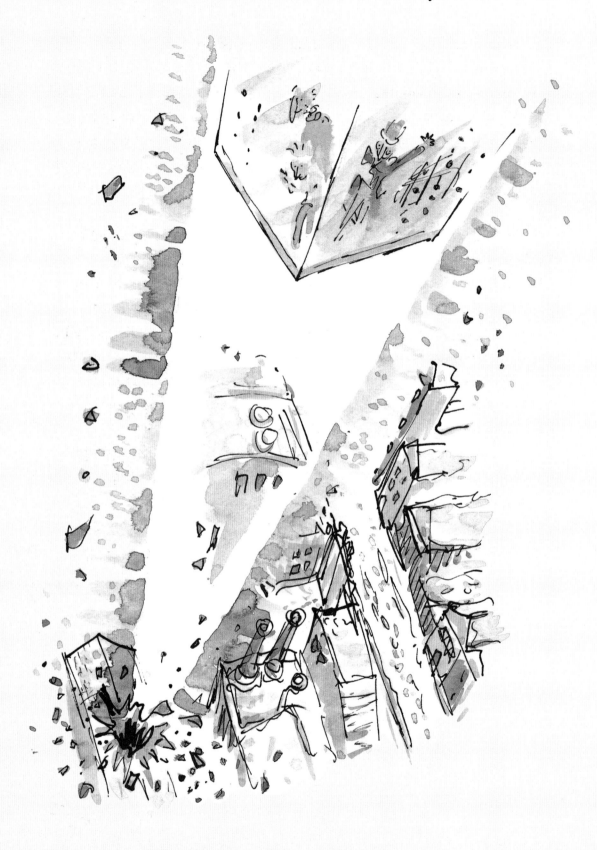

Then suddenly, *CRASH!* – and the most tremendous noise of splintering wood and broken tiles came from directly above their heads, and Grandpa Joe shouted, 'Help! It's the end! We're done for!' and Mr Wonka said, 'No, we're not! We're through! We're out!' Sure enough, the lift had shot right up through the roof of the factory and was now rising into the sky like a rocket, and the sunshine was pouring in through the glass roof. In five seconds they were a thousand feet up in the sky.

'The lift's gone mad!' shouted Grandpa Joe.

'Have no fear, my dear sir,' said Mr Wonka calmly, and he pressed another button. The lift stopped. It stopped and hung in mid-air, hovering like a helicopter, hovering over the factory and over the very town itself which lay spread out below them like a picture postcard! Looking down through the glass floor on which he was standing, Charlie could see the small far-away houses and the streets and the snow that lay thickly over everything. It was an eerie and frightening feeling to be standing on clear glass high up in the sky. It made you feel that you weren't standing on anything at all.

'Are we all right?' cried Grandpa Joe. 'How does this thing stay up?'

'Sugar power!' said Mr Wonka. 'One million sugar power! Oh, look,' he cried, pointing down, 'there go the other children! They're returning home!'

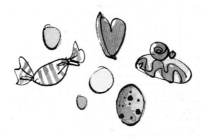

CHAPTER TWENTY-NINE

The Other Children Go Home

'We *must* go down and take a look at our little friends before we do anything else,' said Mr Wonka. He pressed a different button, and the lift dropped lower, and soon it was hovering just above the entrance gates to the factory.

Looking down now, Charlie could see the children and their parents standing in a little group just inside the gates.

'I can only see three,' he said. 'Who's missing?'

'I expect it's Mike Teavee,' Mr Wonka said. 'But he'll be coming along soon. Do you see the trucks?' Mr Wonka pointed to a line of gigantic covered vans parked in a line near by.

'Yes,' Charlie said. 'What are *they* for?'

'Don't you remember what it said on the Golden Tickets? Every child goes home with a lifetime's supply of sweets. There's one truckload for each of them, loaded to the brim. Ah-ha,' Mr Wonka went on, 'there goes our friend Augustus Gloop! D'you see him? He's getting into the first truck with his mother and father!'

'You mean he's *really* all right?' asked Charlie, astonished. 'Even after going up that awful pipe?'

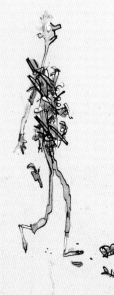

The Other Children Go Home

'He's very much all right,' said Mr Wonka.

'He's changed!' said Grandpa Joe, peering down through the glass wall of the elevator. 'He used to be fat! Now he's thin as a straw!'

'Of course he's changed,' said Mr Wonka, laughing. 'He got squeezed in the pipe. Don't you remember? And look! There goes Miss Violet Beauregarde, the great gum-chewer! It seems as though they managed to de-juice her after all. I'm so glad. And how healthy she looks! Much better than before!'

'But she's purple in the face!' cried Grandpa Joe.

'So she is,' said Mr Wonka. 'Ah, well, there's nothing we can do about that.'

'Good gracious!' cried Charlie. 'Look at poor Veruca Salt and Mr Salt and Mrs Salt! They're simply *covered* with rubbish!'

'And here comes Mike Teavee!' said Grandpa Joe. 'Good heavens! What have they done to him? He's about ten feet tall and thin as a wire!'

'They've overstretched him on the gum-stretching machine,' said Mr Wonka. 'How very careless.'

'But how dreadful for him!' cried Charlie.

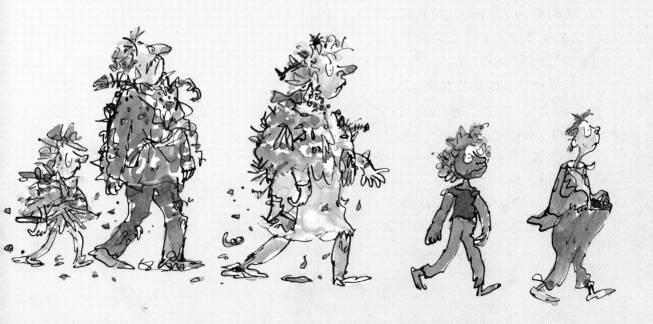

'Nonsense,' said Mr Wonka, 'he's very lucky. Every basketball team in the country will be trying to get him. But now,' he added, 'it is time we left these four silly children. I have something very important to talk to you about, my dear Charlie.' Mr Wonka pressed another button, and the lift swung upwards into the sky.

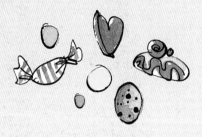

CHAPTER THIRTY

Charlie's Chocolate Factory

The great glass lift was now hovering high over the town. Inside the lift stood Mr Wonka, Grandpa Joe, and little Charlie.

'How I love my chocolate factory,' said Mr Wonka, gazing down. Then he paused, and he turned around and looked at Charlie with a most serious expression on his face. 'Do *you* love it too, Charlie?' he asked.

'Oh, yes,' cried Charlie, 'I think it's the most wonderful place in the whole world!'

'I am very pleased to hear you say that,' said Mr Wonka, looking more serious than ever. He went on staring at Charlie. 'Yes,' he said, 'I am very pleased indeed to hear you say that. And now I shall tell you why.' Mr Wonka cocked his head to one side and all at once the tiny twinkling wrinkles of a smile appeared around the corners of his eyes, and he said, 'You see, my dear boy, I have decided to make you a present of the whole place. As soon as you are old enough to run it, the entire factory will become yours.'

Charlie stared at Mr Wonka. Grandpa Joe opened his mouth to speak, but no words came out.

'It's quite true,' Mr Wonka said, smiling broadly now. 'I really am giving it to you. That's all right, isn't it?'

'*Giving* it to him?' gasped Grandpa Joe. 'You must be joking.'

'I'm not joking, sir. I'm deadly serious.'

'But . . . but . . . why should you want to give your factory to little Charlie?'

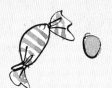

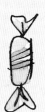

'Listen,' Mr Wonka said, 'I'm an old man. I'm much older than you think. I can't go on for ever. I've got no children of my own, no family at all. So who is going to run the factory when I get too old to do it myself? *Someone's* got to keep it going – if only for the sake of the Oompa-Loompas. Mind you, there are thousands of clever men who would give anything for the chance to come in and take over from me, but I don't want that sort of person. I don't want a grown-up person at all. A grown-up won't listen to me; he won't learn. He will try to do things his own way and not mine. So I have to have a child. I want a good sensible loving child, one to whom I can tell all my most precious sweet-making secrets – while I am still alive.'

'*So that* is why you sent out the Golden Tickets!' cried Charlie.

'Exactly!' said Mr Wonka. 'I decided to invite five children to the factory, and the one I liked best at the end of the day would be the winner!'

'But Mr Wonka,' stammered Grandpa Joe, 'do you really and truly mean that you are giving the whole of this enormous factory to little Charlie? After all . . .'

'There's no time for arguments!' cried Mr Wonka. 'We must go at once and fetch the rest of the family – Charlie's father and his mother and anyone else that's around! They can all live in the factory from now on! They can all help to run it until Charlie is old enough to do it by himself! Where do you live, Charlie?'

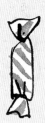

Charlie peered down through the glass floor at the snow-covered houses that lay below. 'It's over there,' he said, pointing. 'It's that little cottage right on the edge of the town, the tiny little one . . .'

'I see it!' cried Mr Wonka, and he pressed some more buttons and the lift shot down towards Charlie's house.

'I'm afraid my mother won't come with us,' Charlie said sadly.

'Why ever not?'

'Because she won't leave Grandma Josephine and Grandma Georgina

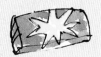

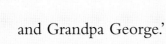
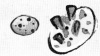
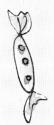

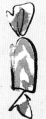

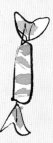

and Grandpa George.'

'But they must come too.'

'They can't,' Charlie said. 'They're very old and they haven't been out of bed for twenty years.'

'Then we'll take the bed along as well, with them in it,' said Mr Wonka. 'There's plenty of room in this lift for a bed.'

'You couldn't get the bed out of the house,' said Grandpa Joe. 'It won't go through the door.'

'You mustn't despair!' cried Mr Wonka. 'Nothing is impossible! You watch!'

The lift was now hovering over the roof of the Buckets' little house.

'What are you going to do?' cried Charlie.

'I'm going right on in to fetch them,' said Mr Wonka.

'How?' asked Grandpa Joe.

'Through the roof,' said Mr Wonka, pressing another button.

'No!' shouted Charlie.

'Stop!' shouted Grandpa Joe.

CRASH went the lift, right down through the roof of the house into the old people's bedroom. Showers of dust and broken tiles and bits of wood and cockroaches and spiders and bricks and cement went raining down on the three old ones who were lying in bed, and each of them thought that the end of the world was come. Grandma Georgina fainted, Grandma Josephine dropped her false teeth, Grandpa George put his head under the blanket, and Mr and Mrs Bucket came rushing in from the next room.

'Save us!' cried Grandma Josephine.

'Calm yourself, my darling wife,' said Grandpa Joe, stepping out of the lift. 'It's only us.'

'Mother!' cried Charlie, rushing into Mrs Bucket's arms. 'Mother! Mother! Listen to what's happened! We're all going back to live in Mr Wonka's factory and we're going to help him to run it and he's given it

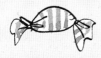

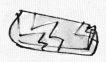
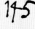

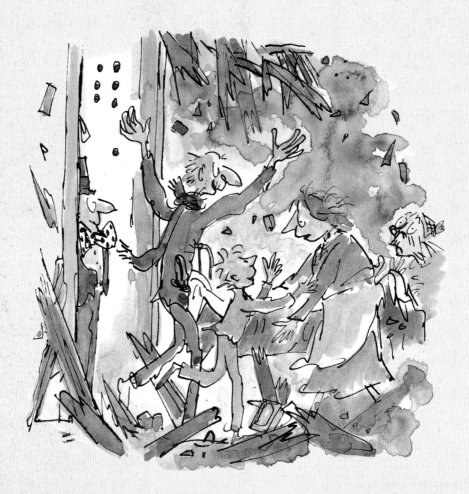

all to me and . . . and . . . and . . . and . . .'

'What *are* you talking about?' said Mrs Bucket.

'Just look at our house!' cried poor Mr Bucket. 'It's in ruins!'

'My dear sir,' said Mr Wonka, jumping forward and shaking Mr Bucket warmly by the hand, 'I'm so very glad to meet you. You mustn't worry about your house. From now on, you're never going to need it again, anyway.'

'Who *is* this crazy man?' screamed Grandma Josephine. 'He could have killed us all.'

'This,' said Grandpa Joe, 'is Mr Willy Wonka himself.'

It took quite a time for Grandpa Joe and Charlie to explain to everyone exactly what had been happening to them all day. And even then they all refused to ride back to the factory in the lift.

'I'd rather die in my bed!' shouted Grandma Josephine.

'So would I!' cried Grandma Georgina.

'I refuse to go!' announced Grandpa George.

So Mr Wonka and Grandpa Joe and Charlie, taking no notice of their screams, simply pushed the bed into the lift. They pushed Mr and Mrs Bucket in after it. Then they got in themselves. Mr Wonka pressed a button. The doors closed. Grandma Georgina screamed. And the lift rose up off the floor and shot through the hole in the roof, out into the open sky.

Charlie climbed on to the bed and tried to calm the three old people who were still petrified with fear. 'Please don't be frightened,' he said. 'It's quite safe. And we're going to the most wonderful place in the world!'

'Charlie's right,' said Grandpa Joe.

'Will there be anything to eat when we get there?' asked Grandma Josephine. 'I'm starving! The whole family is starving!'

'Anything to *eat*?' cried Charlie laughing. 'Oh, you just wait and see!'

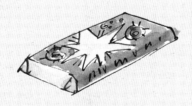

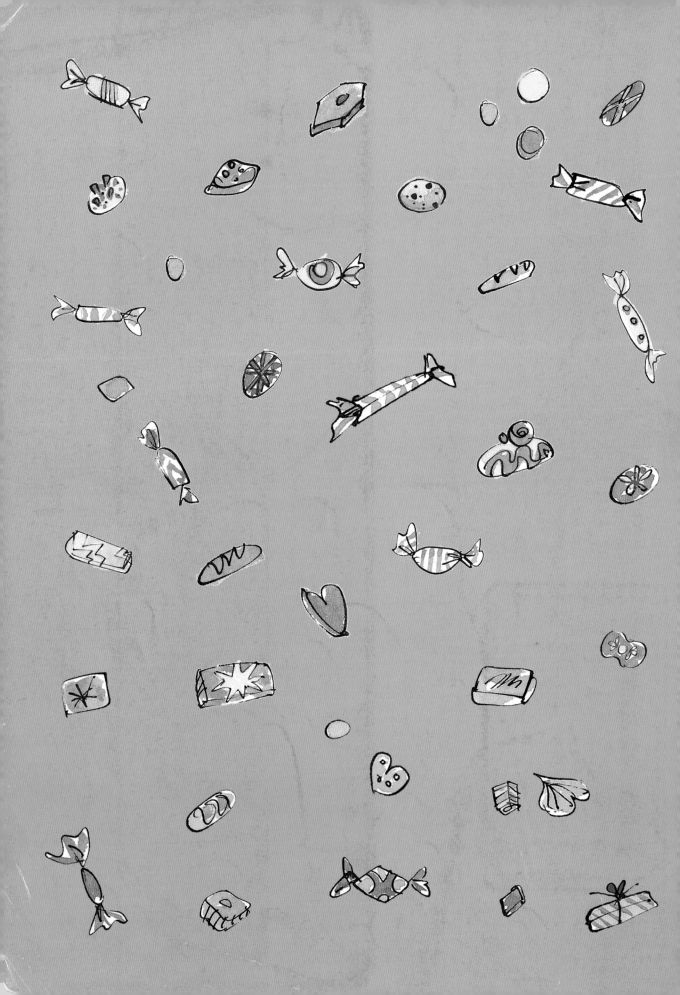

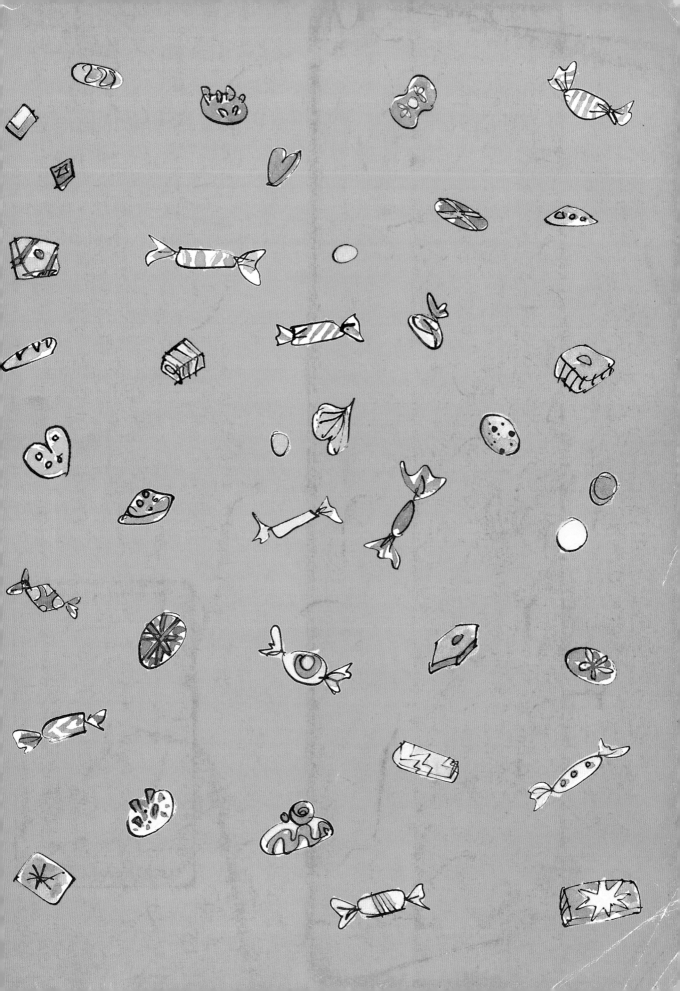

There's more to
ROALD DAHL
than great stories . . .

Did you know that 10% of author royalties* from this book go to help the work of the Roald Dahl charities?

Roald Dahl is famous for his stories and rhymes, but much less well known is how often he went out of his way to help seriously ill children. Today **Roald Dahl's Marvellous Children's Charity** helps children with the severest conditions and the greatest needs. The charity believes every child can have a more marvellous life, no matter how ill they are, or how short their life may be.

Can you do something marvellous to help others?
Find out how at **www.roalddahlcharity.org**

You can find out about Roald Dahl's real-life experiences and how they found their way into his stories at the **Roald Dahl Museum and Story Centre** in Great Missenden, Buckinghamshire (the author's home village). The Museum is a charity that aims to inspire excitement about reading, writing and creativity. There are three fun and fact-packed galleries, with lots to make, do and see (including Roald Dahl's writing hut). Aimed at 6–12-year-olds, the Museum is open to the public and to school groups throughout the year.

Find out more at **www.roalddahlmuseum.org**

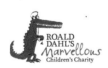